NEUROSCIENCE RESEARCH PROGRESS

MIGRAINE SURGERY

NEUROSCIENCE RESEARCH PROGRESS

Additional books in this series can be found on Nova's website
under the Series tab.

Additional e-books in this series can be found on Nova's website
under the e-book tab.

NEUROSCIENCE RESEARCH PROGRESS

MIGRAINE SURGERY

ANTONIOS MAMMIS, M.D.
EDITOR

NOVA BIOMEDICAL

New York

For permission to use material from this book please contact us:
Telephone 631-231-7269; Fax 631-231-8175
Web Site: http://www.novapublishers.com

Library of Congress Cataloging-in-Publication Data

Library of Congress Control Number: 2014948037
ISBN: 978-1-63321-761-4

Published by Nova Science Publishers, Inc. † New York

This book is dedicated to my wife Georgia, and my children Zara, John, and Tina, who keep me focused on the important things in life; and to the physicians, residents, medical students, and patients who have taught me that there is no nobler calling than the practice of medicine

Contents

Preface

Chronic migraine is a condition which is both prevalent and disabling, and which has great impact on society as a whole. The accurate diagnosis, workup, and treatment of migraine requires a multidisciplinary approach, involving primary care physicians, neurologists, pain management specialists, mental health specialists, alternative practitioners, and surgeons. Across the spectrum of migraine patients, the most challenging are those deemed refractory to conventional therapy. These patients may be surgical candidates, and are best served in a multidisciplinary, patient-centered model of migraine care.

Migraine Surgery should serve as a reference to any practitioner dealing with the migraine patient. The fundamentals of migraine diagnosis and workup are reviewed, in addition to conventional therapies. We review the medical optimization of the migraine patient, and establish what it means to have intractable migraine.

We discuss the role of the allied health professions in the management of chronic migraine, with chapters on psychological considerations, complementary medical management, and exercise. Furthermore, the standard interventional treatment of migraine is presented, in addition to surgical therapies, with an emphasis on patient selection, surgical technique, and complication avoidance.

I hope this book serves to improve the care of the migraine patient, while providing a beacon of hope to intractable migraine patients, their caretakers, and medical providers.

About the Editor

Antonios Mammis, M.D.
Assistant Professor
Department of Neurological Surgery
Rutgers New Jersey Medical School
Newark, New Jersey

Contributors

Nitin Agarwal, M.D.
Resident
Department of Neurological Surgery
University of Pittsburgh School of Medicine
Pittsburgh, Pennsylvania

Michelle C. Armonda, B.S., A.T.C.
Project Manager
Department of Neurological Surgery
Rutgers New Jersey Medical School
Newark, New Jersey

Rachid Assina, M.D.
Resident
Department of Neurological Surgery
Rutgers New Jersey Medical School
Newark, New Jersey

Annapoorna Bhat, M.D., Ph.D.
Resident
Department of Neurology & Neurosciences
Rutgers New Jersey Medical School
Newark, New Jersey

Dawn C. Buse, Ph.D.
Associate Professor
Department of Neurology
Albert Einstein College of Medicine
Bronx, New York

Shabbar F. Danish, M.D.
Assistant Professor
Division of Neurosurgery
Rutgers – RWJ Medical School
New Brunswick, New Jersey

Adam M. Feintisch, M.D.
Resident, Division of Plastic Surgery
Department of Surgery
Rutgers New Jersey Medical School
Newark, New Jersey

BranDee N. Gentile, M.S., A.T.C., L.A.T.
Physician Extender/Athletic Trainer
Department of Neurological Surgery
Rutgers New Jersey Medical School
Newark, New Jersey

Antonio Gonzalez-Fiol, M.D.
Associate Professor
Department of Anesthesiology
Rutgers New Jersey Medical School
Newark, New Jersey

Mark S. Granick, M.D.
Professor and Chief, Division of Plastic Surgery
Department of Surgery
Rutgers New Jersey Medical School
Newark, New Jersey

Dennis Grech, M.D.
Assistant Professor
Department of Anesthesiology
Rutgers New Jersey Medical School
Newark, New Jersey

Jennifer Gyi, D.O.
Assistant Professor
Department of Neurological Surgery
Rutgers New Jersey Medical School
Newark, New Jersey

Aaron F. Hajart, M.S., A.T.C.
Sr. Director of Administration
Department of Neurological Surgery
Rutgers New Jersey Medical School
Newark, New Jersey

Van Le, M.D.
Assistant Professor; Associate Residency Program Director
Department of Anesthesiology
Rutgers New Jersey Medical School
Newark, New Jersey

Edward S. Lee, M.D.
Program Director, Division of Plastic Surgery
Department of Surgery
Rutgers New Jersey Medical School
Newark, New Jersey

Antonios Mammis, M.D.
Assistant Professor
Department of Neurological Surgery
Rutgers New Jersey Medical School
Newark, New Jersey

David A. Marks, M.D.
Associate Professor
Department of Neurology & Neurosciences
Rutgers New Jersey Medical School
Newark, New Jersey

Sarah Jo Mayson, B.A.
Graduate Student
Ferkauf Graduate School of Psychology
Yeshiva University
Bronx, New York

Alon Y. Mogilner, M.D., Ph.D.
Associate Professor
Department of Neurological Surgery
NYU Langone Medical Center
New York, New York

Sam Nia, M.D.
Resident
Department of Anesthesiology
Rutgers New Jersey Medical School
Newark, New Jersey

Tasneem Peeraully, M.B.B.S., B.Sc.
Assistant Professor
Department of Neurology & Neurosciences
Rutgers New Jersey Medical School
Newark, New Jersey

Sascha Qian, M.D.
Resident
Department of Anesthesiology
Columbia University
New York, New York

Christina E. Sarris, B.S.
Medical Student
New Jersey Medical School
Newark, New Jersey

Elizabeth K. Seng, Ph.D.
Assistant Professor
Ferkauf Graduate School of Psychology
Yeshiva University
Bronx, New York

Shelly Sharma, M.D.
Resident
Department of Anesthesiology
Rutgers New Jersey Medical School
Newark, New Jersey

Peter Y. Shin, B.A.
Medical Student
Rutgers New Jersey Medical School
Newark, New Jersey

Anthony N. Sifonios, M.D.
Assistant Professor
Department of Anesthesiology
Rutgers New Jersey Medical School
Newark, New Jersey

Saurabh Sinha, B.S.
Medical Student
Rutgers Robert Wood Johnson
Medical School
New Brunswick, New Jersey

Nomita Sonty, Ph.D.
Associate Clinical Professor
Department of Anesthesiology
Columbia University
New York, New York

Traci Stein, Ph.D., M.P.H.
Clinical Psychologist
New York, New York

Patricia Tsui, Ph.D.
Assistant Professor
Department of Anesthesiology
Stony Brook University
Stony Brook, New York

Katherine J. Zehr, B.A.
Personal Trainer
Synergy Fitness Clubs
Queens, New York

In: Migraine Surgery
Editor: Antonios Mammis
ISBN: 978-1-63321-761-4

Chapter 1

History of Migraine Surgery

Rachid Assina**[*] **and Christina E. Sarris
Department of Neurological Surgery, Rutgers New Jersey Medical School, Newark, New Jersey, US

Introduction

Headache is an entity that has been described and existed as long as human history has been recorded. It can be traced back at least 4000 years ago to the Mesopotamian ritual texts. [1] Throughout history, it made its way into myth, magic, theology and medicine. [2] It has touched ordinary, privileged, and famous people.

Early on it was viewed as a spiritual entity rather than a symptom of various physical diseases. While the first description of migraine was by the ancient Egyptians, where it was described as "sickness of half the head" in the Ebers papyrus, it was Hippocrates who characterized the different types of headaches and attributed them to a real physical pathological state. [3] Even though Hippocrates described many features of migraine, it was Aretaeus of Cappadocia who was the first to accurately described and defined what is today termed migraine as heterocrania. [3] Galen of Pergamon later called it hemicranias, which was then transmuted to the term migraine. Although the earliest documented description of headache only dates back 4000 years ago, its treatment may be traced back to the trepanation of Neolithic skulls 9000 years ago. [4] Surgical treatment for migraine has evolved throughout history and we will highlight in a chronological order the surgical treatments and the rational behind them in each historical era.

[*] Corresponding author: Rachid Assina, M.D. Department of Neurological Surgery, Rutgers New Jersey Medical School 90 Bergen Street, Suite 8100 Newark NJ, 07103, assinara@njms.rutgers.edu.

Prehistoric Period

The prehistoric era was marked by the lack of understanding of the human body, the concept of disease and its origin. This period is also known in the neurosurgical field as the age of trepanation. One of the many theories explaining the rational behind the practice of skull trepanation was the treatment of headaches. It is believed that trephination was used to treat headaches by giving the evil spirit a physical route to leave the ailing head. [4] Some trepanned Neolithic skulls 7000 BC showed evidence of healing, suggesting that the patient survived the procedure. Many unsuccessful attempts have been proposed to explain, based on the trepanation location, if the procedure was used as an elective treatment or a treatment for trauma (Figure 1).

Mesopotamian Period

> "Headache roams over the desert, blowing like the wind. Flashing like lightning, it is loosed above and below; it cuts off like a reed him who fears not his god…This man it has struck, and like one with heart disease he staggers, like one bereft of reason, he is broken…Headache whose course like the dread windstorm none knows, none knows its fulltime or its bond."[5]

Above is a translation of a Mesopotamian tablet dated 3000-4000 BC that may be a clinical description of headache, which was attributed to a demon. Headache was attributed to God and the evil spirits. Tiu was the evil spirit of headache. The treatment for such headache was based on appeasing or releasing the evil spirit with medicinal formulas or trephination.

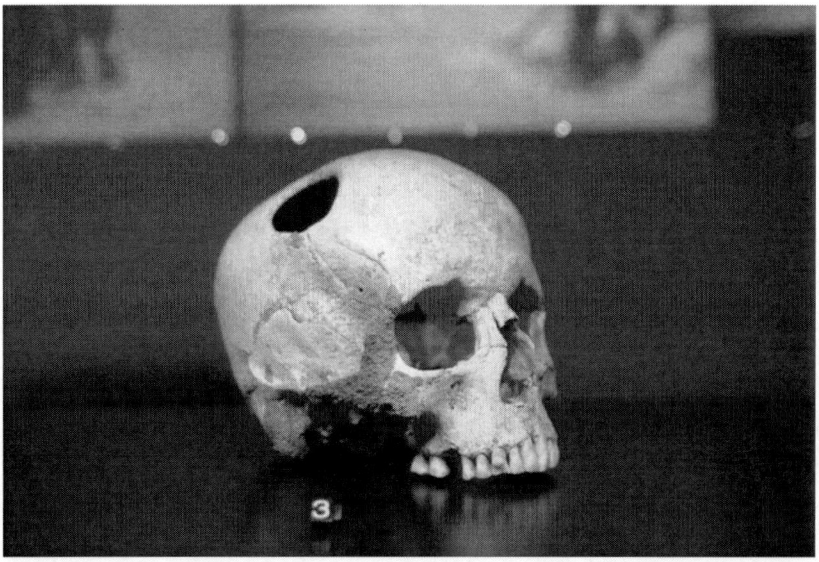

Figure 1. Trepanated female from the Neolithic Era. The trepanation defect shows new bone tissue growth, demonstrating that the patient survived the procedure. This skull is displayed in the Natural History Museum of Lausanne, Switzerland.

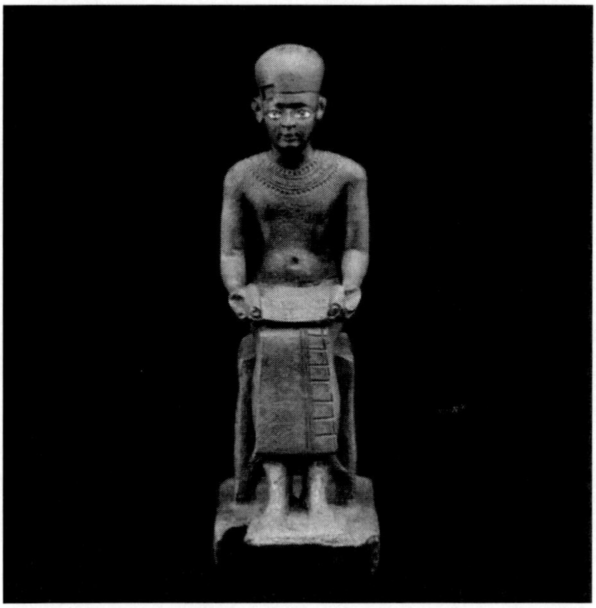

Figure 2. Bronze seated statuette of the architect Imhotep from Egypt, 6th-4th century BC. Imhotep was valued as a god of medicine and learning and was credited with writing many guidelines on the practice of medicine in ancient Egypt. mage courtesy of the Trustees of the British Museum.

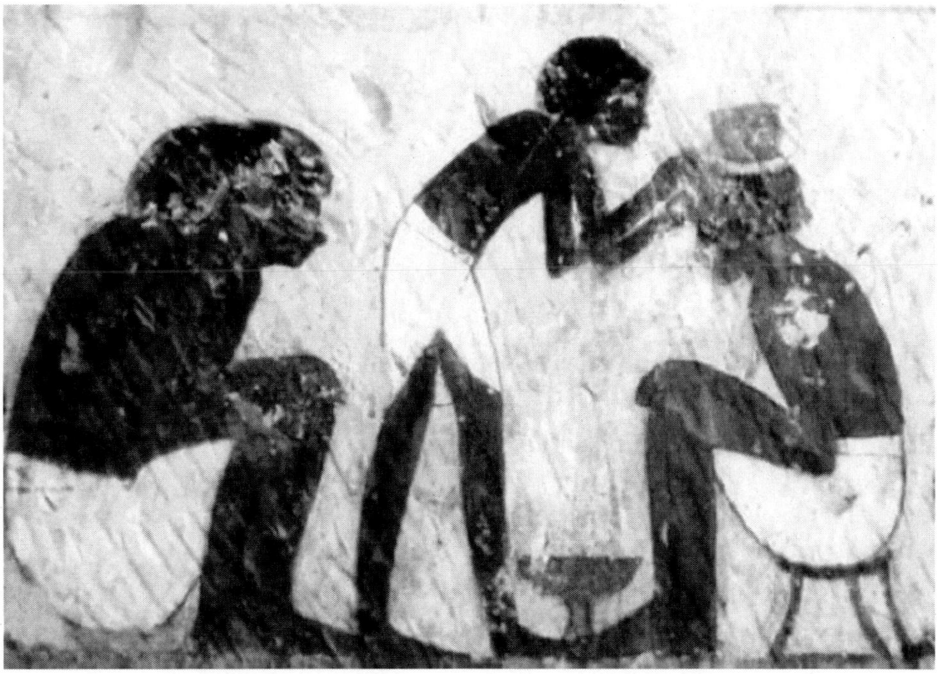

Figure 3. Ancient Egyptian artwork illustrating the treatment of headache. The Ebers Papyrus (1500 BC) outlined diagnoses and cures for migraine headache.

Egyptian and Babylonian Period

This period is considered to be the embryonic era of medicine in which anatomical dissection and surgical procedures were first performed. The Egyptians and Babylonians both introduced the concepts of diagnosis, prognosis, and medical examination. The first recorded evidence of managed health care, legislation and rules governing the ethical and legal practice of medicine also defined this era. The code of Hammurabi, established in 1750 BC by the king of Babylon, Hammurabi, outlined the rules of practice, payments, and punishments in medicine. [6] As well, this epoch gave birth to the first known practicing physician; Imhotep[7] (27th century BC), an Egyptian who authored a medical treatise devoid of magical thinking and containing 48 cases (27 cranial, one spinal) discussing anatomical observation, diagnosis, cures and prognosis (Figure 2). From the surviving papyrus of this treatise, the oldest book on surgery was written around 1700 BC: The Edwin Smith Papyrus. [8] It contains the first description of the cerebrospinal fluid, the meninges, and the cranial sutures. This era also witnessed the birth of the oldest medical text, the Ebers Papyrus around 1500 BC. [9] A case report in this papyrus describing a unilateral headache accompanied by vomiting and malaise titled "Sickness of half the head" has been considered the first documented description, not diagnosis, of migraine headache symptoms (Figure 3). Although the Ebers Papyrus has passages advocating surgical treatment such as removal of tumors and surgical drainage of abscesses, it was not devoid of magical thinking. It contains many magical formulas, incantations, and remedies to cure the disease causing demons. It has 12 prescriptions for the treatments of headaches. [9] The Egyptian healer would take a clay crocodile with herbs stuffed in its mouth and wrap it to the head of the patient with a strip of linen that is engraved with names of the headache healing gods (Figure 4). Rather than the gods, it was the action of compressing the skull, which put pressure on the dilated vessels of the head that alleviated the pain. In addition to the many incantations that were invoked against migraine headaches and its accompanying symptoms such as nausea, trephination was still practiced to release the demons from the suffering heads.

The Greek, Roman, and Byzantine Period

The scholarly and academic development of neurosurgery began during the Greek era. Homer, Herodotus and Thucydides described and recorded plenty of head injuries, but there was no mention of headaches. It was Hippocrates (460-370 BC), the father of modern medicine, who was the first to recognize headache as a symptom of a true disease and not a spell from the demons or the gods. Hippocrates described and distinguished different types of headaches and he is believed to be the first to accurately describe a migraine headache with an aura in his Aphorisms [3]:

> "... He seemed to see something shining before him like a light, usually in part of the right eye; at the end of a moment, a violent pain supervened in the right temple, then in all the head and neck…vomiting, when it become possible, was able to divert the pain and render it more moderate."

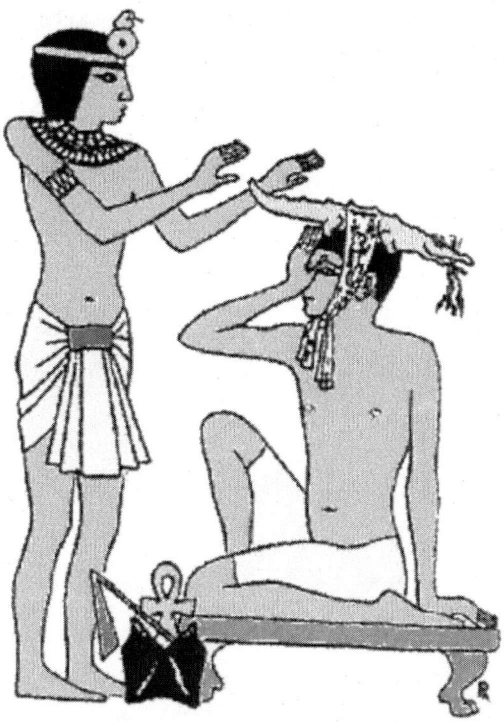

Figure 4. Artwork from ancient Egyptian papyrus illustrating the treatment of migraine headache by bandaging a clay crocodile with herbs stuffed into its mouth onto the head of the ailing patient. Reproduction from a drawing in an Egyptian medical papyrus, date unknown.

The ancient Greeks developed the concept of humoral medicine in which it was believed that disease stems from an unbalance of the four humors within the body: blood, phlegm, yellow and black bile. Treatment for many diseases by withdrawal of body fluid sought to restore the balance of humors within the body. Hippocrates also believed that headache stems from a fluid imbalance, as humors from the liver ascend to the head, and he found that headaches were relieved by vomiting. Although he felt that draining the excess humors would treat the headache, there are few references in his work regarding how to treat the headache except for cupping. [10] Cupping was performed by placing a heated glass tube on the skin, causing blistering which withdraws humors and thus believed to restore humoral balance.

> "For intense pain of the head, whatever of the upper parts that is suffering, apply cupping."[11]

Hippocrates described and provided detailed instruction and clear warning of trepanation in his work "On Injuries of the Head," but never mentions its use for headache treatment. [12]

Although Hippocrates described different types of headache, including migraine, it was Aretaeus of Cappadocia (30-90 AD) who accurately described and named migraine headache as Heterocrania. He introduced the nomenclature of headaches by describing three types of headaches: (a) Cephalalgia, a mild, infrequent, and short-lasting headache that could have been tension headache, (b) Cephalaea, a severe long-lasting headache that was difficult to treat and possibly originates from a structural cause such as hydrocephalus or tumors, and (c)

Heterocrania, a unilateral paroxysmal headache that is usually accompanied by nausea, vomiting, photophobia and osmophobia. [13]

> "... The pain...remains in the half of the head. This is called Heterocrania, an illness by no means mild, even though it appears to be slight...It sets in acutely, it occasions unseemly and dreadful symptoms...nausea; vomiting of bilious matter...there is much torpor, heaviness of the head, anxiety and weariness. For they flee the light; the darkness soothes their disease; nor can they bear readily to look upon or hear anything disagreeable; their sense of smell is vitiated."[13]

One of the two survived works of Aretaeus was on therapy (Detherapia acutorum et chronicorum morborum), "Manual For The Treatment Of Chronic Disease." He also believed in the humoral medicine concepts and advocated bloodletting from veins and arteries and cupping. He reserved cauterization for recurrent headaches and trepanation for persistent severe headaches:

> "The more necessary the head is to life, the more agonizing it may be as a result of disease... Therefore, do not overlook slight pains. In some patients notably, the pains disappear by equally slight treatments. If the pains have been present for a certain period (as complaints of a more serious nature come along), incise the vein at the elbow... Then, order the patient to eat more during three or four days... Then, incise the vein that runs upward in the middle of the forehead, as bleeding here is very important... Next, shave off his hair and place a cup at the crown of the head. Put a second cup between the shoulder blades without bleeding there and carry out a good-sized incision at the crown in order to draw a large quantity of blood and to incise the deep layer. Incisions that get to the bone are beneficial to headache. If the wounds have become scars, then cut out the arteries... One is situated behind the ear... The other lies before the ear... It runs along the tragus... Cut out the bigger arteries where they lie on the bone, because it is very good if one removes these arteries... In all these cases, you have to drive out phlegm after you have emptied the bowels by a laxative or by a clyster. At one time you drive out through the nose by sneezing remedies, at another through the mouth by expectorants... The subsequent day bleed from the inside of the nose. Push the instrument... inside the nose up to the ethmoid bones... a lot of blood will be discharged in a short time, as many small veins end there, and the site is soft and easy to injure... For the ailment usually recurs and remains hidden in its den... cauterize superficially down to the muscles. If you wish to cauterize down to the bone, carry it out at a site where there are no muscles... Some physicians... abrade or chisel the bone down to the diploe... Others perforate the bone down to the meninges. These are hazardous treatments. You have to apply them when the headache persists after all that has been done... Heterocrania may be treated in the same way."[13]

Aulus Cornelius Celsus, (25 BC- 50 AD) the great Roman encyclopedist was the first to use the word cephalagia to describe an acute headache. He also believed in humoral medicine and recommended peripheral bloodletting, cupping, nostril bleeding, and cauterization for acute severe afebrile headaches. [13] He recommended that the trepanation should be performed where the pain is best localized. Rufus of Ephsus (around 100 AD) and Soranus of Ephsus (90-138 AD) both described headaches and made important notes on migraine adding to the work of Hippocrates and Aretaeus, but did not offer any new treatments.

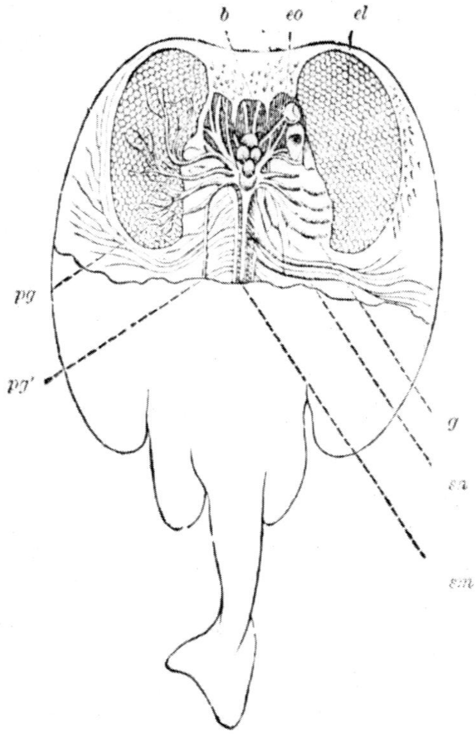

Figure 5. Torpedo fish. These rays are capable of producing electric currents strong enough to stun prey. They were believed to have therapeutic value and were applied to bodies to treat a variety of maladies in ancient times. *b*, brain; *eo*, eye and optic nerve; *el*, electric organs; *sn*, spinal nerves; *sm*, spinal marrow; *pg*, pneumogastric nerves going to the electric organs; *pg',* branch of the preceding; *g*, gills. Illustration from *Odd Forms among Fishes* by Professor Sanborn Tenney, *Popular Science Monthly, Volume 11, September 1877.*

Six centuries after Hippocrates, the state of medicine and neurosurgery reached a second milestone through the work of the Roman physician Claudius Galen of Pergamon (129-200 AD). His contribution to our knowledge of the nervous system, neuroanatomy, neurology, and neurosurgery is vast. It is to him that the word migraine is attributed, as it was transfigured from its original terminology "hemicrania." He described it as a painful disorder affecting half of the head that extends along the longitudinal suture, and he claimed that the headache was kept to one side because of the falx cerebri. [1,3,14] He also subscribed to the school of humoral medicine and recommended the same treatments as Hippocrates and Aretaeus. In addition he mentioned the use of the electric torpedo fish to be applied to the forehead of the patient [1], a method that was originally used by the court physician of the Roman emperor Claudius, Scribonius Largus (about 47 AD). He was the first to recognize the benefits of the torpedo's fish electrical discharge and used it for the treatment of headache and gout (Figure 5). [10]

Later, the Byzantine period following Galen did not witness any major changes in the description of migraine headache nor its treatment. Orobasius (325-403 AD) recommended bloodletting for treatment. [15] Aetius Amidenus (520-575 AD) mentions headache in his writing following Galen guiding principals of diagnosis and treatment. [16] Alexander of

Tralles (525-605 AD) suggested bloodletting from the opposite side of the headache. Paul of Aegina (625-690) advised opening the veins of the nose and designed a trephine bit with conical shape to prevent plunging. [17] They all discussed various types of headaches, referring extensively to the work of Hippocrates, Aretaeus, and Galen without offering anything new in the diagnosis or treatment of headache or advancing medical knowledge significantly.

The Arabic Islamic Period

When the medical and the intellectual development died in Western Europe (Roman Empire) and started fading away in Eastern Europe (Byzantine empire), it was the Islamic civilizations that took over the advancement of knowledge from the eighth century until approximately the beginning of the thirteen century (Figure 6). The Arabic schools translated and systematized the surviving Greek, Roman, and Byzantine texts into Arabic encyclopedias. As guardian to the Hippocratic and Galenic work, Arabic physicians also believed that headache stemmed from an unbalance of the four humors, and similarly prescribed bloodletting, cupping, and cautery (Figures 7 and 8). Abu Bakr Muhammad Ibn Zakariya Al-Razi known as Rhazes (854-925) from Persia was the first to introduce the concept of concussion headache. [18] Abu Ali Al-Husayn Ibn Abdallah Ibn Sina, known as Avicenna (980-1037) from Bukhara (Uzbekistan), used the term "Sodaa" to describe headache and "al-shakika" for migraine. He was the first to address the neurovascular theory of migraine headache in addition to the Hippocratic/Galenic theory of vapors arising from the liver or body to the head. [14] He speculated that migraine pain could be from the skull bone, the dura mater, distant substance reaching the head via veins or arteries, or the brain and it meninges. [19,20]

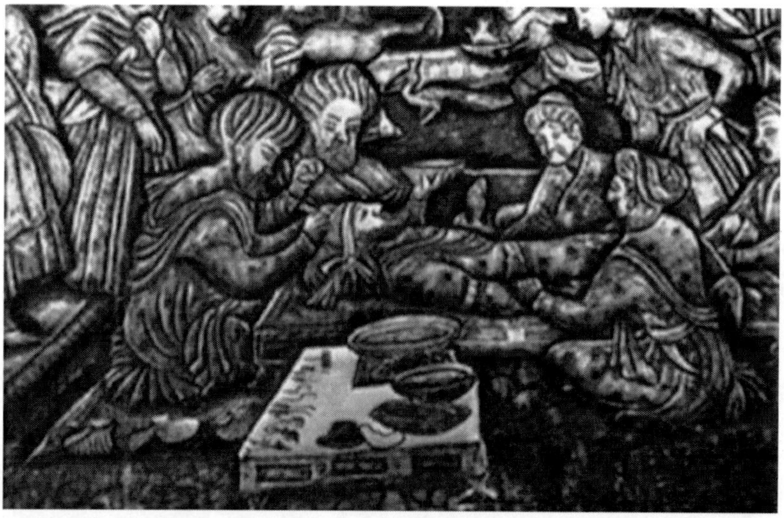

Figure 6. Ibn Sina (Avicenna) performing a neurosurgical procedure; a burr-hole trephination. Part of a miniature copper engraving.

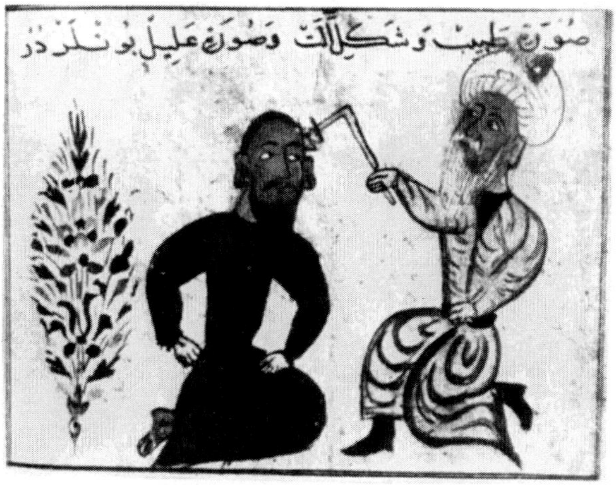

Figure 7. Illustration of medieval Arab doctor treating a patient through wound cauterization.

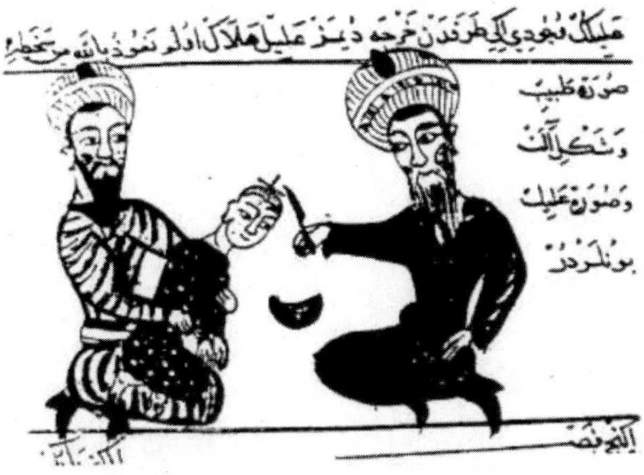

Figure 8. Illustration of medieval Arab doctor performing incision and evacuation of hydrocephalus. The physician uses a reversed T-type incision and wide and sharp pointed scalpel. Illustration from *Cerrahiyyetu'l Haniyye*, a 15th-century medicine book by Serafeddin Sabuncuoglu.

(فنقول هي وجع في أحد جانبي الرأس يهيج ويحدها جالينوس بأنها الساترة المتوسطة وربما كان سببه من داخل القحف وربما كان في الغشاء المجلّل للقحف وأكثر ما يكون يكون في عضل الصدغ وما كان خارجاً فقد يبلغ إلى أن لا يحتمل المس وتكون المواد واصلة إلى موضعه إما من الأوردة والشرايين الخارجة وإما من الدماغ نفسه وحجبه فيصعد أكثر ذلك من طريق الدروز وقد يكون من بخارات تندفع من البدن كله أو عضو من ذلك الشق)

"We say it is pain in one side of the head that rage and what Galen said it is stopped by the falx-cerebri, may be its cause is from inside the skull, may be from the mighty under covering of the skull, and mostly it is (the pain) in the temporalis muscle and if it is outside it may reach no touch tolerance and substances reach it either from the arteries, the exiting veins, from the brain itself, or its meninges and most of that ascend through the cranial sutures or it could be from vapors that get pushed from the whole body or part of it."

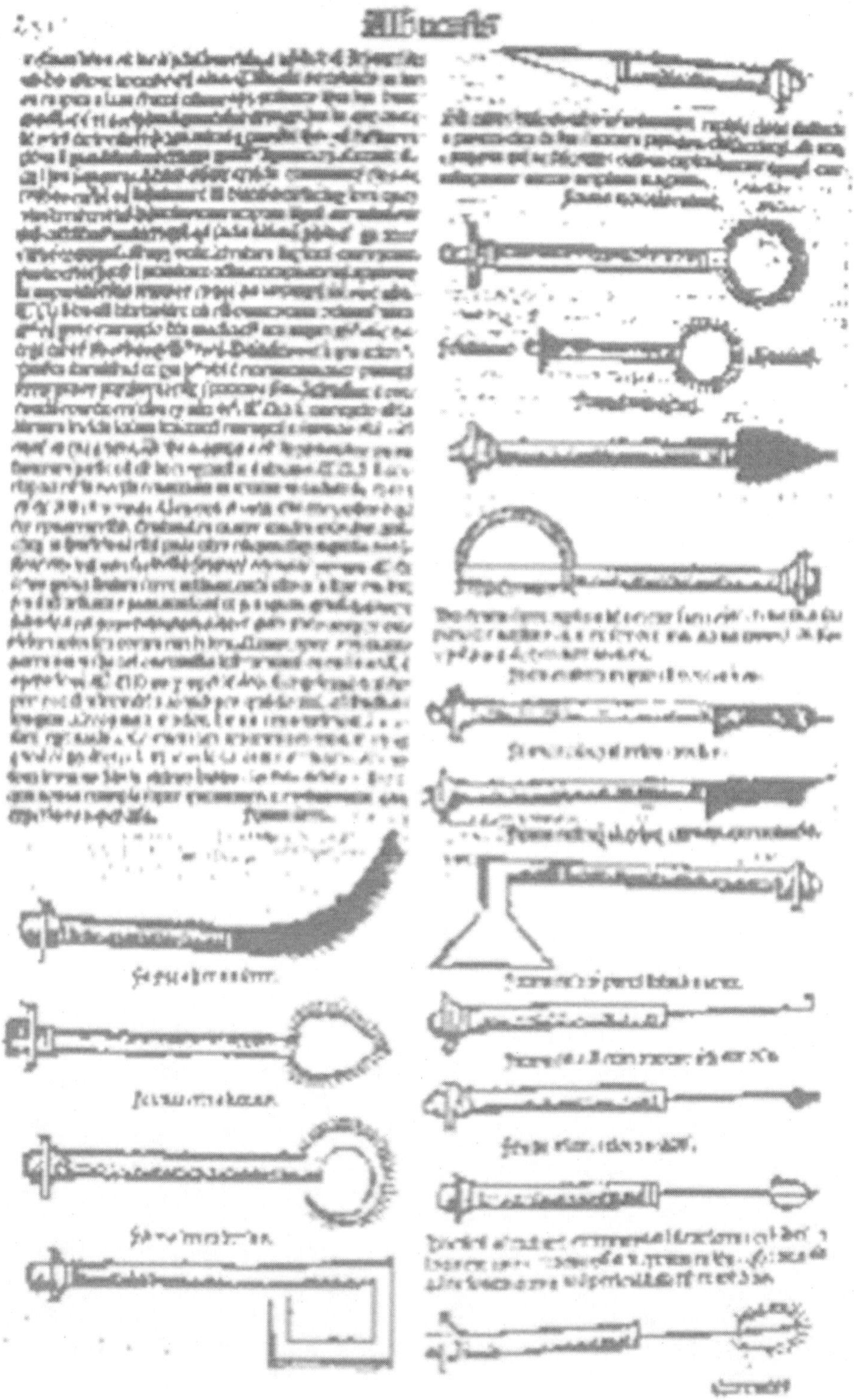

Figure 9. Latin translation of El Zahrawi's treatise by Peter Argellata, which shows many surgical and medical instruments.

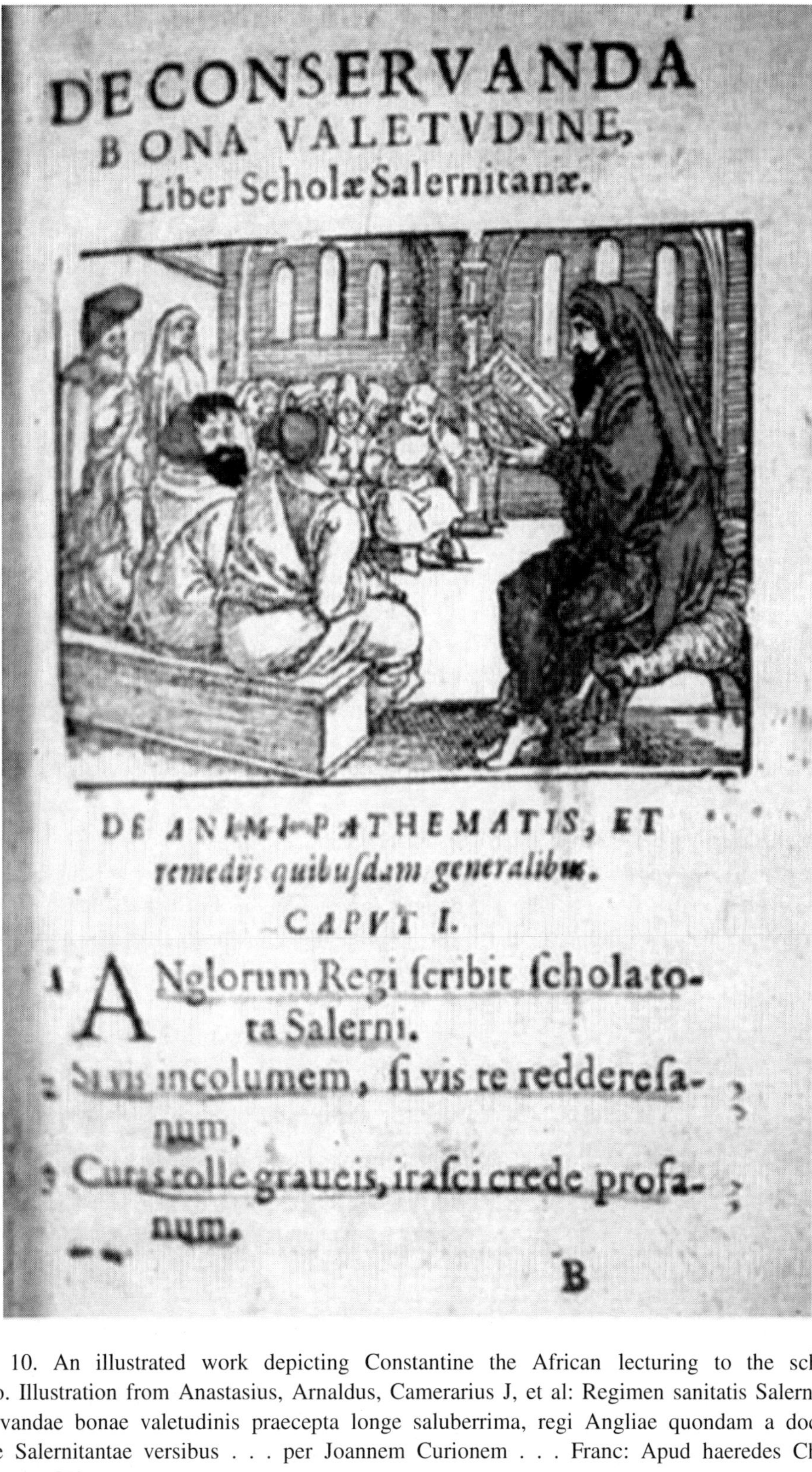
DE CONSERVANDA
BONA VALETUDINE,
Liber Scholæ Salernitanæ.

DE ANIMI-PATHEMATIS, ET
remedijs quibusdam generalibus.
CAPUT I.

1 ANglorum Regi scribit schola tota Salerni.
2 Si vis incolumem, si vis te reddere sanum,
3 Curas tolle graueis, irasci crede profanum.

B

Figure 10. An illustrated work depicting Constantine the African lecturing to the school of Salerno. Illustration from Anastasius, Arnaldus, Camerarius J, et al: Regimen sanitatis Salernitanum. Conservandae bonae valetudinis praecepta longe saluberrima, regi Angliae quondam a doctoribus scholae Salernitantae versibus . . . per Joannem Curionem . . . Franc: Apud haeredes Christiani Egenolphi, 1573.

During the same era, another great surgeon and scholar emerged on the other side of the world: Abu al-Qasim Khalaf ibn al-Abbas Al-Zahrawi, known as Albucasis (936-1013, from Al-andalus Spain). He described the application of cautery for chronic headache treatment by placing a hot iron on the occiput, burning through the skin but not the skull. He also suggested, in another headache treatment, to avulse the temporal artery by hooking it, twisting it then ligating it. He is accredited for inventing the non-sinking trephine, where he placed a collar around the trephine to prevent plunging into the brain (Figure 9). [21]

The Medieval European Period

Advancement of medical knowledge stood still in Western Europe during the medieval European era. It began with the collapse of the Roman Empire in the fifth century and lasted until the renaissance era. Medical knowledge started trickling back to Western Europe in the beginning of the eleventh century by translation of the Arabic books into Latin. Constantine the African (1020-1087) played a bridging role between the Islamic schools and the school of Salerno in Europe as he spearheaded this translation movement (Figure 10). [22] Despite this transfer of knowledge there was no advancement in the description, diagnosis, or treatment of migraine headache. The lack of anatomical knowledge and poor surgical outcomes stalled all surgical treatment of cranial pathology. [23] An important figure during this period was the court physician of Morocco, Abu Imram Musa Ibn Maimun (1135-1204), known as Maimonides who wrote ten medical treasures in Arabic. [24] He, as well, suggested that headaches come from thick viscous humors and described migraine, recommending for its severe cases, bloodletting from the pulsating arteries behind the ear. [25]

Renaissance Period and the Rise of the West (14th-17th Century)

The renaissance period was marked by the reintroduction of the human anatomical dissection and the correction of Greco-Romano-Arab anatomical errors. Leonardo da Vinci (1452-1519), Giacomo Berengario da Carpi (1460-1530), Johannes Dryander (1500-1560), Ambroise Pare (1510-1590), and Andreas Vesalius (1514-1564) were among the great anatomists of this era. The development of new surgical concepts, basic research techniques, and the renewed interest in surgery laid the foundation for modern neurosurgery during this period. Although headache description, characterization, and classification witnessed an enormous advancement during this period, its surgical treatment, unfortunately, did not depart from the ancient beliefs and the humoral theory despite the great anatomical understanding that was achieved. Most cases were explained within the framework of the humoral pathophysiology, so bloodletting and drainage of other body fluids through cupping, blistering and purging were still widely used during this period for the treatment of headaches (Figure 11). Trepanation was reserved for incurable cases. The Dutch Hippocrates, Forestus (1521-1597), used leeches for bloodletting to treat hemicranias, and for incurable headaches he used trepanation. [26]

William Harvey (1578-1657) was an English physician who described in detail the systemic circulation, and he recommended “the opening of the skull with a Trepand iron near the place of the pain” for headache treatment. [27] The Dutch physician Nicholaus Petreus Tulpius (1593-1674) in his “Observationes Medicae” describes various types of headaches and its treatments. [28] He subscribed to the Hippocratic school of thought and believed that if water or blood escaped the body through the nose or the ears it would cure headaches. He also recommended cupping to drain the volatile spirit from the body of the wife of a carpenter who suffered from headaches for years. [28] Thomas Willis [1621-1675] was an English physician who was a pioneer in the nervous system anatomy research and one of the greatest contributors to the 17th century medicine. He described the circle of Willis and introduced the term "neurology". [1] His research on the head pain innervation was significant and he described migraine headache symptoms and its causes in detail. [29] Although, Avicenna was the first to address the neurovascular theory of migraine headache, it is thought that Willis is the first to introduce it. He suggested that congestion of the blood vessels in the head may cause migraine and that its symptoms may be the result of ascending spasms. [30] He proposed spinning the patient around in a centrifuge to force the blood from the head to the feet [31] and also recommended bloodletting by phlebotomy or arteriotomy for chronic headaches, [32] but he did not think that trepanation has much benefit in headache treatment. [27] Johann Jakob Wepfer (1620-1695) was a Swiss pharmacologist who applied cantharides paste to the shaved scalp to induce blistering and withdraw fluid from the head in the treatment of headaches.

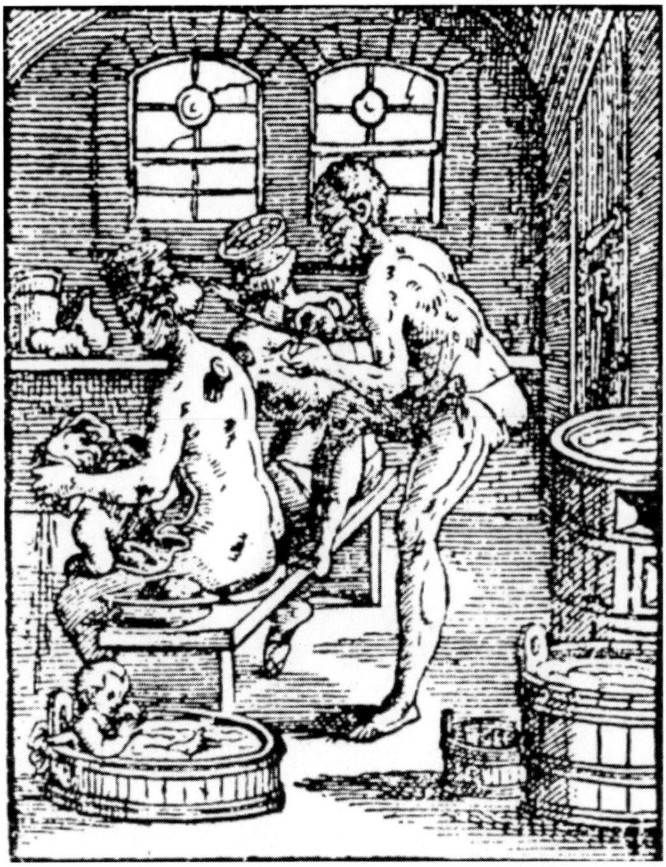

Figure 11. 16th century woodcutting held by the Bibliotheque Nationale that demonstrates cupping during the renaissance. Image courtesy of the National Library of Medicine.

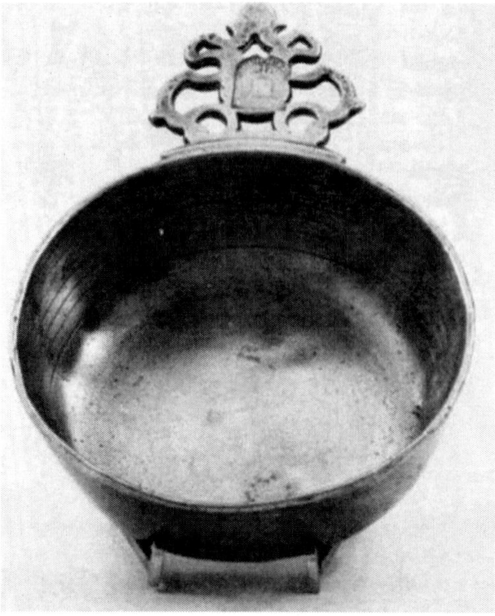

Figure 12. Bowl used for bloodletting, with gradations to allow measurement of blood. Crafted by John Foster of London after 1740. (Held by the Division of Cultural History, Greenwood Collection, Smithsonian Institution, SI photo 61166-C).

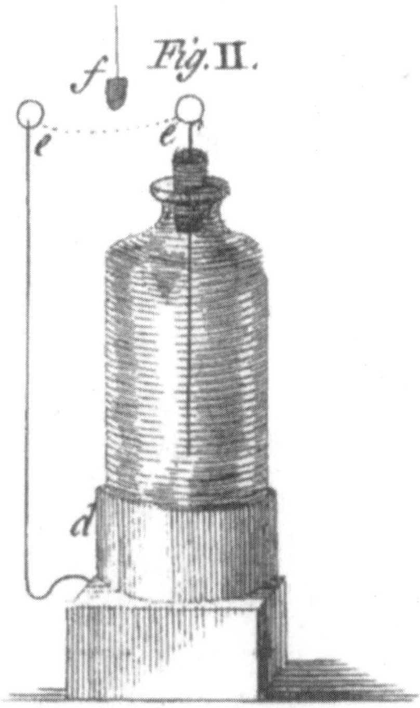

Figure 13. The Leyden Jar, originally known as a condenser, is an instrument capable of storing static electricity between two electrodes on the outside and inside of a glass jar. Illustration from Benjamin Franklin: New Experiments and Observations on Electricity (1754).

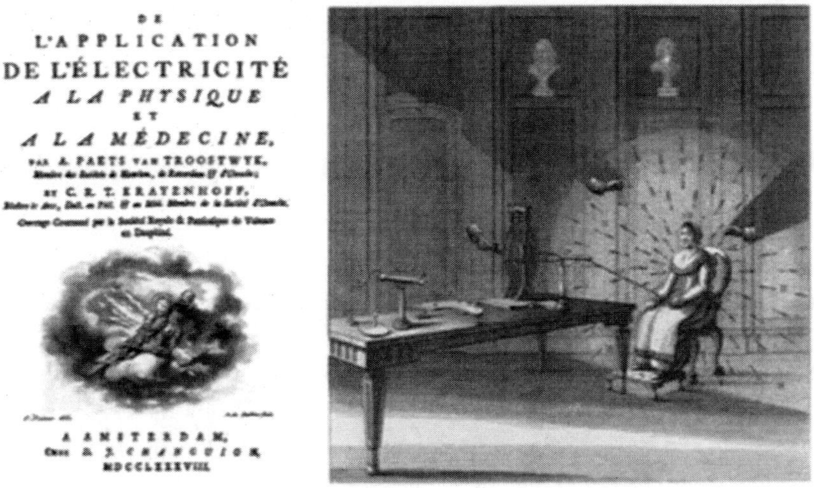

Figure 14. The title page and a picture from a book in French dedicated to the application of electricity in physics and medicine in which headache cases are also described (Paets van Troostwijk and Krayenhoff, 1788).

Modern Period (18th – 19th Century)

A great cultural movement of intellectuals who put emphasis on reason and scientific methods to advance knowledge and challenge the traditional and spiritual doctrines marked the 18th century, known as the Age of Enlightenment or Age of Reason. Clinical bedside medicine was reintroduced with emphasis on diagnostic examination of the patient. Although surgeons during this period became more aggressive in the management of head pathology such as head trauma, bloodletting and fluid drainage from the body was still the main treatment method of headaches (Figure 12). Gerard Van Swieten (1700-1772) used bloodletting, purging, cupping of the neck, and blistering to treat headaches. [33] Robert Whytt (1714-1766) used phlebotomy for bloodletting from vessels of the neck, nose, or ankles. He also applied leeches to the temporal area and for violent headache he did an arteriotomy of an artery of the head. For drainage of other bodily fluids he used purging or blistering of the head or legs. [34] William Heberden (1710-1801) used blistering of the head and bloodletting by cupping between the shoulders to treat headaches that failed pharmacological remedies. [35] Others like Claude Pouteau (1725-1775) used cauterization for rapid humoral drainage. [36]

The middle of the 18th century was marked by the discovery of electricity. The Leyden Jar, the original capacitor, was invented independently but simultaneously in 1745 by the German physicist Ewald Georg von Kleist (1700-1748) and the Dutch scientist Pieter van Musschenbroek (1692-1761) (Figure 13). In 1791, Luigi Galvani (1737-1798) discovered that nerve cells use electrical signals to communicate with muscles. [37] Although, Scribonius Largus was the first who recognized the benefits of the torpedo fish's electrical discharge and used it to treat headaches, it was not until the middle of the 18th century that the cognoscente application of electrical current in medicine and headache treatment was introduced. The Dutch Society of Sciences recognized the electrical effects of the South American fish, the electrical eel, that delivered a powerful shock similar to the Leyden Jar[10] and used it for slaves that suffered from headaches by putting one of their hands on the eel fish and the other hand on their heads claiming immediate help with no exceptions. [38] Electricity from other sources gained a wide use in medicine including the treatment of headaches (Figure 14). Pierre Bertholon (1742-1800) a French physicist who described the use of negative electrical current to cure migraine headache stating that he cured many of his attacks by applying negative electricity to his temporal area. [39]

The 19th century witnessed major advancements in medicine and surgery. Three major innovations: anesthesia, antisepsis, and brain localization made it possible for great advancement in neurosurgery. The practice of medicine changed in the face of the rapid advancement of the scientific method and the disappearance of the humoral theory. Edward Liveing (1832-1919) introduced the "nerve storm" theory as a source of migraine in his treatise of migraine headaches, thereby distinguishing himself from Willis and his vasodilation theory of migraine. [40] The function of the vasomotor nerve was discovered through the competitive and non-collaborative work of Bernard and Brown-Sequard. In 1851, Claude Bernard (1813-1878) demonstrated that sections of the cervical sympathetic nerve caused a marked change in skin temperature. [41] In 1852, Charles Edward Brown-Sequard (1817-1894) showed that electrical stimulation of sympathetic nerve produces blood vessel contraction. [41] These discoveries reinforced and popularized the electrical treatment for migraines and helped the departure from the digestive and humoral theory of headaches. Rudolf Lewandowski, Albert Eulenburg, William Hammond, and Charles Loomis Dana are among the proponent of electrical use for the treatment of migraine. [10] Elizabeth Garrett Anderson (1836-1917), the first female physician in England, advocated the use of electricity to cure migraines in her thesis "Sur la migraine"[42,43] (Figure 15). She wrote:

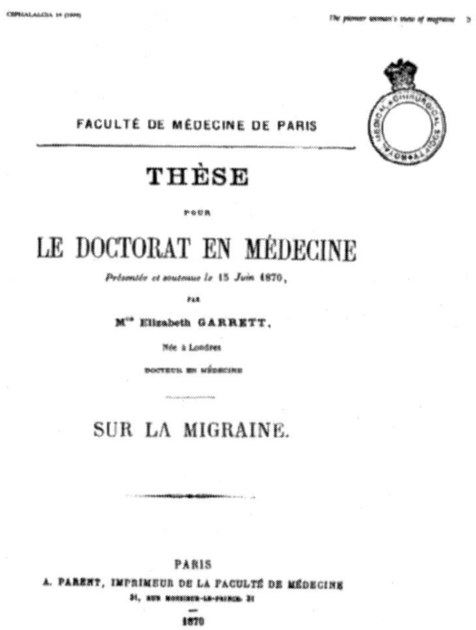

FACULTÉ DE MÉDECINE DE PARIS

THÈSE

POUR

LE DOCTORAT EN MÉDECINE

Présentée et soutenue le 15 Juin 1870,

PAR

Mlle Elizabeth GARRETT,

Née à Londres

DOCTEUR EN MÉDECINE

SUR LA MIGRAINE.

PARIS

A. PARENT, IMPRIMEUR DE LA FACULTÉ DE MÉDECINE

1870

Figure 15. Posting highlighting Elizabeth Garrett Anderson's thesis presentation, "Sur la migraine" which advocated the use of electricity to cure migraine headache.

> "In the treatment of migraine, remedies should be directed against the alteration in the nervous system rather than those of the digestive system…After natural means such air and exercise, the most artificial remedy is without doubt voltaic electricity…It is therefore possible to apply a similar current directed to the brain in cases where, as in migraine, the original fault of innervation is localized in the cranium …There are serious reasons to believe that, in continuous current, we have a curative agent which is more effective than all the remedies known before"

Despite the wide acceptance of the electrical current as a treatment of migraine, many prominent physicians casted major doubt in its usefulness. William Gowers (1845-1915) thought that the voltaic current might give occasional transient relief but rarely a permanent one. [44] William Osler (1849-1919) did not believe that electricity offered any benefits. [45] Edward Flatau (1868-1932) stated that he had never been convinced of electrical current efficacy in headache treatment. [46]

Arterial compression, especially carotid compression, was also practiced during this period. Although it was first practiced in 1786 by the English physician Caleb Hillier Parry (1755-1822) to prevent violent propulsion of blood into the brain in the treatment of headache, it was the vasomotor theory that led to its revival in the 19th century. Mollendorff [10] and Hammond [47] advocated carotid compression during migraine attacks. Romberg and Schroeder recommended the combined compression of the carotid artery and the vagus nerve. [40]

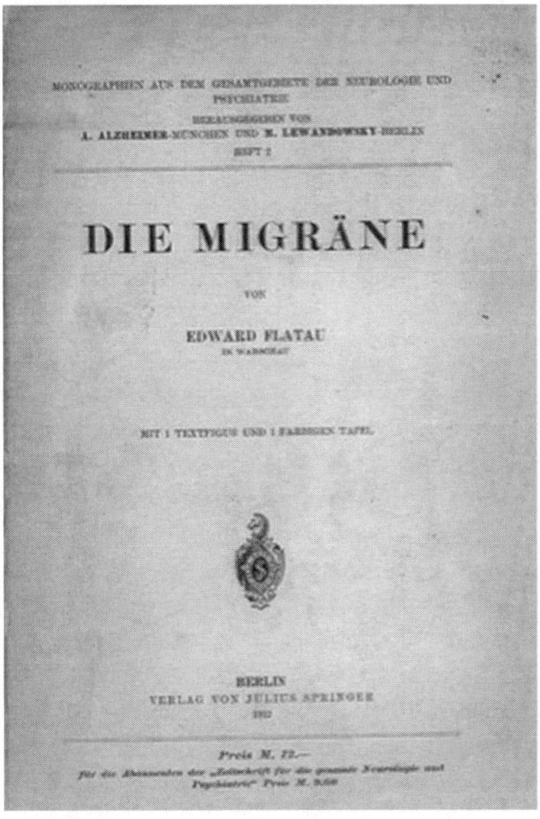
DIE MIGRÄNE

EDWARD FLATAU

BERLIN
VERLAG VON JULIUS SPRINGER

Figure 16. Die Migrane" by Edward Flatau, published in Berlin in 1912.

The 20th Century

The 20th century produced a plethora of discoveries and breakthroughs in all aspects of science. Improved communication through conferences, publications, and the Internet disseminated knowledge rapidly throughout the world among scientists. Medicine witnessed a rapid progression in all fronts during this era. Although it had a slow start, headache treatment was no exception. In the beginning of the century, some famous surgeons reverted to humoral medicine, recommending the use of seton tape. Walter Whitehead (1840-1913), a consulting surgeon at the Manchester Royal Infirmary, described in detailed his successful surgical technique for migraine treatment in 1901 "The Surgical Treatment of Migraine" [48]:

> "I have never failed to treat successfully the most inveterate and severe cases of migraine by the introduction of an ordinary tape seton through the skin at the back of the neck…All the cases have been previously under medical treatment without receiving any material benefits"

William Osler, in the fourth edition of his textbook "The principles and practice of medicine," recommended the use of seton tape under the skin at the back of the neck with reference to Mr. Walter Whitehead. [45]

Attribution of migraine to organic and structural causes arising from the nasopharyngeal, oral, and otic disorders, has led to the surgical removal of adenoids, nasal turbinate, dentures, and mastoid bone with mixed results. [10,49]

The emergence of increased intracranial pressure as a cause of migraine led to the revival of trepanation and newer surgical treatments. Heinrich Irenaeus Quincken (1842-1922) who is accredited for the first lumbar puncture [50], reported migraine attack relief in two of his patients after a lumbar puncture. [10] Wilfred John Harris (1869-1960), the consulting physician to St. Mary's for nervous diseases, believed that migraine pain is caused by increased intracranial pressure secondary to vasodilation of cranial and meningeal vessels and recommended local trepanation and opening of dura, lumbar puncture, or leeches to the scalp. [51] Edward Flatau (1868-1932) recommended lumbar puncture for migraine referring to Quincken report and confirming it benefits in the case of a young boy (Figure 16). [10]. Schuller (1909) stated that increased intracranial pressure could be diagnosed on skull radiographs and suggested trepanation. He even proposed palliative trepanation of the sella and third ventriculostomy. [10] Harvey William Cushing (1969-1993), the father of American neurosurgery, attempted to cure migraine surgically with very limited success. In 1909 and 1910 he performed three decompressive craniotomies with sub-temporal decompression for the treatment of tree females suffering from migraine (Figure 17). [52] Although he favored the increased intracranial pressure theory as a cause of migraine, he never discounted the humoral theory, organic causes, and especially the vasomotor theory since he ligated the temporal artery in one of his migraine patients. [52] The vasomotor hypothesis was based on the combination of vasodilatation and vasospasm from sympathetic stimulation of meningeal branches of the external carotid artery especially the middle meningeal artery. One of the founders of the American neurosurgery, Walter Edward Dandy (1886–1946), considered migraine as a vasospastic disorder and in 1931 he described migraine relief in some of his patients after performing a cervicothoracic sympathectomy. [53] Some surgeons claimed successful migraine relief after sympathectomy but other disclaimed it and called it "capricious". [54] Others argued that migraine is a vasodilatation problem and should be treated with arterial ligation rather than sympathectomy. [10] In 1933, Dickerson reported migraine relief after ligation of the middle meningeal artery in some of his patients. [55] Many other surgeons followed suit and tried to treat migraine by ligating other branches of the external carotid artery with mixed success. [54]

Wilder Graves Penfield (1891–1976) used a direct approach to disrupt the pain fibers associated with cranial vessels that are causing migraine, and in 1940 he reported positive results after partial sectioning of the trigeminal nerve. [56] Others believed that the afferent pain fibers from the carotid artery and the dura are carried via the greater superficial petrosal nerve (GSPN) to the geniculate ganglion then through the nervus intermedius to the somatic sensory pathways of the brain stem. [57] In 1948, James C. White (1895-1981) and William H. Sweet (1910-2001) sectioned the GSPN for the treatment of migrainous neuralgia with varied success. [58] Surgical sectioning, alcohol injection and radiofrequency were used for gangliorhizotomy throughout the second half of the 20th century. [10,59] The greater occipital, the posterior auricular, and the auriculotemporal nerves were also targeted for the treatment of migraine. [60] By the end of the century, targeted anesthetic blockade of some this nerve emerged as a treatment for migraine with some success. [61,62]

The 21st Century

The end of the 20th century and beginning of the 21st century saw the introduction of many innovative methods for attempted treatment of migraine headache. By the 21st century, it was commonly believed that the pathogenesis of primary headache syndromes such as migraine involve afferents from pain-producing cranial structures such as blood vessels and dura. Most commonly, trigeminal structures were implicated in pain pathogenesis. Newer thought also attributes cervically derived nerves in the pathogenesis of migraine pain, as migraine pain is not always constrained within trigeminal innervation territories. With such knowledge in mind, physicians and scholars of this century have been investigating mechanisms to modulate both trigeminal and cervical components of the cranial pain system.

At the beginning of the 21st century, Bahman Guyuron, a plastic surgeon, developed four surgical procedures designed to deactivate migraine headache trigger sites. With the belief that activation of the terminal branches of the trigeminal nerve results in characteristic migraine pain, Guyuron proposed that these nerve branches can be stimulated by contraction of surrounding head and neck muscles, resulting in migraine pain. [63] His surgical procedures are based on the location of the migraine headache: Frontal, occipital, temporal, and nasal. For patients with frontal migraines, the glabellar muscle group (procerus muscle, corrugator supercilli, and depressor supercilli) are removed through a palpebral incision to decompress the supratrochlear and supraorbital nerves that traverse these muscles [Figure 18]. For occipital migraines, a portion of the semispinalis capitis muscle medial to the greater occipital nerve is removed, and the nerve is then protected using a subcutaneous flap to prevent irritation from surrounding muscles. For temporal migraines, segments of the zygomaticotemporal branch of the trigeminal nerve are removed to prevent compression by the temporalis muscle. As well, patients with migraines triggered from intranasal regions have been treated with septoplasties and turbinectomies (Comprehensive surgical treatment of migraine). [64] Five-year follow-up data on these procedures suggests that manipulation of one or more migraine trigger sites can successfully help reduce duration, intensity, and frequency of migraine headaches. [65]

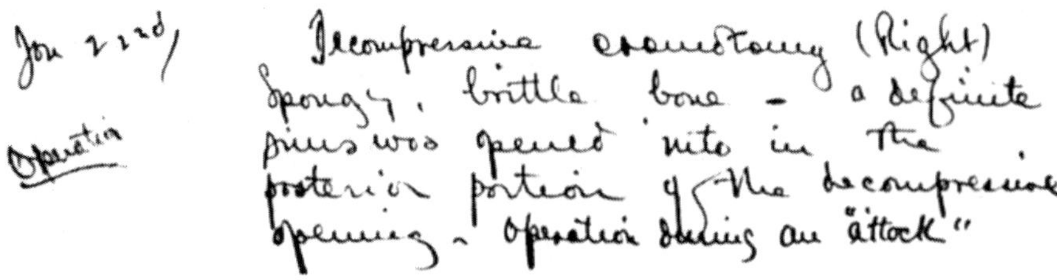
Jan 22nd /
Operation
Decompressive craniotomy (Right)
Spongy, brittle bone - a definite
sinus was opened into in the
posterior portion of the decompressive
opening - Operation during an "attack"

Figure 17. Harvey Cushing's note describing one of his craniotomy procedures for headache treatment, which reads: "Decompressive craniotomy (Right) Spongy, brittle bone – a definite sinus was opened into in the posterior portion of the decompressive opening – Operation during an "attack."" Image from the Alan Mason Chesney Archives.

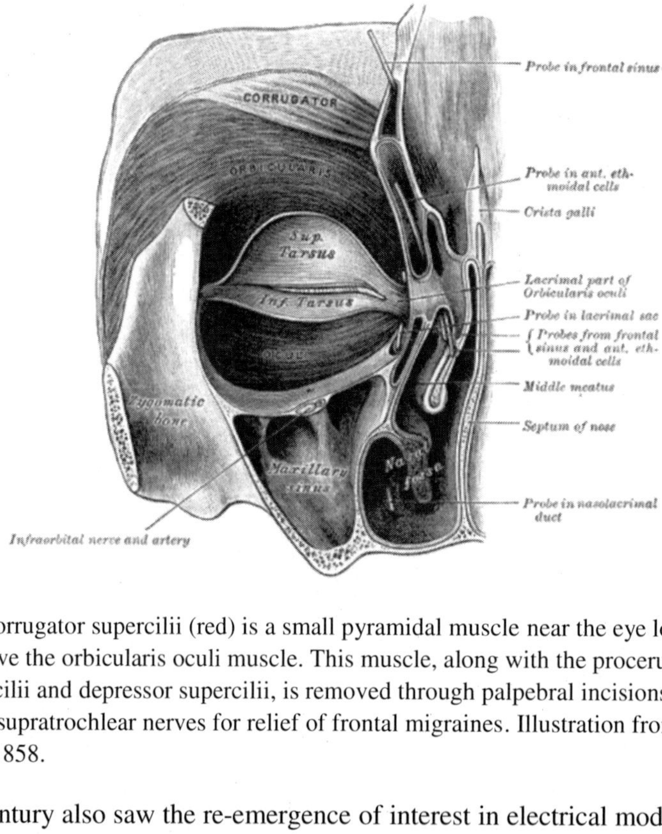

Figure 18. The corrugator supercilii (red) is a small pyramidal muscle near the eye located beneath the frontalis and above the orbicularis oculi muscle. This muscle, along with the procerus muscle, corrugator supercilii and depressor supercilii, is removed through palpebral incisions to decompress the supraorbital and supratrochlear nerves for relief of frontal migraines. Illustration from Gray's Anatomy by Henry Gray, 1858.

The 21st century also saw the re-emergence of interest in electrical modification of neural transmission in treatment of migraine. Known as neuromodulation, this developing field includes use of nerve stimulation in migraine treatment. [10] Most of these procedures are reserved particularly for migraine refractory to medications and patients without medication overuse. Currently, most approaches focus on the stimulation of the occipital nerve, composed of branches of the C2 and C3 spinal roots. The principle underlying success of occipital nerve stimulation rests on the gate control theory of pain, which states that activation of large-fiber afferents involved in proprioception or vibration leads to simultaneous inhibition of small-fiber afferents that are responsible for pain transmission via inhibitory interneurons. [66] The occipital nerve has synapses in the trigeminocervical complex implicated in migraine pain, and thus nerve stimulation is thought to modulate the complex's excitability and thus perception of pain in structures such as the dura and blood vessels responsible for migraine headache. [67]

The first human trials of occipital nerve stimulation for head pain occurred in 1999. [68] In 2004, Matharu et al. described eight cases of chronic migraine that responded successfully to bilateral implanted suboccipital stimulation. Patients reported that stimulation quickly suppresses pain and have been able to discontinue or decrease their intake of preventative and abortive medications for migraine. [69] Follow-up studies have suggested that occipital nerve stimulation can be effective long-term. [66,70 71,72]

The same technology and equipment utilized for spinal cord stimulation is used in occipital nerve stimulation, including electrodes and their leads, anchors for fastening leads to surrounding tissue, and the battery, or internal neurostimulator. [73] Batteries can be rechargeable or non-rechargeable, and are comparable in weight and size to cardiac implantable devices. This battery is coupled to a programmable radiofrequency receiver. [74] The surgical procedure involves placement of subcutaneous leads along the intermastoid line at the C1 arch (Figure 19). [75]

Over the past years, alternative stimulation sites and combinations have been suggested, including combined stimulation of the occipital and supraorbital nerves. [76] Greater auricular nerve stimulation has also been studied for its utility in migraine treatment.

Neuromodulation technology continues to evolve. The Bion microstimulator (Boston Scientific Neuromodulation Corporation) has been studied for its use in chronic migraine. It contains a single anode/cathode configuration, a rechargeable lithium ion battery, and programmable microchip. Its small size allows it to be positioned adjacent to nerves via an introducer needle without needing additional hardware (Figure 20). It is hoped that such technology will minimize risks associated with paddle or percutaneous leads implanted. [77]

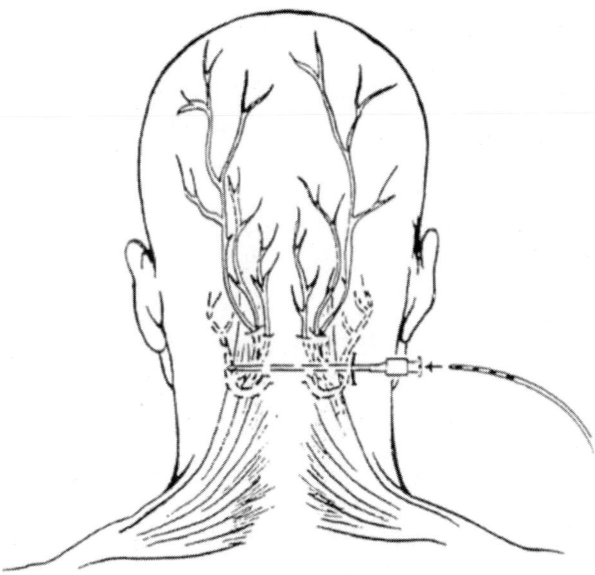

Figure 19. Illustration demonstrating electrode placement for occipital nerve stimulation. Illustration from *Peripheral Neurostimulation for Control of Intractable Occipital Neuralgia* by Richard L. Weiner and Kenneth L. Reid, *Neuromodulation Vol. 2, Number 3, 217-221.* 1999.

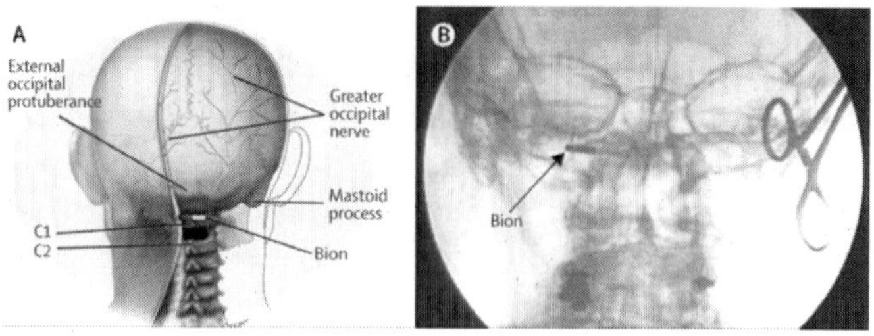

Figure 20. The Bion Microstimulator. A. Diagram of the implanted bion microstimulator for occipital nerve stimulation. B. Intraoperative X-ray of the bion in situ. Image courtesy of *The Lancet Neurology*. Reprinted from "Treatment of hemicrania continua by occipital nerve stimulation with a bion device: long-term follow-up of a crossover study", Burns, B, Watkins, L, Goadsby, P, Vol. 7, Issue 11, p. 1001-1012. Nov. 2008.

The development of the S8 Lamitrode electrode, a narrow electrode designed to minimize trauma during placement, minimize lead migration, and deliver more focused stimulation, is under study for its utility. [78]

The 21st century has also seen heightened interest in the epidemiological relation between patent foramen ovale (PFO) and migraine with aura. Studies have demonstrated that PFO closer may improve or even cure migraine headache in select individuals. However there is currently not enough justification for PFO closure to be used as standard of care. [70]

Conclusion

Mankinds' understanding of headache and migraine has evolved over thousands of years. As greater knowledge of anatomy and pathophysiology has developed, so have newer methodologies for headache treatment, as evidenced by the transformation from the early days of trepanation to modern microstimulation of precise neuronal structures. By tracing the contributions of those clinician scientists throughout historical epochs in human history, our society can better evaluate the mechanisms of headache and therapeutic treatments that are utilized today. Reflection on the vast history of migraine surgery allows us to apply this knowledge towards more effective management of headache disorders in the 21st century.

References

[1] Magiorkinis, E., Diamantis, A., Mitsikostas, D. D. & Androutsos, G. (2009). Headaches in antiquity and during the early scientific era. *Journal of Neurology. 256*(8),1215-1220.

[2] Friedman, A. P. (1972). The headache in history, literature, and legend. *Bulletin of the New York Academy of Medicine. 48*(4), 661-681.

[3] Rose, F. C. (1995). The history of migraine from Mesopotamian to Medieval times. Cephalalgia: *An International Journal of Headache.* 15 Suppl 15,1-3.

[4] Campillo, D. (1984). Neurosurgical pathology in prehistory. *Acta neurochirurgica. 70*(3-4), 275-290.

[5] Garrison, F. H. & McHenry, L. C. (1969). *History of neurology.* Rev. and enl. ed. Springfield, Ill.: Charles C Thomas Pub Ltd.

[6] Hammurabi (1903). The laws of Hammurabi, King of Babylonia. *Washington, D.C.*: Records of the Past Exploration Society.

[7] Shehata, M. (2004). The Father of Medicine: A Historical Reconsideration. Turkiye *Kilikleri Journal of Medical Ethics. 12.*

[8] Sanchez, G. M., Meltzer, E. S., Smith, E. & Harer, W. B. (2012). The Edwin Smith Papyrus: updated translation of the trauma treatise and modern medical commentaries. *Atlanta, Ga.*: Lockwood Press.

[9] Ghalioungui, P. (1987). The Ebers papyrus: a new English translation, commentaries and glossaries. *Cairo*: Academy of Scientific Research and Technology.

[10] Koehler, P. J. & Boes, C. J. (2010). A history of non-drug treatment in headache, particularly migraine. *Brain: a journal of neurology. 133*(Pt 8), 2489-2500

[11] Hippocrates, Verhoofd L. & Marks, E. The aphorisms of Hippocrates. New York,: Collins & Co.; 1818

[12] Missios, S. & Hippocrates, Galen, & the uses of trepanation in the ancient classical world. (2007). *Neurosurgical Focus. 23*(1), E11.

[13] Koehler, P. J. & van de Wiel, T. W. (2001). Aretaeus on migraine and headache. *Journal of the History of the Neurosciences*, *10*(3), 253-261.

[14] Rapoport, A. & Edmeads, J. (2000). Migraine: the evolution of our knowledge. *Archives of Neurology. 57*(8), 1221-1223.

[15] Oribase, C. & Oeuvres d'Oribase. (1873). *Imprimerie Nationale. 5*, 87-89.

[16] Aetius of Amida O. A. (1453). Aetii Amideni Libri medicinales.

[17] Paulus & Adams, F. (1844). The seven books of Paulus Ægineta. London,: Printed for the Sydneham Society.

[18] McCrory, P. R. & Berkovic, S. F. (2001). Concussion: the history of clinical and pathophysiological concepts and misconceptions. *Neurology. 57*(12), 2283-2289.

[19] Abokrysha, N. (2009). Ibn Sina (Avicenna) on pathogenesis of migraine compared with the recent theories. *Headache*, *49*(6), 923-927.

[20] Avicenna & Desparts J. (1498). Canon medicinae. *Lyons,*: Johannes Trechsel.

[21] Albucasis, S., M. S., & Lewis, G. L. (1973). On Surgery and Instruments. London: London Wellcome Institute.

[22] Pasca, M. (1994). The Salerno School of Medicine. *American journal of nephrology. 14*(4-6), 478-482.

[23] Goodrich, J. (2005). Landmarks in the history of neurosurgery. In: Rengachary S, Ellenbogen, RG, ed. Principles of Neurosurgery. 2 ed. Philadelphia, PA, USA: Elsevier Mosby.

[24] Rosner, F. (2010). Moses Maimonides: biographic outlines. *Rambam Maimonides medical journal.1*(1), e0002.

[25] Rosner, F. (1993). Headache in the writings of Moses Maimonides and other Hebrew sages. *Headache*, *33*(6),315-319.

[26] Foreest, V. (1653). Observationum et curatonium medicinalium. Rotho Magi.

[27] Willis, T. & Eugenius, P. (1977). The London practice of physick. *Boston*: Longwood Press.

[28] Tulp, N. (1716). Observationes medicae. 5 ed. *Leiden*: Vivie.

[29] Critchley, M. (1967). Migraine: from Cappadocia to Queen Square. In: Smith R, ed. Background to Migraine. London: Heinemann 28-38.

[30] Willis, T. & Feindel, W. (1978). The anatomy of the brain and nerves. Special ed. *Birmingham, Ala.*: Classics of Medicine Library.

[31] Green, M., Green, L. & Rothrock, J. (2005). Headache for history buffs. In: Green M, Green, L, Rothrock, J, ed. Managing Your Headaches. *New York, NY, USA:* Springer 1-11.

[32] Willis, T. (1674). De Anima Brutorum. *Ammstelodami*: Johannem a Someren;

[33] Isler, H. (1993). Episodic cluster headache from a textbook of 1745: van Swieten's classic description. *Cephalalgia: an international journal of headache. 13*(3), 172-174; discussion 149.

[34] Whytt, R. Observations on the nature, causes, and cure of those disorders which have been commonly called nervous, hypochondriac, or hysteric: to which are prefixed some remarks on the sympathy of the nerves. The 3d ed. *Edinburgh,*: Printed for T. Becket, and P.A. De Hondt, London; etc.;

[35] Heberden, W. (1962). Commentaries on the history and cure of diseases. New York,: Published by Hafner Pub. Co.

[36] Pouteau, C. (1760). Me'langes de chirugie. *Lyon*: Regnault.

[37] Kirby, R. S. (1990) Engineering in history. Dover ed. *New York*: Dover Publications.

[38] Koehler, P., Finger, S. & Picolino, M. (2009). The 'eels' of South America: two mid-eighteenth century letters from the dutch colonies on animal electricity. *Journal of Historical Biology. 42*, 715-763.

[39] Bertholon, P. (1780). Electricite du corps humain dans l'e tat de sante et de maladie. *Paris*: Didot.

[40] Living, E. (1873). Pathology of megrim and allied disorder. On megrim, sick-headache and some allied disorders: A contribution to the pathology of nerve storms. *Churchill, London*: Inter Documentation Company 335-398.

[41] Montastruc, J. L., Rascol, O. & Senard, J. M. (1996). The discovery of vasomotor nerves. Clinical autonomic research: *Official Journal of the Clinical Autonomic Research Society. 6*(3),183-187.

[42] Wilkinson, M. & Isler, H. (1999). The pioneer woman's view of migraine: Elizabeth Garrett Anderson's thesis "Sur la migraine". *Cephalalgia: an international journal of headache. 19*(1), 3-15.

[43] Anderson, E. (1870). Sur la migraine. Paris: Faculte de la medicine.

[44] Gowers, WR. (1970). A manual of diseases of the nervous system. 2d ed. *Darien, Conn.,*: Hafner Pub. Co.

[45] Osler, W. (1892). The principles and practice of medicine: designed for the use of practitioners and students of medicine. *New York*: D. Appleton and Company.

[46] Flatau, E. (1914). Migraine und ihre Abarten. In: Lewandowsky M, ed. Handbuch der Neurologie. Vol 5. Berlin: Springer. 342-426.

[47] Hammond, W. A. & Hammond G. M. (1891). A treatise on the diseases of the nervous system. 9th ed. New York,: D. Appleton and company.

[48] Whitehead, W. (1901). The Surgical Treatment of Migraine. *British medical journal. 1*(2093), 335-336.

[49] Brunton, L. (1899). A Discussion on Headaches and their Treatment. *British Medical Journal.*

[50] Frederiks, J. A. & Koehler, P. J. (1997). The first lumbar puncture. *Journal of the History of the Neurosciences. 6*(2),147-153.

[51] Harris. (1908). An address on the treatment of some of the severer forms of headache. *British Medical Journal. 8*(2), 297-298.

[52] Latimer, K., Pendleton, C., Rosenberg, J., Cohen-Gadol, A. A. & Quinones-Hinojosa, A. Dr. (2011). Harvey Cushing's attempts to cure migraine based on theories of pathophysiology. *Journal of neurosurgery.115*(5), 924-928.

[53] Dandy, W. (1954). Treatment of hemicrania (migraine) by removal of the inferior cervical and first thoracic sympathetic ganglion. J*ohns Hopkins Hospital Bulletin.* 1931, *48*, 357-361.

[54] Bronson, S. The Surgical Treatment of Headache and Atypical Facial Neuralgia. *Journal of Neurosurgery. 11*, 596-606.

[55] Dickerson, D. (1933). The surgical relief of the headache of migraine. *Journal of Nervous and Mental Disease. 77*

[56] Penfield, W. & McNaughton, E. (1940). Dural headache and innervation of the dura mater. *Archives of Neurology & Psychiatry.* 4.

[57] Solomon, S. (1986). Cluster headache and the nervus intermedius. *Headache. 26*(1), 3-8.

[58] White, J. C. & Sweet, W. H. (1969). Pain and the neurosurgeon; a forty-year experience. Springfield, Ill.,: C. C. Thomas.

[59] Morgenlander, J. C. & Wilkins, R. H. (1990). Surgical treatment of cluster headache. *Journal of Neurosurgery. 72*(6), 866-871

[60] Knight, G. (1968). Surgical treatment of migraine. In: Vinken P, Bruyn, GW, ed. Handbook of Clinical Neurology. Vol 5. *Amsterdam*: North-Holland Publishing 104-110.

[61] Bovim, G. & Sand, T. (1992). Cervicogenic headache, migraine without aura and tension-type headache. Diagnostic blockade of greater occipital and supra-orbital nerves. *Pain. 51*(1), 43-48.

[62] Caputi, C. A. & Firetto, V. (1997). Therapeutic blockade of greater occipital and supraorbital nerves in migraine patients. *Headache. 37*(3), 174-179.

[63] Guyuron, B., Tucker, T. & Davis, J. (2002). Surgical treatment of migraine headaches. *Plastic and Reconstructive Surgery. 109*(7), 2183-2189.

[64] Guyuron, B., Kriegler, J. S., Davis, J. & Amini, S. B. (2005). Comprehensive surgical treatment of migraine headaches. *Plastic and reconstructive surgery. 115*(1),1-9.

[65] Guyuron, B., Kriegler, J.S., Davis J. & Amini, S.B. (2011) Five-year outcome of surgical treatment of migraine headaches. *Plastic and reconstructive surgery. 127*(2), 603-608.

[66] Mammis, A. & Sinclair, G. L. (2012). 3rd, Mogilner AY. Peripheral neuromodulation for headache and craniofacial pain: indications, outcomes, and complications from a single center. *Clinical neurosurgery. 59*, 114-118.

[67] Goadsby, P. J. & Sprenger, T. (2010). Current practice and future directions in the prevention and acute management of migraine. *Lancet neurology. 9*(3), 285-298.

[68] Weiner, R. L. & Reed, K. L. (1999). Peripheral neurostimulation for control of intractable occipital neuralgia. *Neuromodulation: Journal of the International Neuromodulation Society. 2*(3), 217-221.

[69] Matharu, M. S., Bartsch, T., Ward, N., Frackowiak, R. S., Weiner, R. & Goadsby, P. J. (2004). Central neuromodulation in chronic migraine patients with suboccipital stimulators: a PET study. *Brain: A Journal of Neurology. 127*(Pt 1), 220-230.

[70] Brewer, A. C., Trentman, T. L., Ivancic, M. G., et al. (2012). Long-Term Outcome in Occipital Nerve Stimulation Patients With Medically Intractable Primary Headache Disorders. *Neuromodulation: Journal of the International Neuromodulation Society.*

[71] Palmisani, S., Al-Kaisy, A., Arcioni, R., et al. (2013). A six year retrospective review of occipital nerve stimulation practice--controversies and challenges of an emerging technique for treating refractory headache syndromes. *The Journal of Headache and Pain. 14*(1), 67.

[72] Verrills, P., Rose, R., Mitchell, B., Vivian, D. & Barnard, A. (2013). Peripheral Nerve Field Stimulation for Chronic Headache: 60 Cases and Long-Term Follow-Up. Neuromodulation.

[73] Lambru, G. & Matharu, M. S. (2012) Occipital nerve stimulation in primary headache syndromes. *Therapeutic advances in neurological disorders. 5*(1), 57-67.

[74] Freeman, J. A. & Trentman, T. L. (2013). Clinical utility of implantable neurostimulation devices in the treatment of chronic migraine. *Medical devices. 6*, 195-201.

[75] Trentman, T. L., Zimmerman, R. S. & Dodick, D. W. (2011). Occipital nerve stimulation: technical and surgical aspects of implantation. *Progress in neurological surgery. 24*, 96-108.

[76] Reed, K. L., Black, S. B. & Banta, C. J. 2nd & Will K. R. (2010). Combined occipital and supraorbital neurostimulation for the treatment of chronic migraine headaches: initial experience. *Cephalalgia: an international journal of headache. 30*(3), 260-271.

[77] Trentman, T. L., Rosenfeld, D. M., Vargas, B. B., Schwedt, T. J., Zimmerman, R. S. & Dodick, D. W. (2009). Greater occipital nerve stimulation via the Bion microstimulator: implantation technique and stimulation parameters. Clinical trial: NCT00205894. *Pain physician. 12*(3), 621-628.

[78] Kumar Abhinav, M., Nicholas, D., Park, F. R. C. S., Savithru, K., Prakash, M. R. C. S., Sarah Love-Jones, F. R. C. A., Nikunj, K. & Patel, F. R. C. S. (2012). Novel Use of Narrow Paddle Electrodes for Occipital Nerve Stimulation-Technical Note. Neuromodulation.

In: Migraine Surgery
Editor: Antonios Mammis

ISBN: 978-1-63321-761-4

Chapter 2

Fundamentals of Migraine

Annapoorna Bhat and David Marks*
Department of Neurology and Neurosciences
Rutgers New Jersey Medical School, Newark, New Jersey, US

Definition, Epidemiology and Genetics

Migraine is the 2nd most common type of primary headache and is one of the most common complaints in office based neurology practice [1]. Migraine can be defined as episodic neurological disorder that manifests as recurrent attacks of typically throbbing and unilateral, often severe headache lasting hours to days, with certain associated features such as nausea, photophobia, and phonophobia and worsened by routine physical exertion. In US population studies, the prevalence of migraine is approximately 18% in women and 6% in men [2,3]. In European population, 17% women and 8% men are affected by migraine [4]. Approximately 90% of the migraineurs have moderate or severe pain, three quarters have a reduced ability to function during the headache attacks, and one-third require bed rest during their attacks. According to World Health Organization (WHO) migraine is one of the twenty most disabling diseases [5]. Hence, it is a public health problem of great impact on both the individual and society.

In one of the major epidemiological studies done by Lipton et al., in 2007, a total of 120,000 households were contacted, encompassing 257,399 household members. Response was obtained from 77,879 households (65% response) yielding data for 162,576 household members aged 12 years or older [6]. This study found that migraine prevalence was highest in those aged 30 to 39 years for both men (7.4%), and women (24.4%). Prevalence was lowest in those aged 60 years or older at 1.6% in men and 5.0% in women. At the other end of the lifespan, prevalence was 4.0% in men and 6.4% in women aged between 12 and 17 years. For both men and women, prevalence was significantly higher in whites than in blacks (women,

* Corresponding author: Dr. David Marks, Department of Neurology and Neurosciences, Rutgers New Jersey Medical School , MSB H-506, 185 South Orange Avenue Newark, NJ, Ph: 973-972-5209, Fax: 973-972-5059, E-mail: marks@njms.rutgers.edu.

17.3% vs 13.7%; men, 5.7% vs 4.1%). Finally, for both sexes, the prevalence of migraine was higher in those of lower income. The majority of the migraineurs (62.7%) had 1 to 4 headache days per month. During migraine attacks, most migraineurs reported severe impairment or the need for bed rest (53.7%); and 7.2% reported no attack related impairment. During a 3-month period, 35.1% of the migraineurs had at least 1 day of activity restriction related to headache [6]. Migraine is a complex genetic disorder with heritability estimates as high as 50% and with a likely polygenic multi-factorial inheritance. Most of our present molecular understanding of migraine comes from studies of familial hemiplegic migraine (FHM), a rare, monogenic, autosomal dominant form of migraine with aura. The first three types of familial hemiplegic migraine are channelopathies numbered according to the gene involved. FHM1 is caused by mutations in the CACNA1A gene, which codes for a calcium channel [7]. The mutations of this calcium channel can result in gain of function that increases excitatory neurotransmitter release. FHM2 is caused by mutations in the ATP1A2 gene, causing alterations in the Na/K ATPase gene. It reduces the function of the enzyme and thereby leading to an increase in extracellular potassium, which increases neuronal excitability [8,9]. FHM3 is caused by mutations in the SCN1A gene, Na channel gene mutations may change the kinetics of the channel such that action potentials can fire with increased frequency [10]. Mutations in the PRRT2 gene also cause some cases of familial hemiplegic migraine [11]. The known types of familial hemiplegic migraine account for only a small proportion of cases. Large national registry-based twin studies have confirmed a consistently higher concordance of migraine in monozygotic twins versus dizygotic twins [12]. One of the early general population based study found that the risk of migraine in relatives of migraineurs was three times greater than that of relatives of non-migraine control subject [13]. However segregation analysis does not identify any single Mendelian pattern of inheritance in the common forms of migraine [14]. It is still uncertain which candidate loci and genes are truly implicated in the pathogenesis of migraine. The eventual identification of the genes that underlie migraine in an individual patient is extremely important, as it may be predictive of the type of prophylactic treatment to which the patient will respond.

Types and Classification

Migraine is the second most common type of primary headache. The other primary headaches being tension-type headache, trigeminal autonomic cephalalgias and other primary headache disorders

Migraine has two major subtypes.

A. Migraine without aura is a clinical syndrome characterized by headache with specific features and associated symptoms.
B. Migraine with aura is primarily characterized by the transient focal neurological symptoms that usually precede or sometimes accompany the headache. Some patients also experience a premonitory phase, occurring hours or days before the headache, and a headache resolution phase. Premonitory and resolution symptoms include hyperactivity, hypoactivity, depression, cravings for particular foods, repetitive yawning, fatigue and neck stiffness and/or pain.

Table 2.1. ICHD-3 classification of migraine [15]

1. Migraine
    - 1.1. Migraine without aura
    - 1.2. Migraine with aura
        - 1.2.1. Migraine with typical aura
            - 1.2.1.1. Typical aura with headache
            - 1.2.1.2. Typical aura without headache
        - 1.2.2. Migraine with brainstem aura
        - 1.2.3. Hemiplegic migraine
            - 1.2.3.1. Familial hemiplegic migraine (FHM)
                - 1.2.3.1.1. Familial hemiplegic migraine type 1 (FHM1)
                - 1.2.3.1.2. Familial hemiplegic migraine type 2 (FHM2)
                - 1.2.3.1.3. Familial hemiplegic migraine type 3 (FHM3)
                - 1.2.3.1.4. Familial hemiplegic migraine, other loci
            - 1.2.3.2. Sporadic hemiplegic migraine
        - 1.2.4. Retinal migraine
    - 1.3. Chronic migraine
    - 1.4. Complications of migraine
        - 1.4.1. Status migrainosus
        - 1.4.2. Persistent aura without infarction
        - 1.4.3. Migrainous infarction
        - 1.4.4. Migraine aura-triggered seizure
    - 1.5. Probable migraine
        - 1.5.1. Probable migraine without aura
        - 1.5.2. Probable migraine with aura
    - 1.6. Episodic syndromes that may be associated with migraine
        - 1.6.1. Recurrent gastrointestinal disturbance
            - 1.6.1.1. Cyclical vomiting syndrome
            - 1.6.1.2. Abdominal migraine
    - 1.6.2. Benign paroxysmal vertigo
    - 1.6.3. Benign paroxysmal torticollis

ICHD III Migraine Classification

The International Headache Society classifies migraine as in Table 2.1 [15].

A. Migraine without Aura

Recurrent headache disorder manifesting in attacks lasting 4-72 hours. Typical characteristics of the headache are unilateral location, pulsating quality, moderate or severe intensity, aggravation by routine physical activity and association with nausea and/or photophobia and phonophobia.

Diagnostic Criteria

A. At least five attacks fulfilling criteria B–D
B. Headache attacks lasting 4-72 hours (untreated or unsuccessfully treated)
C. Headache has at least two of the following four characteristics:

1. unilateral location
2. pulsating quality
3. moderate or severe pain intensity
4. aggravation by or causing avoidance of routine physical activity (e.g., walking or climbing stairs)

D. During headache at least one of the following:
1. nausea and/or vomiting
2. photophobia and phonophobia

E. Not better accounted for by another ICHD-3 diagnosis.

B. Migraine with Aura

Recurrent attacks, lasting minutes, of unilateral fully reversible visual, sensory or other central nervous system symptoms that usually develop gradually and are usually followed by headache and associated migraine symptoms.

Diagnostic Criteria

A. At least two attacks fulfilling criteria B and C

B. One or more of the following fully reversible aura symptoms:
1. visual
2. sensory
3. speech and/or language
4. motor
5. brainstem
6. retinal

C. At least two of the following four characteristics:
1. at least one aura symptom spreads gradually over 5 minutes, and/or two or more symptoms occur in succession
2. each individual aura symptom lasts 5-60 minutes
3. at least one aura symptom is unilateral
4. the aura is accompanied, or followed within 60 minutes, by headache

D. Not better accounted for by another ICHD-3 diagnosis, and transient ischemic attack has been excluded.

Basilar migraine is classified under migraine with aura. Basilar-type migraine predominantly affects young women and children. Symptoms may include any combination of dysarthria, vertigo, diplopia, tinnitus, decreased hearing, ataxia, simultaneous bilateral paresthesias, and altered consciousness. Visual symptoms may be difficult to distinguish from a classic migraine aura, although basilar-type migraine is more likely to cause simultaneous visual symptoms in both temporal and nasal fields. The occurrence of decreased level of consciousness followed by headache sometimes results in diagnostic difficulty. It is important to remember that basilar-type migraine is rare and that there must be another brainstem symptom in addition to decreased consciousness to make the diagnosis. In the absence of a second brainstem localizing symptom, other causes of unexplained loss of consciousness such as seizure and cardiogenic syncope must be considered and appropriately investigated.

Basilar-type migraine should be diagnosed only when weakness is absent, since about 60 percent of patients with familial hemiplegic migraine have basilar-type symptoms.

Other types of migraine with aura include ocular migraine and vestibular migraine. These can often can be mistaken for stroke. A detailed history and physical exam often helps to differentiate migraine for stroke.

Approximately 75% patients have at least one trigger for acute migraine attacks. The most common ones are emotional stress, sleep disturbances, missing meals, specific odors, smoke, to name a few [16].

Obesity has been associated with an increased frequency and severity of migraine [17]. Migraine headaches are often worsened by rapid head motion, sneezing, straining, constant movement, or physical exertion.

There has been lot of interest in relation between migraine and PFO. One meta-analysis found that there is evidence of a low grade for an increased prevalence of migraine in patients with PFO, perhaps limited to patients with a large PFO. Although an overall association was evident between PFO and migraine with aura, no association was found between PFO and migraine without aura [18]. It has been postulated that PFO may allow venous-circulating, migraine-triggering, vasoactive chemicals to bypass the pulmonary filter and reach the cerebral circulation to induce a migraine attack [18].

Pathophysiology

The discussion of migraine pathogenesis over the past century has been dominated by two competing theories: the vasogenic theory and the neurogenic theory [19].

The vasogenic theory dominated the debate until the 1980s. It viewed migraine as a form of vascular dysregulation and assumed that the aura was due to a transiently induced ischemia. The aura symptoms were hypothesized to be due to vasoconstriction. The headache was claimed to be due to a rebound vasodilation that caused a mechanical depolarization of primary nociceptive neurons within the walls of engorged intra and extracerebral vessels [20]. The vasogenic theory was consistent with the known vasoconstrictive effects of the ergotamines. Thus far, unpublished reports of lack of efficacy in nonvasoconstrictive selective 5-HT1D agonists in acute migraine also seem to favor the vasogenic hypothesis [19].

The alternative neurogenic theory viewed migraine as a disorder of the brain in which vascular changes followed neuronal dysfunction. Proponents of this theory pointed to the fact that multiple neurological symptoms that are difficult to localize within one neurovascular territory may occur during a single aura. Also in favor of the neurogenic theory are findings from neuroimaging studies conducted during spontaneous, classical visual auras that indicated that the decreases in cortical blood flow observed during aura are not sufficient to cause ischemia and that subsequent vasodilation does not take place until well after the onset of headache [21]. fMRI studies have shown activation of brainstem especially dorsolateral pons during migraine attacks [22, 23, 24]. Unfortunately, neither theory alone can account for all of the clinical and treatment response characteristics of migraine.

The central feature of the migraine syndrome is the recurrent activation of the trigeminocervical pain system [25]. In the physiological setting, this activation occurs when peripheral terminals of nociceptive neurons are depolarized and then, in turn, transmit the depolarization to the central terminals causing a trans-synaptic activation of second-order neurons in the medulla and cervical spinal cord. Dura-sensitive VPM thalamic neurons project mainly in the trigeminal primary and secondary somatosensory (S1 and S2) cortices and the insular cortex (components of the so-called pain matrix) and are thus likely to play a role in the perception of headache [26]. The trigeminovascular projections to specific hypothalamic and brain stem nuclei likely contribute to other aspects of the complex migraine symptomatology, such as loss of appetite, fluid retention, sleepiness, irritability, stress, pursuit of solitude, and autonomic symptoms [27].

A large fraction of migraineurs experience exacerbation of headache by light (photophobia). Investigators recently uncovered a neural mechanism for migraine photophobia. Dura-sensitive thalamic neurons in the rat posterior thalamus receive monosynaptic input from retinal ganglion cells (mainly intrinsically photosensitive cells involved in non-image-forming functions), and light enhances the activity of dura-sensitive thalamic neurons located in the same area. The idea that a non-image-forming retinal pathway is involved in migraine photophobia is supported by the finding that exacerbation of headache by light was preserved in blind migraineurs who could sense light in the face of severe degeneration of rod and cone photoreceptors [28].

On the basis of a large body of indirect evidence from both clinical and animal studies, a sterile meningeal inflammation is considered one key mechanism that may underlie the sustained activation and sensitization of perivascular meningeal afferents during migraine attacks [29]. In experimental animals, activation of meningeal nociceptors in vivo leads to release of vasoactive proinflammatory peptides such as CGRP and SP from their peripheral nerve endings; these peptides produce vasodilation of meningeal blood vessels (due mainly to CGRP), plasma extravasation, and local activation of dural mast cells (MCs), with ensuing release of cytokines and other inflammatory mediators [30]. Dural mast cell degranulation can produce a long-lasting activation and sensitization of rat dural nociceptors [31] as well as cephalic tactile hypersensitivity [32].

Thus far, a single mechanism of trigeminal activation common to all migraineurs has not been identified. For example, sumatriptan (the prototype of the highly effective 'triptan' class of migraine abortive agents) does not avidly cross the blood-brain barrier, suggesting that it acts at peripheral sites [25]. Furthermore, during acute migraine attacks levels of calcitonin gene-related peptide (CGRP), which is released from the peripheral terminals of activated peripheral nociceptive neurons, rise in external jugular blood [33].

In migraineurs who experience aura, there is increasing evidence to suggest that the cortical events responsible for the aura symptoms may also be capable of activating trigeminal nociceptors [34,35]. Blood flow studies in patients also have shown that a focal hyperemia tends to precede the spreading oligemia and again this is similar to what would be expected with spreading depression [35]. After this passage of oligemia, the cerebrovascular response to hypercapnia in patients is blunted, while autoregulation remains intact. The mechanisms by which trigeminal and cervical nociceptive neurons are activated during migraine without aura are not well understood. The possibility that a CSD-like phenomenon may occur in non-eloquent areas of the cortex during migraine without aura cannot at this point be excluded; however, preliminary evidence from PWI does not support this view [36]. There may be one or (perhaps, more likely) several mechanisms of activation in migraine without aura that remain to be detected and elucidated. Bolay and coworkers [35] have reported experimental data from animal models that demonstrate that induced spreading depression can cause vasodilation in meningeal vessels by a reflex dependent on intact trigeminal and parasympathetic neurons.

Cortical spreading depression (CSD) is thought to be related to massive depolarization of neuronal membranes in the gray matter and extraordinary excitability in ion change status [36]. Neuronal firing induced by cortical spreading depression reaches its peak in 20 minutes following cortical spreading depression [37, 38, 39]. A direct nociceptive effect of CSD was demonstrated by the finding that a single CSD can lead to a long lasting increase in ongoing activity of dural nociceptors and central trigeminovascular neurons in superficial and deep laminae of the trigemino-cervical complex (TCC) CSD-induced CGRP release from perivascular trigeminal fibers contributes to the transient dilation of pial vessels measured during CSD [41, 42, 43]. CSD was also found to have an important role in trigeminovascular activation and neurogenic edema [44]. CSD causes an increase in the blood flow in the arteries supplying the dura mater by way of the trigeminal nerve. Trigeminal neurons innervate the meninges in many ways including visceral sensory neurons. The idea that CSD is noxious and may trigger headache is indirectly supported by the finding that the electrical stimulation threshold for induction of CSD in the rat cortex increases after chronic treatment with five different migraine prophylactic drugs that are equally effective in reducing the frequency of MA and MO attacks [44]; in contrast, two drugs ineffective in migraine prophylaxis do not affect susceptibility to experimental CSD [45]. In addition to the prolonged activation of TCC neurons, there are other significant CSD-driven central effects, including gene upregulation in the TCC and dilation and increase in blood flow within the middle meningeal artery mediated by trigeminally evoked brain stem reflexes [46]. Despite the strong support provided by animal studies, the idea that CSD may initiate the headache mechanisms in migraine is not generally accepted [47, 48].

The molecular and cellular mechanisms underlying the abnormal regulation of cortical function and its periodicity remain largely unknown. Possible hypothetical mechanisms include (*a*) alterations in the cortical circuits that dynamically maintain the excitation/inhibition balance and are essential for correctly processing sensory information and for preventing over-excitation [49, 50] and (*b*) alterations of cortical neuromodulation by serotonergic, noradrenergic, or cholinergic inputs from the brain stem. The extent to which some of the cortical and/or subcortical alterations are affected by disease duration (e.g., repetitive CSDs) is unclear. Equally unclear is the extent to which the abnormal processing of trigeminal nociceptive input reflects a primary dysregulation of central sensory processing or central sensitization persisting outside the attack [51, 52]. The relation between triggering of sensory neurons by specific stimuli and occurrence of migraine pain is not clear. Additional factors may also be responsible; mechanical compression, ion changes in the extracellular space (increased potasssium, increased osmolarity, decreased pH), neuropeptides (bradykinin, substance P, endothelin, calcitonin gene related peptide (CGRP), neurotransmitters (glutamate, serotonin, histamine, adenosine triphosphate (ATP), adenosine) eicosanoids and NO [53].

The whole clinical picture of migraine can also be explained by a dysfunction of neuromodulatory structures in the brainstem, such as the locus coeruleus or periaqueductal grey matter. The locus coeruleus, the major noradrenergic nucleus, has a critical role in the regulation of cortical function and is known to modulate responses to afferent traffic. [41]. Its connections are widely distributed throughout the neocortex and in positron emission tomography (PET) studies investigating acute migraine attacks, activation of an area of the dorsolateral brainstem that included the locus coeruleus has been shown [54]. Compared to other hypothesis on migraine neurobiology, dysfunction of such brainstem structures and networks could not only account for the somatosensory component of migraine (headache) but also for the auditory, olfactory and visual components [41].

Medical Management

Once the diagnosis has been confirmed, management process is started by explaining the condition to provide an understanding of the problem and to set realistic expectations. A headache diary will often be instructive in the planning and evaluation of therapy. Recording affected days, pain severity, and medication use and response, as well as obvious triggers (e.g., days of menstrual flow) can be extremely helpful to determine the need for preventive strategies and for considering therapeutic outcomes [55, 56]. Goals of treatment include restoration of function, reduction of disability and suffering, and, possibly, reduction in disease progression and future episodes.

Acute treatment

Initially, acute migraine-specific management was based on the vascular model of headache advanced by Wolff and Graham. Thus, vasoconstricting agents were sought that could terminate an attack. As a result, ergot preparations were developed and were efficacious, but with significant side effects. The 1990s saw a major advance with the introduction of sumatriptan. This serotonin receptor 5-hydroxytryptamine 1 (5-HT1) agonist was as effective as ergots but generally produced fewer concerning side effects [57]. Early management requires diligence and can be challenging. Migraine may not always begin as pain, but instead may present as a prodrome of mood change, fatigue, muscle tension, yawning, cognitive dysfunction, or other vague symptoms. One measure of success is the frequency with which the patient returns to a headache-free, fully functional state within 2 hours of treatment, with no recurrence within 24 hours.

Current attack treatments fall into two categories: disease non-specific analgesics and NSAIDS; and more disease specific ergot-related compounds and triptans.

NSAIDS

Nonsteroidal anti-inflammatory drugs (NSAIDs), such as acetylsalicylic acid (ASA), ibuprofen, naproxen sodium, indomethacin, diclofenac, and ketoprofen, have long been used alone or in combination with other agents for the acute treatment of migraine. Naproxen 500–1000 mg orally or rectally, with an anti-emetic [59-62], ibuprofen 400–800 mg orally [63, 64], or tolfenamic acid 200 mg orally [65] can be extremely effective in migraine if used adequately. Selective cyclo-oxygenase 2 inhibitors have also proven effective in migraine treatment with similar efficacy to NSAIDs [66]. The addition of anti-emetics or prokinetics, such as domperidone 10 mg orally [67-69] or metoclopramide 10 mg orally [70, 71], to analgesics or NSAIDs might improve the efficacy of these drugs with an independent antinociceptive effect and help patients to deal with migraine-associated nausea. Compound analgesics (i.e., those containing aspirin, acetaminophen, and caffeine) have been shown to be more effective than single analgesics [72, 73].

Ergotamines and Triptans

When analgesic measures fail to avert disability, more specific and more effective anti-migraine treatments are required [74]. Ergotamine, previously the mainstay of acute treatment, can no longer be considered the treatment of choice in acute migraine [75]. There are particular situations in which ergotamine is very helpful, such as in the treatment of very long attacks with headache recurrence, but dosing must be carefully monitored because ergotamine overuse can produce severe headache in addition to many vascular problems [76]. Dihydroergotamine (DHE) is currently the only widely available ergot alkaloid. Available preparations include DHE nasal spray (1 puff [0.5 mg] in each nostril, repeat in 15 minutes, 2-mg maximum daily dose) and injection. The nasal spray is cumbersome to use but is efficacious and preferred by some patients [57].

The triptans, which are serotonin 5-HT1B/1D receptor agonists [77], have revolutionized the lives of many patients with severe migraine attacks, and are clearly the most powerful option available to stop a migraine attack. The three postulated mechanisms of action [57]: intracranial vessel vasoconstriction (5-HT1B), peripheral neuronal inhibition (5-HT1D), and presynaptic dorsal horn stimulation (5-HT1D) producing second-order brainstem neuronal inhibition.

Triptans may also enhance descending inhibitory pain pathways and influence the function of 5-hydroxytryptamine 1F (5-HT1F) receptors. Although head-to-head comparisons between triptans are not exhaustive [78], it is widely acknowledged that the seven licensed compounds differ with regard to their effectiveness, side-effect rate, and frequency of headache recurrence [79] (Table 2.2). The 6 mg subcutaneous injection of sumatriptan appears to be the most efficacious dosage formulation; however, patients often prefer oral formulations. Current evidence outlined by Loder suggests nearly equivalent efficacy among the oral formulations, except for frovatriptan, which is less efficacious but has a longer duration of action [58].

Best results with triptans are achieved by taking an adequate dose early in the attack. Oral triptans take effect within 20 to 60 minutes and, if needed, the dose may be repeated in 2 to 4 hours. Recurrence of headache after initial response does seem to occur frequently, in as many as one-third of patients. Triptans may be combined with NSAIDs or antiemetic drugs [57].

Oral triptans are somewhat less efficacious than the parenteral versions and, in some studies, are comparable in efficacy to nonsteroidal agents or other analgesics. Thus, clinicians should discuss with patients the potential benefits of a non-oral acute treatment for use when oral medications are ineffective. Widespread clinical experience suggests that failure with one triptan does not predict failure with another [80, 81]. Each triptan should probably be tried for three attacks, because after three unsuccessful trials, the probability of success will be low, based on extrapolation from consistency studies [82, 83].

Table 2.2. Different triptans and their characteristics. Modified from Rizzoli PB. and Loder E

Drug	Dose/Formulation	Half-Life (Hours)	Selected Drug Interactions	Maximum Daily Dose
Group 1 Fast-Onset Triptans				
Almotriptan	6.25-mg and 12.5-mg tablets	3 to 4	Contains a sulfa group Dose reduction to 6.25 mg suggested when used with potent CYP3A4 inhibitors[b]	25 mg
Eletriptan	20-mg and 40-mg tablets	4	Avoid with potent CYP3A4 inhibitors[b]	80 mg
Rizatriptan	5-mg and 10-mg tablets 5-mg and 10-mg orally dissolving wafers	2 to 3	Dose reduction to 5 mg recommended in patients using propranolol Do not use within 2 weeks of a monamine oxidase inhibitor (MAOI)	30 mg (15 mg if on propranolol)
Sumatriptan	25-mg, 50-mg, and 100-mg tablets 5 mg and 20 mg intranasal Single dose vial, 6 mg/0.5 mL for subcutaneous injection 4-mg and 6-mg cartridges for autoinjector 6-mg needle-free single-use devices for subcutaneous injection Fixed-dose combination tablet of 85-mg sumatriptan with 500-mg naproxen sodium	3	Do not use within 2 weeks of an MAOI	200 mg oral 40 mg intranasal 12 mg subcutaneous
Zolmitriptan	2.5-mg and 5-mg tablets 2.5-mg and 5-mg orally dissolving wafers 5 mg intranasal	3	Do not use within 2 weeks of an MAOI	Two tablets or 10-mg maximum oral daily dose Two sprays or 10 mg intranasal
Group 2 Slower-Onset Triptans				
Frovatriptan	2.5-mg tablet	26		7.5 mg
Naratriptan	1-mg and 2.5-mg tablets	6		5 mg

Triptans are contraindicated in patients with known fixed or spastic coronary artery disease or with risk factors for coronary artery disease [57]. Caution has also been advised with the combination of triptans and selective serotonin reuptake inhibitors (SSRIs) owing to the possible production of the potentially life-threatening serotonin syndrome, with symptoms such as tremor, palpitations, flushing, hypertension, and agitation [84, 85].

Preventive Treatment

Preventive therapy is a crucial component of the management strategy to reduce migraine disability, and is indicated in about a third of patients with migraine [6]. The notion of preventing headaches began with the introduction of methysergide in the 1960s. Preventive treatment not only changed the management of migraine it also caused a paradigm shift toward viewing migraine as a biological rather than a psychiatric entity [57]. The goals of prevention are to reduce attack frequency and severity, reduce associated disability, return the patient to normal function, and improve response to treatment of future acute attacks. Consensus guidelines differ substantially with regard to recommendations about when to start pharmacological migraine prophylaxis [55]. In the US guidelines, treatment is recommended when attacks regularly exceed two times per week [86], whereas European guidelines suggest migraine prophylaxis for two attacks or more per month [87]. Patient preference is certainly a major factor in deciding whether to start a preventive treatment. Unfortunately, the mechanisms of action of current preventive treatments are not well understood. Possible therapeutic mechanisms include stabilization of reactive nervous system centers, enhancement of antinociceptive pathways, inhibition of central and peripheral sensitization, and inhibition of cortical spreading depression[57].

The classes of preventive medications are antiepileptic drugs, beta-adrenergic blockers, antidepressants, calcium channel antagonists, serotonin antagonists and neurotoxins. Selected examples are summarized in Table 2.3. Apart from these, the class of drugs such as alpha adrenergic agonists (clonidine), guanfacine, tizanidine, ACE inhibitors (lisinopril), Angiotensin II receptor antagonists (candesartan), Riboflavin have also been used in migraine prevention with variable evidence [57].

Table 2.3. Different classes of preventive medications, dose and side effects. Modified from Goadsby PJ, Sprenger T

	Dose	Common side effects
Anti-epileptic drugs		
Valproate	250-1500 mg daily	Drowsiness, weight gain, tremor, hair loss, fetal abnormalities, hamatological or liver abnormalities
Topiramate	50-200 mg daily	Paraesthesias, cognitive dysfunction, weight loss, care with a family history of glaucoma, nephrolithiasis
Gabapentin	900-3600 mg daily	Dizziness, sedation
Beta-adrenergic blockers		
Propranolol	80-240 mg daily	Reduced energy, tiredness, postural symptoms; contraindicated in asthma
Metoprolol	50-200 mg daily	Reduced energy, tiredness, postural symptoms; contraindicated in asthma
Antidepressants		
Amitriptyline/Nortriptyline	25-75 mg every night	Drowsiness, urinary retention, arrhythmias; note that some patients are very sensitive and might only need a total dose of 10 mg, although generally 1–1·5 mg/kg bodyweight is required
Venlafaxine	25–100 mg twice daily	Drowsiness, urinary retention, arrhythmias;
Calcium channel antagonists		
Verapamil	120 mg and 480 mg daily	constipation, dizziness, hypotension, and, at higher doses, cardiac conduction blocks
Serotonin antagonists		
Pizotifen	0.5–2 mg daily	Weight gain, drowsiness
Methysergide	1–6 mg daily	Drowsiness, leg cramps, hair loss, retroperitoneal fibrosis; 1 month drug holiday is required every 6 months
Neurotoxins		
Onabotulinumtoxin A	repeated set of injections every 3 months	clinical effect may be delayed or transient after the first set of injections and that a second set of injections is warranted before concluding that the therapy is unhelpful

Guideline principles suggest starting with low doses of medication and increasing slowly. A good practice approach is to increase doses about every 2 weeks, allowing time for assessment between increases. A slow titration can help patients adjust to the effects of a new medication. An adequate trial duration of 2 to 3 months is often necessary to determine efficacy. Patients should monitor headache response with a calendar or diary. Reviewing all medications and doses with patients at follow-up visits can help prevent medication interactions. Tapering the preventive treatment after a 6-month period of headache control is often feasible [88]. Co-morbid conditions, such as stroke and other vascular conditions, epilepsy, and affective disorders, can influence preventive treatment decisions in migraine. When practical, an agent can be selected that treats two co-morbid conditions, such as migraine and hypertension; migraine and epilepsy. Alternatively, avoiding agents that could worsen a co-morbid condition is also important, as is monitoring for medication interactions. Pregnancy issues can add another layer of complexity to appropriate medication selection [57].

With regard to the efficacy of preventive agents in studies, a 25% increase in responders (i.e., patients with a 50% reduction in migraine days) can typically be expected in the active drug group compared with those on placebo [89]. In clinical practice, this translates into a 50% reduction in migraine days for half the patients who use them, and usually a more obvious reduction in severity with some concomitant opportunity to provide better control of residual attacks [90].

Alternative Management Strategies

Migraine is clearly an inherited disposition to headache that is triggered by change: too much or too little sleep, skipping meals, weather change, change in exertion patterns, or change in stress. Thus a balanced, regular lifestyle seems desirable, although it has not been proven by evidence-based medicine that education of patients and other adjustments to lifestyle truly reduce the frequency or severity of headaches. The same applies to the careful intake of recognized aggravating substances, such as caffeine [58].

Two large multicentre RCTs of acupuncture for the prevention of migraine have been done [91, 92]. One study showed similar effectiveness of the acupuncture interventions to standard medical treatment with beta blockers, calcium-channel blockers, or antiepileptic drugs. However, there was no difference between verum and sham acupuncture, indicating that exact adherence to the traditional acupuncture concepts might not be important [91]. The other study also showed no difference between verum and sham acupuncture, but both interventions were clearly superior to a waiting-list group [92]. Therefore, there are good reasons to include acupuncture in a multimodal setting of migraine prevention. By contrast, there is no evidence to recommend homoeopathy.

Taken together, there is increasing evidence for the efficacy of some non-pharmacological approaches. These interventions are usually very well tolerated and provide an important measure to combine with pharmacological approaches in multidisciplinary care to achieve optimum responses.

References

[1] Lipton, R. B., Stewart, W. F. & Simon, D. (1998). Medical consultation for migraine: results from the American Migraine Study. *Headache*, *38*, 87.

[2] Lipton, R. B., Stewart, W. F., Diamond, S., Diamond, M. L. & Reed, M. (2001). Prevalence and burden of migraine in the United States: data from the American Migraine Study II. *Headache*, *41*, 646.

[3] Lipton, R. B., Diamond, S., Reed, M., Diamond, M. L. & Stewart, W. F. (2001). Migraine diagnosis and treatment: results from the American Migraine Study II. *Headache*, *41*, 638.

[4] Stovner, L. J. & Hagen, K. (2006). Prevalence, burden, and cost of headache disorders. *Curr. Opin. Neurol. 19*, 281.

[5] Leonardi, M., Steiner, T. J, Scher, A. T., Lipton, R. B. (2005). The global burden of migraine: measuring disability in headache disorders with WHO's Classification of Functioning, Disability and Health (ICF). *J. Headache Pain*, 6, 429.

[6] Lipton, R. B., Bigal, M. E., Diamond, M., et al. (2007). Migraine prevalence, disease burden, and the need for preventive therapy. Neurology, *68*, 343.

[7] van den Maagdenberg, A. M. J. M., Pietrobon, D., Pizzorusso, T., et al. (2004). A CACNA1a knockin migraine mouse model with increased susceptibility to cortical spreading depression. *Neuron*, *41*, 701.

[8] Vanmolkot, K. R. J., Kors, E. E, Turk, U., et al. (2006). Two de novo mutations in the Na,K-ATPase gene ATP1A2 associated with pure familial hemiplegic migraine. *Eur J Hum Genet*, *14*, 555.

[9] Tavraz, N. N., Friedrich, T., Durr, K. L., et al. (2008). Diverse functional consequences of mutations in the Na/K-ATPase alpha2-subunit causing familial hemiplegic migraine type 2. *J Biol Chem*, *283*, 31097.

[10] Dichgans, M., Freilinger. T., Eckstein, G., et al. (2005). Mutation in the neuronal voltage-gated sodium channel SCN1A in familial hemiplegic migraine. *Lancet*, *366*, 371.

[11] Dale, R. C., Gardiner, A., Antony, J. & Houlden, H. (2012). Familial PRRT2 mutation with heterogeneous proxysmal disorders including torticollis and hemiplegic migraine. *Dev Med Child Neurol*, *54*, 958.

[12] Honkasalo, M. L., Kaprio, J., Winter, T., et al. (1995). Migraine and concomitant symptoms among 8167 adult twin pairs. *Headache*, *35*, 70.

[13] Merikangas, K. R., Risch, N. J., Merikangas, J. R., et al. (1988). Migraine and depression: association and familial transmission. *J Psychiatr Res.*, *22*, 119.

[14] Devoto, M., Lozito, A., Staffa, G., et al. (1986). Segregation analysis of migraine in 128 families. *Cephalalgia*, *6*,101.

[15] Headache Classification Committee of the International Headache Society (IHS). (2013). The International Classification of Headache Disorders, 3rd edition (beta version) *Cephalalgia*, *33*, 629.

[16] Kelman, L. (2007). The triggers or precipitants of the acute migraine attack. *Cephalalgia*, *27*, 394.

[17] Bigal, M. E., Liberman, J. N. & Lipton, R. B. (2006). Obesity and migraine: a population study. *Neurology*, *66*, 545.

[18] Schwedt, T. J., Demaerschalk, B. M. & Dodick, D. W. (2008). Patent foramen ovale and migraine: a quantitative systematic review. *Cephalalgia*, *28*, 531.
[19] Cutrer, F. M. (2010). Pathophysiology of Migraine. *Semin Neurol. 30*, 120.
[20] Wolff, H. G. (1963). Headache and Other Head Pain. 2nd ed. New York: Oxford University Press.
[21] Cutrer, F. M., Sorensen, A. G., Weisskoff, R. M., et al. (1998). Perfusion weighted imaging defects during spontaneous migrainous aura. *Ann Neurol. 43*, 25.
[22] Bahra, A., Matharu, M. S., Buchel, C., Frackowiak, R. S. & Goadsby, P. J. (2001). Brainstem activation specific to migraine headache. *Lancet. 357*, 1016.
[23] Afridi, S. K., Matharu, M. S., Lee, L., Kaube, H., Friston, K. J., Frackowiak, R. S. & Goadsby, P. J. (2005). A PET study exploring the laterality of brainstem activation in migraine using glyceryl trinitrate. *Brain*, *128*, 932.
[24] Denuelle, M., Fabre, N., Payoux, P., Chollet, F. & Geraud, G. (2007). Hypothalamic activation in spontaneous migraine attacks. *Headache*, *47*, 1418.
[25] Pietrobon, D. & Moskowitz, M. A. (2013). Pathophysiology of Migraine. *Annu Rev Physiol.*, *75*, 365.
[26] Noseda, R., Jakubowski, M., Kainz, V., Borsook. D. & Burstein, R. (2011). Cortical projections of functionally identified thalamic trigeminovascular neurons: implications for migraine headache and its associated symptoms. *J. Neurosci. 31*,14204.
[27] Akerman, S., Holland, P. R. & Goadsby, P. J. (2011). Diencephalic and brainstem mechanisms in migraine. *Nat. Rev. Neurosci. 12*, 570.
[28] Noseda, R., Kainz, V., Jakubowski, M., Gooley, J. J., Saper, C. B., et al. (2010). A neural mechanism for exacerbation of headache by light. *Nat. Neurosci. 13*, 239.
[29] Waeber, C. & Moskowitz, M.A. (2005). Migraine as an inflammatory disorder. *Neurology*, *64*, S9
[30] Levy, D. (2009). Migraine pain, meningeal inflammation, and mast cells. *Curr. Pain Headache Rep.*; *13*, 237.
[31] Levy, D., Burstein, R., Kainz, V., Jakubowski, M. & Strassman, A. M. (2007). Mast cell degranulation activates a pain pathway underlying migraine headache. *Pain*, *130*, 166.
[32] Levy, D. (2012). Endogenous mechanisms underlying the activation and sensitization of meningeal nociceptors: the role of immuno-vascular interactions and cortical spreading depression. Curr. *Pain Headache Rep.*, *16*, 270.
[33] Goadsby, P. J., Edvinsson, L. & Ekman, R. (1990). Vasoactive peptide release in the extracerebral circulation of humans during migraine headache. *Ann Neurol*, *28*, 183.
[34] Olesen, J., Larsen, B., Lauritzen, M. (1981). Focal hyperemia followed by spreading oligemia and impaired activation of rCBF in classic migraine. *Ann Neurol*, *9*, 344.
[35] Bolay, H., Reuter, U., Dunn, A. K., Huang, Z., Boas, D. A. & Moskowitz, M. A. (2002). Intrinsic brain activity triggers trigeminal meningeal afferents in a migraine model. *Nat Med*, *8*, 136.
[36] Sanchez del Rio, M., Bakker, D., Wu, O., et al. (1999). Perfusion weighted imaging during migraine: Spontaneous visual aura and headache. *Cephalalgia*, *19*, 701.
[37] Smith, J. M., Bradley, D. P., James, M. F. & Huang, C. L. (2006) Physiological studies of cortical spreading depression. *Biol Rev*, *81*, 457.
[38] Bolay, H. & Moskowitz, M. A. (2005). The emerging importance of cortical spreading depression in migraine headache. *Rev Neurol (Paris)*, *161*, 655.

[39] Kraig, R. P. & Nicholson, C. (1978). Extracellular ionic variations during spreading depression. *Neuroscience*, *3*, 1045.

[40] Obrenovitch, T. P., Urenjak, J. & Wang, M. (2002). Nitric oxide formation during cortical spreading depression is critical for rapid subsequent recovery of ionic homeostasis. *J Cereb Blood Flow Metab*, *22*, 680.

[41] Boran, H. E. & Bolay, H. (2013). Pathophysiology of Migraine. *Arch of Neuropsych*, *50*, S1:1.

[42] Zhang, X., Levy, D., Noseda, R., Kainz, V., Jakubowski, M. & Burstein, R. (2010). Activation of meningeal nociceptors by cortical spreading depression: implications for migraine with aura. *J. Neurosci.*, *30*, 8807.

[43] Zhang, X., Levy, D., Kainz, V., Noseda, R., Jakubowski, M. & Burstein, R. (2011). Activation of central trigeminovascular neurons by cortical spreading depression. *Ann. Neurol.*, *69*, 855.

[44] Charles, A. (2010). Does cortical spreading depression initiate a migraine attack? May be not. *Headache*, *50*, 731.

[45] Ayata, C., Jin, H., Kudo, C., Dalkara, T. & Moskowitz, M. A. (2006). Suppression of cortical spreading depression in migraine prophylaxis. *Ann. Neurol.*, *59*, 652.

[46] Hoffmann, U., Dilekoz, E., Kudo, C. & Ayata, C. (2011). Oxcarbazepine does not suppress cortical spreading depression. *Cephalalgia*, *31*, 537.

[47] Bolay, H., Reuter, U., Dunn, A.K., Huang, Z., Boas, D.A. & Moskowitz, M. A. (2002). Intrinsic brain activity triggers trigeminal meningeal afferents in a migraine model. *Nat. Med.*, *8*, 136.

[48] Pietrobon, D. & Striessnig, J. (2003). Neurobiology of migraine. *Nat. Rev. Neurosci.*, 2003, *4*, 386.

[49] Shu, Y., Hasenstaub, A. & McCormick, D. A. (2003). Turning on and off recurrent balanced cortical activity. *Nature*, *423*, 288.

[50] Monier, C., Chavane, F., Baudot, P., Graham, L. J. & Fregnac, Y. (2003) Orientation and direction selectivity of synaptic inputs in visual cortical neurons: a diversity of combinations produces spike tuning. *Neuron*, *37*, 663.

[51] Mainero, C., Boshyan, J. & Hadjikhani, N. (2011) Altered functional magnetic resonance imaging resting-state connectivity in periaqueductal gray networks in migraine. *Ann. Neurol.*, *70*, 838.

[52] Moulton, E. A., Becerra, L., Maleki, N., Pendse, G., Tully, S., et al. (2011). Painful heat reveals hyperexcitability of the temporal pole in interictal and ictal migraine states. Cereb. *Cortex*, *21*, 435.

[53] Levy, D. & Strassman, A. M. (2002). Mechanical response properties of A and C primary afferent neurons innervating the rat intracranial dura. *J Neurophysiol*, *88*, 3021.

[54] Aurora, S. K., Barrodale, P. M., Tipton, R. L. & Khodavirdi, A. (2007). Brainstem dysfunction in chronic migraine as evidenced by neurophysiological and positron emission tomography studies. *Headache*, *47*, 996.

[55] Goadsby, P. J. & Sprenger, T. (2010). Current practice and future directions in the prevention and acute management of migraine. *Lancet Neurol*. *9*, 285.

[56] Sprenger, T. & Goadsby, P. J. (2009). Migraine pathogenesis and state of pharmacological treatment options. *BMC Med.*, *7*, 71.

[57] Rizzoli, P. B. (2012). Acute and preventive treatment of migraine. *Continuum Lifelong Learning Neurol*, *18*, 764.

[58] Loder, E. (2010). Triptan therapy in migraine. *N Engl J Med. 363*, 63.
[59] Brandes, J. L., Kudrow, D., Stark, S. R., et al. (2007). Sumatriptan-naproxen for acute treatment of migraine: a randomized trial. *JAMA*, *297*, 1443.
[60] Smith, T. R., Sunshine, A., Stark, S. R., Littlefi eld, D. E., Spruill, S. E. & Alexander, W. J. (2005). Sumatriptan and naproxen sodium for the acute treatment of migraine. *Headache*, *45*, 983.
[61] Welch, K. M. A. (1986). Naproxen sodium in the treatment of migraine. *Cephalalgia*, *6*, 85.
[62] Wentz, A. L., Jimenez, T. B., Dixon, R. M., Aurora, S. K. & Gold, M. (2008). A doubleblind, randomized, placebo-controlled, single-dose study of the cyclooxygenase-2 inhibitor, GW406381, as a treatment for acute migraine. *Eur J Neurol*, *15*, 420.
[63] Kellstein, D. E., Lipton, R. B., Geetha, R., et al. (2000). Evaluation of a novel solubilized formulation of ibuprofen in the treatment of migraine headache: a randomized, double-blind, placebo-controlled, dose-ranging study. *Cephalalgia*, *20*, 233.
[64] Codispoti, J. R., Prior, M. J., Fu, M., Harte, C. M. & Nelson, E. B. (2001). Efficacy of nonprescription doses of ibuprofen for treating migraine headache. A randomized controlled trial. *Headache*, *41*, 665.
[65] Myllyla, V. V., Havanka, H., Herrala, L., et al. (1998). Tolfenamic acid rapid release versus sumatriptan in the acute treatment of migraine: comparable effect in a double-blind, randomized, controlled, parallel-group study. *Headache*, *38*, 201.
[66] Silberstein, S., Tepper, S., Brandes, J., et al. (2004). Randomized, placebo-controlled trial of rofecoxib in the acute treatment of migraine. *Neurology*, *62*, 1552.
[67] Macgregor, E. A., Wilkinson, M. & Bancroft, K. (1993). Domperidone plus paracetamol in the treatment of migraine headache. *Cephalalgia*, *13*, 124.
[68] Cottrell, J., Mann, S. G. & Hole, J. (2000). A combination of ibuprofen lysine (IBL) and domperidone maleate (DOM) in the acute treatment of migraine: a double-blind study [abstract]. *Cephalalgia*, *20*, 269.
[69] Dowson, A., Ball, K. & Haworth, D. (2000) Comparison of a fixed combination of domperidone and paracetamol (domperamol) with sumatriptan 50 mg in moderate to severe migraine: a randomized UK primary care study. *Curr Med Res Opin*, *16*,190.
[70] Oral Sumatriptan and Aspirin plus Metoclopramide Comparative Study Group. (1992). A study to compare oral sumatriptan with oral aspirin plus metaclopramide in the acute treatment of migraine. *Eur Neurol*, *32*,177.
[71] Geraud, G., Compagnon, A. & Rossi, A., (2002). Cozam Study Group. Zolmitriptan versus a combination of acetlysalicylic acid and metaclopramide in the acute oral treatment of migraine: a doubleblind, randomised, three-attack study. Eur Neurol 47:88.
[72] Goldstein, J., Hoff man, H. D., Armellino, J. J., et al. (1999). Treatment of severe, disabling migraine attacks in an over-the-counter population of migraine sufferers: results from three randomized placebo controlled studies of the combination of acetaminophen, aspirin and caffeine. *Cephalalgia*, *19*, 684.
[73] Lipton, R. B., Stewart, W. F., Ryan, R. E., Saper, J., Silberstein, S. & Sheftell, F. (1998). Efficacy and safety of acetaminophen, aspirin, and caffeine in alleviating migraine headache pain—three double-blind, randomized, placebo-controlled trials. *Arch Neurol*, *55*, 210.

[74] Goadsby, P. J., Lipton, R. B. & Ferrari, M. D. (2002). Migraine—current understanding and treatment. *N Engl J Med*, *346*, 257.

[75] Tfelt-Hansen, P., Saxena, P. R., Dahlof, C., et al. (2000). Ergotamine in the acute treatment of migraine—a review and European consensus. *Brain*, *123*, 9.

[76] Silberstein, S. D. & McCrory, D. C. (2003). Ergotamine and dihydroergotamine: history, pharmacology, and efficacy. *Headache*, *43*, 144.

[77] Ferrari, M. D., Goadsby, P. J., Roon, K. I. & Lipton, R. B. (2002). Triptans (serotonin, 5-HT1B/1D agonists) in migraine: detailed results and methods of a meta-analysis of 53 trials. *Cephalalgia*, *22*, 633.

[78] Adelman, J. U., Lipton, R. B., Ferrari, M. D., et al. (2001) Comparison of rizatriptan and other triptans on stringent measures of efficacy. *Neurology*, *57*, 1377.

[79] Ferrari, M. D., Roon, K. I., Lipton, R. B. & Goadsby, P. J. (2001). Oral triptans (serotonin, 5-HT1B/1D agonists) in acute migraine treatment: a metaanalysis of 53 trials. *Lancet*, *358*, 1668.

[80] Farkkila, M., Olesen, J., Dahlof, C., et al. (2003). Eletriptan for the treatment of migraine in patients with previous poor response or tolerance to oral sumatriptan. *Cephalalgia*, 23, 463.

[81] Diener, H. C., Gendolla, A., Gebert. I. & Beneke, M. (2005) Almotriptan in migraine patients who respond poorly to oral sumatriptan: a double-blind, randomized trial. *Headache*, *45*, 874.

[82] Kramer, M. S., Matzura-Wolfe, D., Polis, A., et al. (1998). A placebo-controlled crossover study of rizatriptan in the treatment of multiple migraine attacks. *Neurology*, *51*, 773.

[83] Dahlof, C. G. H., Lipton, R. B., McCarroll, K. A., Kramer, M. S., Lines, C. R. & Ferrari, M. D. (2000). Within-patient consistency of response of rizatriptan for treating migraine. *Neurology*, *55*, 1511.

[84] Shapiro, R. E., Tepper, S. J. (2007). The serotonin syndrome, triptans, and the potential for drug-drug interactions. *Headache*, *47*, 266.

[85] Gillman, K. (2008), Serotonin toxicity. *Headache*, *48*, 640.

[86] Silberstein, S. D., Holland, S., Freitag, F., Dodick, D. W., Argoff, C., Ashman, E. (2012). Quality Standards Subcommittee of the American Academy of Neurology and the American Headache Society. Evidence-based guideline update: pharmacologic treatment for episodic migraine prevention in adults: report of the Quality Standards Subcommittee of the American Academy of Neurology and the American Headache Society. *Neurology.*, *78*, 1337.

[87] Evers, S., Afra, J., Frese, A., et al. (2006). EFNS guideline on the drug treatment of migraine—report of an EFNS task force. *Eur J Neurol*, *13*, 560.

[88] Evans, R. W., Loder, E. W. & Biondi, D. (2004). When can successful migraine prophylaxis be discontinued? *Headache*, *44*, 1040.

[89] Bussone, G., Diener. H. C, Pfeil, J. & Schwalen, S. (2005). Topiramate 100 mg/day in migraine prevention: a pooled analysis of double-blind randomised controlled trials. *Int J Clin Pract*, *59*, 961.

[90] Nelles, G., Delbruck, A., Schulze, L., et al. (2009). Topiramate for migraine prevention in a naturalistic setting: results from an open label, flexible dose study. *Headache*, *49*, 1454.

[91] Diener, H. C., Kronfeld, K., Boewing, G., et al.(2006). Efficacy of acupuncture for the prophylaxis of migraine: a multicentre randomized controlled clinical trial. *Lancet Neurol*, *5*, 310.

[92] Linde, K., Streng, A., Jurgens, S., et al. (2005). Acupuncture for patients with migraine: a randomized controlled trial. *JAMA*, *293*, 2118.

[93] Whitmarsh, T. E., Coleston-Shields, D. M. & Steiner, T. J. (1997). Double-blind randomized placebo-controlled study of homoeopathic prophylaxis of migraine. *Cephalalgia*, *17*, 600.

In: Migraine Surgery
Editor: Antonios Mammis

ISBN: 978-1-63321-761-4

Chapter 3

Medical Optimization of the Migraine Patient: What is Refractory Migraine?

Shelly Sharma, Peter Y. Shin and Vanny Le*
Rutgers New Jersey Medical School, Newark, New Jersey, US

Migraines pose a significant burden on public health affecting 35 million Americans or 1 out of 4 households in the United States. [1] Over 50% of patients who suffer from migraines report severe impairment requiring the need for bed rest while the debilitation accompanying migraine attacks can bring significant disruption to both family and work life. It is imperative to quickly and effectively treat acute migraines to prevent the progression to chronic migraines or refractory migraines. Chronic migraine is defined by the International Headache Society as a "headache occurring on 15 or more days per month for more than 3 months, which has the features of migraine headache on at least 8 days per month". [2] Unfortunately, there is no consensus for the categorization of refractory migraines which makes it more difficult to understand the pathophysiology or risk factors of refractory migraines as well as provide evidence-based treatment and recommendations. [3, 4]

A proposed definition for refractory migraines by the Refractory Headache Special Interest Section (RHSIS) includes that the headaches meet the criteria of the International Classification of Headache Disorders (ICHD) of migraines or refractory migraines. In addition, patients' function or quality of life must be considerably hindered despite modification of triggers, lifestyle factors and adequate trials of acute and preventive medications. The RHSIS delineates that an adequate trial of a medication is at least 2 months at optimal or maximum-tolerated doses. Patients should have tried at least 2 of 4 drug classes of preventive treatments including beta-blockers, anticonvulsants, tricyclics and calcium channel blockers. They must have also failed adequate trials of abortive drugs such as a triptan and dihydroergotamine (DHE), a nonsteroidal anti-inflammatory medication or a combination of analgesics. [3,4] Furthermore, many of the risk factors associated with

* Corresponding author: Vanny Le, M.D. Department of Anesthesiology 90 Bergen Street, Suite 8100 Newark, NJ 07103 leva@njms.rutgers.edu.

chronic migraine may also contribute to refractory migraine. These include a monthly attack frequency of 3 or more headaches, obesity, stress, medication overuse headache (MOH), sleep disorders, and caffeine excess. [3] In addition, patients should be assessed for mood and personality disorders as well as abuse and mistreatment.

Treating patients with migraines, whether it is acute, chronic or refractory, is a challenging task. Some patients respond very well to single rescue therapy while others necessitate chronic preventive medications. The goals of treatment are to improve the overall wellness of the patient. This includes developing good sleep hygiene, reducing stress, avoiding triggers and addressing any mood disturbances. Patients should be educated on having realistic expectations for treatment since finding a combination of medications and/or interventions may take months. In addition, complete freedom from headache pain may be unattainable. An acceptable goal may be a 50% decrease in pain and to improve functionality. They should be encouraged to actively participate in their care and keep a headache journal which is crucial to understanding headache triggers and patterns. Patients need to understand the risks of overmedicating and the potential of developing MOH. Often times, patients have co-existing psychiatric disorders, such as anxiety, panic disorder, depression, bipolar disorder, and obsessive-compulsive disorder. These patients would benefit from a multidisciplinary approach and require psychiatric consultation.

Finding a successful rescue and/or preventive medication involves a balance between efficacy and tolerability of side effects. Patients should allow at least a trial period of 2 months on an appropriate dose of medication before switching to another anti-migraine medication. Rescue medication should be limited to 2 days a week. If more frequent, patients can develop MOH or chronic daily headaches, both of which can hinder improvement and worsen symptoms.

In this chapter, we will discuss the medical management of migraine patients using various types of pharmacological treatments for rescue therapy as well as preventive medications.

Pharmacological Treatments

NSAIDS

Non-steroidal anti-inflammatory drugs (NSAIDs) are the first line treatment for acute mild to moderate migraines due to their proven efficacy and tolerability. [5] NSAIDs inhibit the neuroinflammatory cascade, prostaglandin release and platelet aggregation that occurs during a migraine. [6] Usually given as an oral medication, these drugs are also available as parenteral and intramuscular preparations. The most commonly used drugs are naproxen, celecoxib, ibuprofen, ketorolac, and indomethacin. [3] Ketorolac IV or IM is often given in the emergency room as an abortive medication. While effective as a single medication for mild to moderate migraines, NSAIDs are often given in combination with other analgesics for moderate to severe migraines. Studies have shown that ketorolac effectively treats acute migraines with cutaneous allodynia in patients who do not respond to sumatriptan subcutaneous injections. [6] However, ketorolac seems to less efficacious then prochlorperazine or DHE with reglan. [6]

NSAIDs are contradicted in patients with gastrointestinal bleeding, renal impairment and nursing mothers. [6] One of the beneficial profiles of NSAIDs is that they are non-sedating and have tolerable side effects. Most patients will complain of gastrointestinal discomfort. Some patients have a high risk of bleeding and developing a cardiovascular event. [3]

Triptans

Triptans are often given to patients with moderate to severe or refractory migraines. [5] Triptans are very selective serotonin receptor agonists at the $5HT_{1B/1D}$ receptor and work by three mechanisms: vasoconstriction of cerebral vessels, peripheral trigeminal inhibition, and inhibition of transmission through second order neurons of the trigeminocervical pathway. [7] Triptans also inhibit the release of inflammatory peptides in the meninges. [8] They are often used as first line therapy because of their selective pharmacological activity, well-established efficacy, tolerable side effects, and favorable safety profile. [9]

While there are many different triptans available for use, the most commonly prescribed are naratriptan, rizatriptan, zolmitriptan, almostriptan, and sumatriptan. All are prepared as oral formulations except sumatriptan which can be administered subcutaneously, rectally, and intranasally. [9] If a patient fails to have migraine relief with one triptan, they should be switched to another triptan medication. At least three different triptans should be tried at tolerable maximum dosages before labeling a patient as a triptan non-responder. (G)

Contraindications to triptan therapy include vascular disease due to the potential for coronary vasoconstriction, uncontrolled hypertension, pregnancy, or the use of a different triptan or ergotamine in the past 24 hours. Common side effects include chest pressure, neck tightness, limb heaviness, dizziness and flushing. [8] Prior to initiating therapy, the patient must be informed that chest pressure may occur and can resemble symptoms of angina. However, the underlying mechanism of chest pain is not related to myocardial ischemia. [7] Fortunately, due of triptan's selective pharmacology, there is no risk of serotonin syndrome because triptans do not affect $5HT_{2a}$ receptors. [8]

Dihydroergotamine

Dihydroergotamine (DHE) is a type of ergot that activates not only the $5HT_{1B/1D}$ receptors like triptans but also $5HT_{1A}$, $5HT_{2A}$, $5HT_{1F}$, $5HT_{2C}$, $5HT_3$, $dopamine_1$ and $dopamine_2$ receptors. [8] DHE is often used as a rescue medication for refractory migraines as either first or second line therapy. Its increasing popularity is due to the fact that it is well studied, inexpensive, non-sedating and produces a decrease in migraine recurrence rate. However, DHE has a complex pharmacology by activating many receptors which leads to a moderate side effect profile and increased risk of overuse syndrome and rebound headache. [9]

Commonly, DHE is prescribed as a nasal spray, subcutaneous or intravenous injection. Ergotamine is an oral preparation combined with caffeine. [3] DHE causes less nausea and vomiting than ergotamine. [3]

DHE can cause nausea, vomiting, diarrhea, abdominal cramping and leg pain. [8] If the patient experiences nausea, then $5HT_2$ and $5HT_3$ receptors have been activated, indicating the dose may be too high for the patient. [8] DHE is contraindicated in patients with uncontrolled hypertension, pregnancy, cardiovascular disease, and prior use of a triptan or ergot in the past 24 hours. [3] Unfortunately, there is a risk for serotonin syndrome because DHE activates $5HT_{2a}$ receptors. [8]

Dopamine Antagonist

Since dopamine has a significant role in the pathogenesis of migraines in the limbic system and basal ganglia, dopamine antagonists are emerging as an alternative therapy for acute refractory migraines. In fact, patients with migraines have an increased frequency of the dopamine D2 receptor allele gene. [10] Usually dopamine antagonists are used as an adjunct to triptan or DHE therapy.

Frequently used dopamine antagonists are promethazine, prochlorperazine, metoclopramide, and chlorpromazine. They are available as parenteral, intramuscular, rectal or oral preparations. [3] Multiple studies have shown that prochlorperazine is more effective as a single agent then ketorolac, magnesium, or sumatriptan. Among the dopamine antagonists, prochlorperazine is more effective then promethazine or metoclopramide [10].

The side effect profile for dopamine antagonists are variable, ranging from mild to severe. Most commonly patients complain of drowsiness. However, some patients do experience extrapyramidal symptoms such as dystonia and akathisia which is often seen with prochlorperazine. Giving anticholinergics such as benztropine and diphenhydramine can prevent these types of symptoms. [10] Droperidol can cause QT prolongation and therefore an EKG should be obtained prior to use. Other less common side effects include hyperprolactinemia, dry mouth, hypotension and weight gain. [3]

Opioids

The use of opioids as first line treatment for acute migraines is very controversial. There are no randomized controlled trials that have shown opioids to have a significant effect on terminating migraine attacks when complete relief of pain was the primary end point. [11] However, opioids are often used in the emergency room as first line rescue therapy for patients with refractory migraines that are unresponsive to their home anti-migraine medications.

Commonly prescribed opioids are oxycodone, morphine, tramadol, hydrocodone/ acetaminophen, meperidine, and nalbuphine. Meperidine is a weak kappa-receptor agonist and because of its poor oral bioavailability, it is given parenterally in the emergency room to treat acute migraines. [6] Nalbuphine is a mixed agonist-antagonist that has low abuse potential due to its analgesic ceiling effect. [6] Tramadol is a weak mu receptor agonist but also inhibits serotonin and norepinephrine reuptake. Due to tramadol's mild side effects, it is often well tolerated by most patients. [6] When compared to placebo trials, meperidine, tramadol and nalbuphine were effective at relieving migraine pain. [6] While meperidine 75 mg IV seems to be more effective then ketorolac 30 mg IM, it seems to the have same efficacy as ketorolac 60 mg IM when combined with an antihistamine. Meperidine seems to be less effective than DHE 1 mg IV. Tramadol 100 mg IM seems to be as effective as diclofenac 75 mg IM. [6]

Opioids have many side effects that can have a detrimental impact on quality of life. Symptoms can range from sedation, sleep disturbance, nausea, vomiting, and gastrointestinal irritability, respiratory depression, withdrawal, addition and dependency. [6] The latter side effects make opioids a very undesirable drug for first line therapy.

While opioids seem to have a significant role as rescue medications, opioids can lead to headache recurrence. This may be due to medication tolerance, medication overuse headache or the conversion of episodic migraines to chronic daily headaches. [11] In fact, many studies have shown that migraine patients are prone to developing chronic daily headaches from overuse of opioids. Using opioids just eight days per month is a risk factor for medication overuse headache. [11] Furthermore, opioids seem to play a role in peripheral and central sensitization of migraine pain. Because of this, there does not seem to be an increase in a patient's daily function or decrease in pain response due to the development of drug tolerance and hyperalgesia. [3] Therefore, patients with refractory migraines should not be on long term opioid therapy because of the potential of worsening the frequency and quality of the migraine as well as developing tolerance and dependence.

Steroids

Steroids act by reducing the propagation of inflammation involved in migraines. While steroids are not used as a first-line agent, they are effective in alleviating exacerbations when used with other anti- migraine medications. There is some debate whether or not steroids can prevent headache recurrence. Steroids seem to reduce recurrence in patients with migraine symptoms lasting longer than 72 hours and have been on a steroid taper for a few days. [6] The optimal regimen likely involves IV doses in the emergency department followed by oral dosing for several days post-discharge.

Commonly prescribed steroids are dexamethasone and prednisone. While dexamethasone can be given orally or intravenously, it is commonly used in the emergency department as a parenteral medication. Prednisone is available as an oral medication and typically tapered over a week. [6]

While side effects are few, patients do complain of sleep disturbance, anxiety and emotional irritability. [3] Long term use is associated with increased risk of osteoporosis and aseptic osteonecrosis of the femoral head. Caution should be used when giving steroids to patients with diabetes mellitus as it can lead to uncontrolled hyperglycemia. [3]

Propofol

Propofol, a short-duration anesthetic agent, has been found to be useful in abortive treatment of migraines and migraine symptoms such as nausea and vomiting refractory to other modes of treatment such as metoclopramide, promethazine, dexamethasone, and meperidine. [12] Propofol is thought to relieve acute migraine by suppressing cortical spreading depression and diminishing central sensitization. [12] A study in 2000 found that subanesthetic doses of propofol monotherapy completely resolved intractable headaches in 63 of 77 patients with the remaining 14 patients reporting 50-90% improvement in headache pain measured by visual analog scale. [13]

Propofol is available as a 10mg/mL aqueous emulsion of 1% propofol in 10% soybean oil, 2% glycerol, and 1.2% egg phosphatide. Propofol is administered via IV injection. The injection of aqueous emulsion may cause local pain which can be alleviated by prior injection of lidocaine or mixing 1mL of 2% lidocaine per 10 mL of propofol emulsion.

Propofol has shown to be effective at alleviating intractable migraines when administered in 20 to 30 mg or 2 to 3 mL IV boluses in fixed time intervals of 3 to 5 minutes. [13] Average propofol dosage in headache relief and abolition was 110 mg or 11 mL with average time to maximum reduction of headache severity taking 20 to 30 minutes. [13]

Side effects observed in migraine patients treated with low dose propofol include transient slurred speech, drowsiness, and spontaneous motor movements of the fingers. [13] Other common side effects include hyperlipidemia, rash, and pruritus. Contraindications to propofol include hypersensitivity to the components of propofol emulsion preparation including eggs, glycerol, or soybean products. Propofol is a pregnancy category B drug and has been shown to be excreted in breast milk. Caution should be used in breastfeeding patients.

Nitrous Oxide

Nitrous oxide is an inhalation anesthetic agent that has been shown to have good short-term efficacy in reducing migraine pain. Using a visual analog pain scale, patients treated with 50% nitrous oxide and 50% oxygen mixture showed significant decrease in pain compared to patients treated solely with 100% oxygen. [3] Furthermore, 60% of patients treated with nitrous oxide did not require rescue treatment at the end of treatment intervention. Reduction of headache pain has been demonstrated in patients treated with a 50% nitrous oxide and 50% oxygen mixture for a total of 20 minutes, with the patient determining level of access to the treatment gas over that time period.

Short-term side effects include transient decreases in mental performance, manual dexterity, and audiovisual ability. Long-term exposure can cause vitamin B_{12} deficiency, numbness, and reproductive side effects.

Contraindications to nitrous oxide treatment relate to its property of rapidly diffusing into air-containing cavities. Therefore, chronic obstructive pulmonary disease, pneumothorax, emphysema, sinusitis, bowel obstruction, and middle ear disease are contraindications to nitrous oxide use. Asthma is not a contraindication unless the patient is undergoing an acute episode. Due to its depressive effect on the CNS, nitrous oxide should be used cautiously in patients treated with opioids and sedative-hypnotics. Nitrous oxide can readily cross the placental barrier and may be toxic to cells undergoing mitosis. Therefore, nitrous oxide should only be considered for emergency use in pregnant patients.

Antihistamines

First-generation antihistamine medications such as diphenhydramine, dimenhydrinate, and hydroxyzine have been used for their antiemetic and sedative properties to alleviate nausea and vomiting that may accompany migraine headaches. [15] They are also used to prevent akathisia and dystonic reactions from other medications used to treat migraine headaches such as dopamine antagonists. They are often used in combination with analgesics and may decrease further peripheral inflammation by preventing mast cell degranulation. Studies indicate that they are not suitable for monotherapy of migraine headaches. [15]

Common side effects of first-generation histamine blockers include weakness, drowsiness, dizziness, impaired coordination, dry mucous membranes, blurred vision, and tachycardia. Serious reactions include agranulocytosis, pancytopenia, arrhythmias, seizures, and heat stroke.

Contraindications to diphenhydramine include known hypersensitivity. Due to the anticholinergic effects of diphenhydramine, caution should be used in patients with concomitant CNS depressant use, closed angle glaucoma, increased intraocular pressure, cardiovascular disease, asthma, COPD, and hypertension. Diphenydramine and dimenhydrinate are classified as pregnancy category B drugs. They are excreted into breastmilk and are contraindicated in breastfeeding patients.

Serotonin Antagonists

Similar to antihistamine use, serotonin antagonists such as granisetron, a 5-HT_3 antagonist, have been used for their antiemetic effects to treat migraine symptoms of nausea and vomiting. 5-HT_3 antagonists have also been shown to decrease inflammatory pain in rats. [14] They are used in conjunction with other rescue treatments. Studies comparing granisetron to placebo show efficacy in reducing nausea and vomiting, but no improvement in headache pain. [14] As such, they are used as adjunct medications rather than monotherapy.

Common side effects reported during granisetron include gastrointestinal symptoms, dizziness, and altered taste. [14] Other common reactions to granisetron include headache and asthenia. One of the adverse reactions of granisetron is QT prolongation and must be used cautiously in patients with arrhythmias, cardiac conduction defects, or QT prolongation risk.

Experimental

One of the newer medications in development for migraine headache is a calcitonin gene-related peptide (CGRP) receptor antagonist. [15] CGRP is involved in sensory neurotransmission and is found in most sensory nerves. CGRP is also a very potent vasodilator and is found to be elevated in patients after migraine and cluster headaches. [15] Telcagepant, the first reported oral formulation of a CGRP receptor antagonist, has been found to be as effective as zolmitriptan in a randomized, double-blind trial. Telcagepant has been shown to not have a vasoconstrictive effect in animal models, making it a possible treatment modality for patients with cardiovascular disease and peripheral vascular disease. However, after progessing to phase III study, Merck & Co. discontinued development of Telcagepant due to reports of liver toxicity. CGRP however still remains a topic of interest in migraine medication research.

Other developments in medical treatment of migraine headaches include devising new routes of delivery for existing classes of medication. An iontophoretic sumatriptan patch delivers sumatriptan utilizing a small electric current to drive transdermal delivery. [15] A linear relationship between the voltage of applied current and drug delivery allows more precise control over medication than the oral route. Randomized, double-blind trials have shown that the iontophoretic patch had similar efficacy as the oral and injected routes and had decreased adverse effects of pain and pressure sensations. Zelrix, an ionteophoretic sumatriptan patch developed by NuPathe was approved for acute migraine treatment by the FDA in January 2013.

Table 1. Acute/Refractory Migraine Treatment

	Dose/Route	Contraindications	Side Effects
NSAIDs			
Naproxen	500 mg PO	Peptic ulcer disease, anticoagulation, renal disease, nursing mothers	GI irritability, kidney impairment
Celecoxib	200 mg PO		
Ibuprofen	200-800 mg PO		
Idomenthacin	25-50 mg PO/PR		
Ketorolac	15-30 mg IV 30-60 mg IM		
Triptans			
Sumatriptan	4-6 mg SC 50-100 mg PO 20 mg NS	Uncontrolled hypertension, coronary vasoconstriction, pregnancy, use of triptan or ergot in the past 24 hours	Chest pressure, neck tightness, limb heaviness, dizziness, flushing
Zolmitriptan	5 mg PO 5 mg NS		
Rizatriptan	10 mg PO		
Naratriptan	2.5 mg PO		
Almotriptan	12.5 mg PO		
Dihydroergotamine (DHE)			
DHE	0.5 mg NS 0.5- 1 mg IV/SC	Uncontrolled hypertension, coronary vasoconstriction, pregnancy, use of triptan or ergot in the past 24 hours	Nausea, vomiting, diarrhea, abdominal cramps, leg pain
Ergotamine/ caffeine	1-2 mg/100 mg PO		
Dopamine Antagonists			
Promethazine	25-50 mg PO 25 mg PR	Pheochromocytoma, pyloric stenosis, porphyria, Parkinson's disease, epilepsy, renal or hepatic impairment, preexisting QT prolongation	Dystonia, akathisia hyperprolactinemia, dry mouth, hypotension, weight gain Droperidol: QT prolongation
Prochlorperazine	5-10 mg IV/IM/PO 25 mg PR		
Metoclopramide	5 -10 mg IV/IM/PO		
Chlorpromazine	25-50 mg PO 10-50 mg IV		
Opioids			
Oxycodone	5-10 mg PO	Allergy to opioids, significant respiratory disease, opioids in combination with other sedatives/hypnotics,	Tolerance, Addiction, Dependency
Morphine	2 mg IV, 10 mg PO		
Tramadol	100 mg PO		
Meperidine	12.5-25 mg PO		
Nalbuphine	10 mg IV		

	Dose/Route	Contraindications	Side Effects
Steroids			
Dexamethasone	4-20 mg IV		Weight gain, hyperglycemia in diabetics, mood irritability
Prednisone	100 mg PO – taper dosing		
Antihistamines			
Diphenhydramine	25-50 mg IV Q6-8 hours PRN	Concomitant CNS depressant use, closed angle glaucoma, increased intraocular pressure, cardiovascular disease, COPD	Weakness, drowsiness, dizziness, impaired coordination, dry mucous membranes, blurred vision, and tachycardia
Dimenhydrinate	50-100 mg IV Q4-6 hours PRN		
Hydroxyzine	25-100 mg IM Q4-6 hours PRN		
Serotonin Antagonist			
Granisetron	40-80 μg/kg IV	Arrhythmias, cardiac conduction defects, or QT prolongation risk	Gastrointestinal symptoms, dizziness, and altered taste
Propofol	20-30 mg IV Q3-5 minutes	Hypersensitivity to eggs, glycerol, or soybean	Slurred speech, drowsiness, spontaneous motor movements
Nitrous Oxide	50% Nitrous Oxide 50% Oxygen via face mask	Pneumothorax, COPD, emphysema, sinusitis, bowel obstruction	Transient decreases in mental performance, manual dexterity, and audiovisual ability

OptiNose is a nasal delivery system that seeks to isolate the nasal cavity from the oropharynx to ensure that the nasally delivered medication is mostly absorbed through the nasal mucosa. [16] Traditional nasal delivery methods resulted in much of the drug being swallowed and subsequently absorbed through the GI tract. OptiNose is seeking FDA approval for nasal delivery of sumatriptan for acute migraine treatment. Phase II trial comparison to placebo showed good efficacy with the most common adverse event being dysgeusia. [15]

Inhaled routes of delivery are being investigated for DHE, prochlorperazine, and loxapine. Levadex is an inhaled DHE that has been shown to have slightly lower efficacy but similarly low 2 day recurrence rates as injected DHE. [15] An inhaled form would enable at home treatment of migraine headaches, which may lead to improved treatment as triptans have been shown to be more effective when applied earlier in the migraine headache period. Levadex is currently still awaiting approval.

Other Medications

Acetaminophen as a single agent is not recommended for migraine treatment. [5] However, when used as an adjunct with other anti-migraine medications, acetaminophen seems to be very effective in alleviating pain. A recent study found that acetaminophen combined with aspirin and caffeine was very effective in relieving migraine headaches as well as the nausea, photophobia, and functional disability that is associated with the attack. [16]

Barbiturates like butalbital often come in combinations with aspirin and caffeine. They are frequently used as first line medications for moderate to severe migraines. However, their use is limited due to addiction and tolerance potential. Furthermore, medication overuse headache may occur when taking these medications chronically.

Prevention Therapy

Preventative therapy should be reserved for patients who require rescue medication more than twice a week, refractory migraines resistant to rescue medication, and/or symptoms of uncommon migraine condition (hemiplegic migraine, migraine with prolonged aura, or migrainous infarction). [17]

Major goals with prevention therapy include decreasing attack frequency, duration and intensity, improving responsiveness to rescue therapy, improving function and preventing occurrences of medication overuse headache and chronic daily headache [17,18]. Current guidelines recommend starting preventive medications at a low dose for a trial period for at least two months. Follow-up and re-evaluation is necessary and important to finding an appropriate regimen [17,18]. Noncompliance to daily therapy seems to be a major obstacle for many patients and often linked to poor outcomes.

Pharmacological Treatments

Beta Blockers

Beta blockers are widely used in migraine prevention because their effectiveness has been shown in multiples studies producing a 50% reduction in the frequency of migraine attacks. [17] It has been proposed that beta blockers reduce overall adrenergic tone by centrally blocking presynaptic noradrenergic receptors, inhibiting norepinephrine release and synthesis, and decreasing activity in the locus ceruleus. [18]

Propanolol, metoprolol, nadolol and atenolol are the most frequently prescribed medications and are available as oral dosing. Beta blockers with sympathomimetic activity like acebutolol, pindolol, and alprenolol are not effective for prevention. [17] Metoprolol has shown to be as effective as aspirin or nebivolol in migraine prevention. Metoprolol 200 mg daily reduces migraine frequency by half when compared to aspirin 300 mg daily. [18] Propranolol 80 mg daily was as effective as cyproheptadine in reducing migraine reoccurrence.

While the side effect profile of beta blockers can be mild, there are many. They include sleep disturbance, weight gain, fatigue, othrostatic hypotension, decrease exercise tolerance, bradycardia and impotence [17,18]. Contraindications include asthma, chronic obstructive lung disease and congestive heart failure among others.

Table 2. Migraine Prophylaxis

	Dose/Route	Contraindications	Side Effects
Antiepileptics			
Divalproex sodium	DR: Initiated at 250 mg PO BID Maximum dosage 500 mg PO BID ER: Initiated at 500 mg PO Maximum dosage 1000 mg PO	Pregnancy, hepatic disease or impairment, or urea cycle disorders	Drowsiness, alopecia, tremor, gastrointestinal disturbance, weight gain
Topiramate	Initiated at 25 mg PO QHS Increase by 25 mg per week Maximum dosage 200 mg PO	Pregnancy or alcohol usage within the past 6 hours	Convulsions, drowsiness, speech disturbance, blurred vision, diplopia, lethargy, hypotension, and abdominal pain
Tricyclic Antidepressants			
Amitriptyline	10-25 mg PO Maximum dosage is 150 mg PO	Acute myocardial infarction recovery Caution: closed angle glaucoma, increased intraocular pressure	Drowsiness, xerostomia, dizziness, constipation, blurred vision, and tachycardia
SNRI			
Venlafaxine	Initiated at 37.5 mg once daily Titrate upwards every 3 days Maximum dosage 150 mg once daily	Caution: Hepatic or renal impairment, seizure history, hypertension, closed angle glaucoma, or increased intraocular pressure	Nausea, drowsiness.
Beta Blockers			
Propranolol	40-400 mg PO	Congestive heart failure, atrioventricular conduction disease, asthma, COPD	Bradycardia, fatigue, drowsiness, gastrointestinal discomfort, impotence
Atenolol	50-200 mg PO		
Metroprolol	100-200 mg PO		
Calcium Channel Antagonists			
Verapamil	120-640 mg PO	Atrioventricular conduction defects, allergy to medication, bradycardia	Weight gain, somnolence, dry mouth, dizziness, hypotension
Flunarizine	5-10 mgPO		

Antiepileptic Medications

Antiepileptic medications have been shown to be effective in lowering migraine headache occurrence rates. Divalproex sodium and topiramate are two antiepileptic medications that have shown efficacy in multiple randomized clinical trials. [18] Data on gabapentin is incomplete and lamotrigine and oxcarbazepine studies show they may be ineffective in migraine prophylaxis. [18] Antiepileptic medications are thought to exert their effect by increasing GABA levels in the CNS and suppressing cortical spreading depression. [18]

Divalproex sodium may cause drowsiness, alopecia, tremor, and gastrointestinal disturbance. Long-term use may also result in weight gain. Serious side effects include bone marrow dysfunction, pancreatitis, hepatitis, and kidney dysfunction. Contraindications to divalproex sodium include known hypersensitivity, hepatic disease or impairment, or urea cycle disorders.

Signs of excessive topiramate ingestion include convulsions, drowsiness, speech disturbance, blurred vision, diplopia, lethargy, hypotension, and abdominal pain. Contraindications to topiramate include known hypersensitivity and alcohol usage within the past 6 hours. Abrupt withdrawal should be avoided with topiramate.

Divalproex sodium and topiramate are classified under pregnancy category D medications and are contraindicated in pregnancy.

Tricyclic Antidepressants

Amitriptyline has been shown to have efficacy in multiple randomized clinical trials. [18] Other tricyclic antidepressants such as clomipramine have been shown to be possibly or probably ineffective for migraine prophylaxis. Amitriptyline is believed to prevent migraines due to its blockade of 5HT receptors, up-regulation of GABA-B receptors, and down-regulation of beta-adrenergic receptors, leading to decreased neuronal excitation. [18]

Amitriptyline can be started at 10 to 25 mg PO at bedtime and then titrated slowly upwards for desired efficacy. Maximum dosage is 150 mg per day, although usually lower doses are effective in migraine prophylaxis.

Due to anticholinergic activity of amitriptyline, common side effects include drowsiness, xerostomia, dizziness, constipation, blurred vision, and tachycardia. Serious reactions include QT prolongation, ventricular arrhythmias, and AV blockage. Amitriptyline is contraindicated in known hypersensitivity and acute myocardial infarction recovery. Caution should be used in patients with closed angle glaucoma, increased intraocular pressure, cardiovascular disease, asthma, prostatic hypertrophy, and hypertension.

SSRI/SNRI

Randomized clinical trials for SSRI medications such as fluoxetine have conflicted efficacy in migraine prophylaxis. However, as migraines may involve a mood disorder component, SSRIs may play a role in an integrated approach to migraine prophylaxis. Venlafaxine, an SNRI, has been shown in randomized clinical trials to reduce migraine occurrence and have superior efficacy compared to SSRI medications. [19] Other SNRI medications have inadequate or insufficient data to recommend use for migraine prophylaxis at this time. [18] One reason for the superior efficacy of venlafaxine compared to SSRIs may be due to its effect on noradrenergic uptake. Venlafaxine also offers a more limited side effect profile than amitriptyline.

Venlafaxine should be started at 37.5 mg PO once daily, and the dosage should be increased every 3 days until desired efficacy is achieved. Maximum dosage is 150 mg per day. Trials have shown that headache occurrence reduction is achieved at 150 mg per day, and that 75 mg per day was ineffective as prophylaxis. [18]

Common side effects include nausea and drowsiness. Serious reactions include suicidality, seizures, serotonin syndrome, hypertension, arrhythmias, and pancreatitis. Contraindications to venlafaxine include known hypersensitivity. Caution should be used for patients with hepatic or renal impairment, seizure history, hypertension, closed angle glaucoma, or increased intraocular pressure.

Venlafaxine is classified as a class C pregnancy drug and should only be used if medication is clearly needed and benefits outweigh risks. Venlafaxine metabolites have been found in breast milk although no adverse effects were reported in infants.

Calcium Channel Antagonists

Once widely used, recently calcium channel antagonists have been downgraded as a preventive medication. [18] Recent studies and guidelines have shown that calcium channel antagonists mainly verapamil may not be as beneficial as once thought. [18,19] Calcium channel antagonists may act by inhibiting serotonin and glutamate release. [18] Most common side effects include dry mouth, dizziness, weight gain, hypotension and sedation. [17]

References

[1] Bigal, ME; Lipton, RB. The epidemiology, burden, and comorbidities of migraine. *Neurologic clinics*, 2009, 27, 321-34.

[2] The International Classification of Headache Disorders, 3rd edition (beta version). Cephalalgia: *an international journal of headache,* 2013, 33, 629-808.

[3] Schulman, E; McGeeney, BE. Current concepts in refractory migraine. *Current treatment options in neurology,* 2013, 15, 40-55.

[4] Shulman, E. Refractory migraine – a review. *Headache,* 2013, 53, 599-613.

[5] Silberstein, SD. Practice parameter: evidence-based guidelines for migraine headache (an evidence-based review): report of the Quality Standards Subcommittee of the American Academy of Neurology. *Neurology,* 2000, 55, 754-62.

[6] Kelly, Nancy, E; and Tepper Deborah, E. Rescue Therapy for Acute Migraine, Part 3: Opioids, NSAIDs, Steroids, and Post Discharge Medications. *Headache,* 2012, 467-482

[7] Ferrari, MD; Roon, KI; Lipton, RB; Goadsby, PJ. Oral triptans (serotonin 5-HT(1B/1D) agonists) in acute migraine treatment: a meta-analysis of 53 trials. *Lancet*, 2001, *358*, 1668-75.

[8] Kelley, NE; Tepper, DE. Rescue therapy for acute migraine, part 1: triptans, dihydroergotamine, and magnesium. *Headache*, 2012, 52, 114-28.

[9] Goadsby, PJ; Lipton, RB; Ferrari, MD. Migraine--current understanding and treatment. *The New England journal of medicine*, 2002, 346, 257-70.

[10] Kelly, Nancy, E; and Tepper Deborah, E. Rescue Therapy for Acute Migraine, Part 2: Neuroleptics, Antihistamine, and others. *Headache*, 2012, vol 12, 292-306

[11] Casucci, G; Cevoli, S. Controversies in migraine treatment: opioids should be avoided. Neurological sciences: *official journal of the Italian Neurological Society and of the Italian Society of Clinical Neurophysiology*, 2013, 34, Suppl 1:S125-8

[12] Mohseni, M; Fatehi, F. Propofol alleviates intractable migraine headache: a case report. *Anesthesiology and pain medicine*, 2012, 2, 94-6.

[13] Krusz, JC; Scott, V; Belanger, J. Intravenous propofol: unique effectiveness in treating intractable migraine. *Headache*, 2000, 40, 224-30.

[14] Triner, WR; Bartfield, JM; Birdwell, M; Raccio-Robak, N. Nitrous oxide for the treatment of acute migraine headache. *The American journal of emergency medicine*, 1999, 17, 252-4.

[15] Rapoport, A. New frontiers in headache therapy. Neurological sciences: *official journal of the Italian Neurological Society and of the Italian Society of Clinical Neurophysiology*, 2011, 32 Suppl *1*, S105-9.

[16] Lipton, RB; Stewart, WF; Ryan, RE. Jr.; Saper, J; Silberstein, S; Sheftell, F. Efficacy and safety of acetaminophen, aspirin, and caffeine in alleviating migraine headache pain: three double-blind, randomized, placebo-controlled trials. *Archives of neurology*, 1998, 55, 210-7.

[17] Siberstein, Stephen. Preventive Migraine Treatment. *Neurologic Clinics*, 2009, *27*(2), 429-443.

[18] Estemalik, E; and Tepper, S. Preventive Treatment in Migraine and the New US Guidelines. *Neuropsychiatr Dis Treat*, 2013, *9*, 709-720.

[19] Ozyalcin, SN; Talu, GK; Kiziltan, E; Yucel, B; Ertas, M; Disci, R. The efficacy and safety of venlafaxine in the prophylaxis of migraine. *Headache*, 2005, 45, 144-52.

In: Migraine Surgery
Editor: Antonios Mammis

ISBN: 978-1-63321-761-4

Chapter 4

Psychological Considerations in the Migraine Patient

Elizabeth K. Seng[1, 2*], Sarah Jo Mayson[1], Nomita Sonty[3], Traci Stein[4], Patricia Tsui[5], Sascha Qian[3] and Dawn Buse[1,2,6]

[1]Ferkauf Graduate School of Psychology at Yeshiva University, Bronx, New York, US

[2]Department of Neurology, Albert Einstein College of Medicine of Yeshiva University, Bronx, New York, US

[3]Department of Anesthesiology of Columbia University, New York, New York, US

[4]Private Practice

[5]Stony Brook Medicine Department of Anesthesiology, Stony Brook, New York, US

[6]Montefiore Headache Center, Bronx, New York, US

Abstract

Migraine is a prevalent, disabling disorder that reduces functioning in social and work spheres. Psychological factors can influence the presentation and course of migraine. Psychological assessment of people with migraine includes self-administered questionnaires of migraine-related quality of life, a psychosocial history, coping with headaches, and psychiatric comorbidities. Psychological factors that are particularly important to consider in medical and surgical treatment of migraine include medication adherence and attitudinal factors. Behavioral treatments are efficacious to treat migraine, and can include relaxation training, biofeedback, and cognitive behavioral therapy.

[*] Corresponding author: Elizabeth K. Seng, Ph.D., 1300 Morris Park Avenue, 130 Rousso Building, Bronx, NY 10461. Telephone: 718-430-3813; Email: Elizabeth.Seng@einstein.yu.edu.

Keywords: Migraine, Behavioral Treatment, CBT, Biofeedback, Relaxation, Psychiatric Comorbidity, Quality of Life, Disability, Adherence, Psychological Assessment, Mindfulness, Hypnosis

Migraine and Quality of Life

Migraine is an episodic and painful disorder that is both prevalent and disabling. Characterized by recurrent headaches and episodes of moderate to severe, unilateral, pulsing pain, migraine is associated with nausea, vomiting and sensitivity to light and sound and may last anywhere from four hours to three days, if left untreated. [1] Migraine may be divided into two categories: episodic and chronic. Episodic migraine is marked by less than15 headache days per month, while 15 or more headache days per month defines chronic migraine. Episodic migraine affects an estimated 12 percent of the population, including 18 percent of females and 6 percent of males. [2, 3] Chronic migraine affects one to two percent of the population, with a similar female preponderance. [4] Approximately two and a half percent of persons with episodic migraine develop chronic migraine over the course of one year. [5] One in every four households in the United States includes someone who suffers from migraine. [6]

Across the world, migraine is associated with great disability, with chronic migraine linked to larger impact than episodic migraine. [4, 7] According to a recent report by The World Health Organization, migraine ranks seventh in specific causes of disability worldwide. [8] A global, epidemiological study of the burden of disease found that migraine accounted for more than one percent of years lived in disability. [9] Unfortunately, the middle—and most productive—years of life are those most positively correlated with migraine, a pattern most pronounced in women. [10] Thus, interference in functioning associated with migraine is ill timed, co-occurring with expectations of individuals to perform at their peak capacity. The burden occurs both during (i.e., ictally) and between (i.e., interictally) attacks. [11] Ictal burden can include head pain, nausea, vomiting, and sensitivity to environmental stimuli while interictal burden often comprises fear of the next attack and limitation in real or perceived ability to make plans, among other elements.

Nearly all individuals with migraine experience reductions in functioning in both social and work spheres. This is not hard to imagine when considering that more than half of people with migraine report that the ictal burden involves needing to lie down and completely abstain from activity. [2] In addition, studies have consistently found that people with migraine experience general impairment as well, from inferior social and emotional functioning to impaired sleep, when compared to people without migraine. [12]

Effects on social functioning appear to be particularly insidious. As migraine attacks often occur without warning, they can lead people both to break and to withdraw from making social and work commitments. Even family members are negatively impacted through factors like worry, emotional distress, [13] perceived increase in arguments and dissatisfaction about heightened responsibility to compensate for the migraine patient's disability. [14] Relatedly, migraine patients report greater disease-related stigma than patients with epilepsy, particularly around issues of work productivity. [15] Finally, expectations about social and work roles appear to interfere with migraine patients' ability to make optimal decisions about acute migraine treatment. [16]

Migraine also carries substantial economic implications for both individuals and communities. Studies consistently demonstrate that people with migraine are underdiagnosed and undertreated, leading to financial burden for individuals, employers and healthcare systems. [17] One study found that individuals with migraine demonstrated significantly higher average, yearly, medical costs than controls ($7,089 vs. $2,923)[18], with outpatient prescription drug costs contributing significantly to this discrepancy ($2,968 vs. $685).

Chronic migraine is a particularly disabling variant of migraine experienced by 1.4% – 2.2% of the population. [1, 19] National surveillance studies examining migraine have consistently demonstrated higher levels of disability for individuals with chronic migraine compared to those with episodic migraine. [10] For example, an analysis of 24,000 individuals with "severe" headache who responded to the 2005 American Migraine Prevalence and Prevention (AMPP) Study survey identified 655 respondents with chronic migraine and 11,249 respondents with episodic migraine. Respondents with chronic migraine (relative to episodic migraine) had statistically significant lower levels of household income, were less likely to be employed full time, were more likely to be occupationally disabled, and had higher rates of self-reported headache-related disability. [20] Chronic migraine has been associated with greater number of days disabled due to migraine and lower health-related quality of life and well-being. [21] One study found that chronic migraine was associated with a loss of nearly $200 per week for men and $90 per week for women compared to episodic migraine. [22]

Together, these data indicate that migraine is a prevalent disorder with high individual, societal, and economic costs. Improved diagnosis and treatment is essential to reduce the burden of migraine.

Psychological Assessment in Migraine

Psychological assessment in migraine headaches can be performed via face-to-face interviews and self-report questionnaires. These approaches may also be integrated in order to paint the most accurate profile possible of an individual with migraine. The biopsychosocial model posits that multiple factors impact the experience of pain and interact in a complex fashion. [23] From this perspective, a thorough understanding of such factors is crucial to optimal care. Psychosocial elements include emotion, social and environmental context, socio-cultural background, the meaning the affected individual ascribes to the pain, beliefs, attitudes and expectations. These variables interact with biological factors and collectively influence the overall experience of pain. Numerous questionnaires have been developed to aid in capturing the complexity of this web of information.

Due to the scope of this chapter, several instruments that measure migraine disability and headache related quality of life will be discussed. Buse, Sollers, Steiner, and colleagues (2012), however, present a more thorough review of the literature surrounding the instruments available for the assessment of migraine. [24]

Patient Self-Administered Questionnaires

The Migraine Disability Assessment (MIDAS) is comprised of five questions and measures headache-related disability over a three month period. [25] Respondents are asked to assess 1) missed days of work or school due to headaches; 2) reduced productivity by half at work or school due to headaches; 3) inability to do household work due to headaches; 4) reduced household-related productivity by at least half due to headaches; and 5) missed family, social, or leisure activities due to headaches. Respondents are also asked to assess the number of days that included headache pain in the last three months and pain intensity on a scale from 0 to 10, where zero represents no pain at all and 10 represents the highest possible level of pain. Significant correlations were found between headache diary scores (taken over a thirteen week period) and MIDAS scores, with correlations ranging from .41 to .76. [26] This questionnaire is not copyrighted and is available to use free of charge (http://www.americanheadachesociety.org/midas/). The instrument demonstrates good test-retest reliability (Pearson's r = 0.80). It has been correlated with daily headache diary summary scores (Spearman's r = 0.63) and has good internal consistency (Chronbach's alpha = 83). [27]

The Headache Impact Test or HIT-6 is a six-item questionnaire measuring interference due to migraine and migraine severity. The HIT-6 was created using Item Response Theory, and can be administered as a Computer Adaptive Test or as a paper-and-pencil self-report. [28] The questions were developed using Item Response Theory with an item pool of 53 questions from several questionnaires that include the Headache Disability Inventory, Headache Impact Questionnaire, MIDAS, and Migraine Specific Questionnaire. The six-items measure pain severity, impact on "usual daily activities" (including work, school or social activities), overall fatigue, desire to lie down, frustration and difficulty with concentration. Confirmatory factor analysis demonstrated that a single headache impact factor was adequate. [29] The HIT-6 has demonstrated good test-retest reliability (average Pearson's r = 0.77). [30]

The Migraine-Specific Quality of Life Questionnaire (MSQ, version 2.1) is a 14-item questionnaire that assesses headache-related quality of life. The MSQ was administered to patients with chronic migraine and a confirmatory factor analysis revealed three subscales: role function-restrictive, role function-preventive, and emotional function [31], which were similar to the results for individuals with episodic migraine. [32] These three factors demonstrate high internal consistency, with Cronbach's alpha ranging from 0.86-0.96. [33]

The Medical Outcomes Study 36-Item-Short-Form-Health-Survey (SF-36; [34, 35] and a shorter version, the Medical Outcomes Study 12-Item-Short-Form-Health-Survey (SF-12; [36]), are assessments developed to measure physical and mental components of health status for a variety of health conditions such as heart disease, diabetes, as well as chronic pain. The survey was designed for use in clinical settings and research. Eight health concepts measured include: 1) limitations in physical activities due to health problems; 2) limitations in social activities because of physical or emotional problems; 3) limitations in usual activities because of physical health problems; 4) bodily pain; 5) general mental-health (psychological distress and well-being); 6) limitations in usual activities because of emotional problems; 7) vitality, i.e., levels of energy and fatigue; and 8) General health perceptions. This survey was designed for a wide variety of medical conditions and age ranges. For the SF-36, internal consistency for each subscale is equal to or greater than .76; physical functioning, role limitations, and bodily pain were strongly correlated with the physical component (*r*s = .77-.88), and general mental heatlh and role limitations were strongly correlated with the mental component (*r*s = .71-.81). [37] Where the SF-36 was constructed to be highly internally consistent, items for the SF-12 were selected to be more heterogenous to maintain satisfactory reliability while reducing the number of items. Selected items each demonstrated unique reliable variance in prediction. [36] The mental and physical component scales of the SF-36 and SF-12 have demonstrated high correlations (*r*s = 0.97 and 0.95, respectively). One limitation is that floor effects may exist especially for severely ill individuals.

The Migraine Interictal Burden Scale (MIBS) is a 4-item, self-administered questionnaire that assesses impairment and burden for the period between migraine headaches. [38] The MIBS measures impairment in four domains: impairment in work or school, impairment in family and social life, difficulty making plans or commitments, and emotional affective and cognitive distress. People with migraine have reported poorer subjective well-being and reduced health-related quality of life during pain-free periods compared to age and sex matched individuals who do not suffer from migraines. Assessing interictal burden and impairment is important for optimizing treatment. The MIBS has demonstrated positive associations with measures of ictal disability (MIDAS [Spearman r = 0.40], HIT-6 [Spearman r = 0.44]), depression (r = 0.41), and measures of workplace productivity (absenteeism [r = 0.18], presenteeism [r = 0.25]). [11]

The Headache Under-Response to Treatment or HURT questionnaire [24] is an eight-item self-administered instrument that assesses multiple dimensions of headache that include headache frequency, disability, medication use and its effects, perceptions of headache "control," and knowledge of diagnosis. Sample items include: "On how many days in the last month did you have a headache?" "On how many days in the last 3 months did your headaches make it hard to work, study or carry out household work?" One of the benefits of using this questionnaire is that it measures many different aspects of care. Psychometric data on this measure is still being collected. A two-factor model has emerged: a) headache frequency, headache-attributed disability, and medication use, and b) medication efficacy and headache control items. There is evidence to support reliability in at least four languages and different countries, cultures, and settings. The HURT questionnaire is sensitive to changes in headache over time. [24]

Psychosocial History

Chronic stress has been found to impact headache severity and frequency. Stressors can arise from various factors. A chaotic family upbringing has been identified as a risk factor for developing chronic migraines. Tietjen, Brandes, Peterlin, and colleagues [39] obtained electronic survery data from 1348 people with migraine at 11 outpatient headache centers. They found that childhood maltreatment, either from abuse or neglect, was reported by 58% of the study population. Using the cutoff score for the Childhood Trauma Questionnaire, 21% of the sample were physically abused, 25% were sexually abused, 38% were emotionally abused, 22% were physically neglected, and 38% were emotionally neglected. The authors concluded that childhood maltreatment, particularly emotional abuse was a risk factor for chronic migraine and the association of emotional abuse with headache frequency and transformation to chronic migraine appears to be independent of other factors, including depression and anxiety, which were also related to both childhood abuse and chronic headache. Having headaches during childhood also seems to be related to increased odds of experiencing stress during adolescence. Waldie [40] found that participants who had a history of childhood headache were 1.4 times more likely to report moderate stress and 1.5 times more likely to report high stress in mid-adolescence compared to those who did not have a history of headache in childhood. Study members with combined headache (migraine and tension type) at aged 26 also reported multiple stress symptoms in adolescence, including changing schools, feeling left out (typically males), feeling overweight, and feeling sick. Interestingly, feeling overweight did not necessarily mean a high Body Mass Index; it was primarily the perception of being overweight. The association between stress and combined headache was strongest among those who suffered frequent headaches in childhood.

Socio-economic status has also been found to impact migraine headache frequency and intensity. Winter, Berger, Buring, and Kurth [41] conducted a cross-sectional study and found that women with self-reported low SES, using annual household income and education, had increased risk for migraine and non-migraine headaches. Data from AMPP study [42] also found that migraine prevalence increased as household income decreased. The authors speculated that social selection and social causation were possible explanations for increased migraine prevalence. According to social selection, higher levels of disability from migraine headaches will tend to interfere with greater academic or occupational achievement. Additionally, social causation, suggests that individuals in lower SES groups experience increased life stressors that will impact headache frequency and intensity.

Coping with Headaches

In order to adapt to the ongoing stress of migraine headache pain, individuals will often develop coping strategies. Based on a cognitive-behavioral therapy framework, there are two types of coping: cognitive and behavioral. Adaptive forms of cognitive coping include developing disputing or correcting erroneous beliefs about pain, focusing attention on the sensory (as opposed to affective or suffering) qualities of the stimulus, and reinterpreting pain sensations in an emotionally detached manner. [43] Although focusing on the sensations of pain may appear to be counterintuitive, the way one focuses on the pain is what is important. Developing coping statements can help to increase self-efficacy and promote an internal locus of control. Self-efficacy refers to confidence in one's ability to engage successfully in migraine management. An internal locus of control refers to beliefs that an individual has personal control over his or her environment including pain and pain-related stressors. Minimizing maladaptive forms of cognitive coping such as catastrophizing (overestimating the likelihood of a possible, exaggerated negative future event) have also been found to be beneficial. Participants in a cognitive-behavioral treatment program focused on reducing catastrophizing had significant reductions in catastrophizing, anxiety, headache frequency, and intensity and increased self-efficacy when compared to a waitlist control. [44] Furthermore, it has also been found that catastrophizing is associated with impaired functioning and quality of life, independent of migraine characteristics and other demographic and psychological variables. [45]

The Coping Strategies Questionnaire [46] is often used to assess how individuals cope with chronic pain. The CSQ is composed of 48-items that the respondent rates on a 7-point rating scale. There is also a revised version [47] that consists of 27 items. The score is a summation of all the items in the scale divided by the number of items. There is also a computerized version of the revised scale.

Pain diaries can also be utilized to assess how people with migraine cope with their headache pain. For instance, many individuals who suffer from migraine headaches take medications as a way of preventing and managing headache pain; however, "Rebound headaches" can occur when medications are overused. Many people with migraine also try to avoid triggers for headaches that include activities, foods, and environmental conditions (e.g., excessive light, odors, or noise) that can cause migraines. Pain diaries can be utilized to determine the frequency with which on uses pain medications and what tends to trigger headaches. Pain diaries can be used in paper and pencil form or on electronic devices.

Psychiatric Comorbidities

"Comorbidity" refers to the occurrence of two conditions in the same individual at a frequency greater than would be expected by chance. Several psychiatric comorbidities and psychological conditions and experiences are comorbid with migraine. Routinely screening and monitoring patients for common psychiatric comorbidities of migraine can aid in management and is the ethical course of treatment. (See Buse et al., for a review of instruments to help in migraine management. [24]) The Patient Health Questionnaire (PHQ or PRIME-MD) is a free, well validated relatively brief, paper-pencil instrument to assess and monitor a range of psychiatric disorders as well as important psychological issues. [5] Briefer versions of assessment instruments are also available, including the Patient Heath Questionniare-9 (PHQ-9) for depression and the GAD-7 for anxiety. The PHQ-4 is an ultra-brief screen for depression and anxiety. All are in the public domain and available for use free of charge. Scoring information, clinical advice, and psychometric development manuscripts can be found at www.depression-primarycare.org.

Psychiatric Comorbidity in Migraine

Migraine is comorbid with a range of medical and psychiatric comorbidities. [20, 48, 49] Associated burden and disability is even greater for persons with chronic migraine as seen in headache-related disability/impact, socioeconomic status, health-related quality of life, medical and psychiatry comorbidities, healthcare resource utilization and direct and indirect costs. [4]

Psychiatric Disorders Common in Migraine

In terms of psychiatric comorbidities of migraine, several large-scale population based studies have confirmed comorbidity between migraine and major depression, anxiety disorders, posttraumatic stress disorder [50], substance abuse, bipolar disorder, suicide attempts, and childhood maltreatment and abuse. Much research involving migraine and mood disorders, including numerous prospective, large- scale, population-based studies, have focused on depression. Population based studies examining the prevalence of depression in migraine patients report ranges from 3.8% to 57.0% compared to the general population lifetime rates of 16%. [20, 51-53]

Additionally, anxiety disorders have been found to be significantly associated with migraine in both clinical and community based studies. [54] Both Generalized Anxiety Disorder and Panic Disorder are found to independently have a higher prevalence among people with migraine. A population-based study found that anxiety disorders were almost twice as likely to be diagnosed in people with migraine than in the general population (> 50% vs. 27% of the general population). [55] Researchers have also found a three-fold increase in migraine prevalence in patients with bipolar spectrum disorders. [56].

Both clinic and population-based studies have demonstrated higher rates of comorbid medical and psychiatric conditions in persons with chronic migraine (relative to episodic migraine). [20, 57] An analysis of 24,000 individuals with "severe" headache from the 2005 AMPP Study survey identified 655 respondents with chronic migraine and 11,249 respondents with episodic migraine. [20] Relative to episodic migraine, respondents with chronic migraine were approximately twice as likely to have depression and anxiety. The International Burden of Illness study revealed a similar pattern. [58] Data were collected on comorbid medical and psychiatric conditions. Participants were asked, "Have you been told by a doctor or any other health professional that you have any of the following health problems?" Conditions were divided into five categories: psychiatric, pain, vascular risk factors, vascular disease events, and other. Almost one-half (45.2%) of US chronic migraine participants reported a psychiatric disorder, compared to approximately one-third (29.0%) of episodic migraine participants (P = .003). Comorbidity profiles were also examined among patients with episodic migraine and chronic migraine in the Taiwan National Health Insurance Research Database. [57] Compared with patients with "other migraines" (n = 2,226), patients with chronic migraine (n = 681) had higher risk of psychiatric comorbidities: depression (RR = 1.88; P≤0.0001), bipolar disorder (RR = 1.81; P = 0.022) and anxiety disorders (RR = 1.48; P ≤0.0001).

Frequent headache has been associated with adverse childhood experiences including emotional abuse, sexual abuse and physical abuse study. [59] Adverse childhood events and childhood maltreatment has been associated with severe headache and migraine in a range of studies. [39, 53, 59-63] An analysis of data from the AMPP Study found that rates of adverse childhood events were higher among respondents with migraine (n=8,305) than those with tension-type headache (n=1,429) for emotional neglect (24.5% versus 21.5%), emotional abuse (22.5% versus 16.7%) and sexual abuse (17.7% versus 13.3%.). [64] Among participants with migraine, all three forms of maltreatment were associated with higher headache day frequency category but results lost significance after adjusting for depression and anxiety, which could be attributed to mediation, confounding or a common brain substrate.

An analysis of AMPP Study data demonstrated that major life events/stressful events are more common among persons with chronic migraine compared to those with episodic migraine. [65] Major life events assessed included change of residence, employment status, marital status, changes related to their children, deaths of relatives or close friends, and "extremely stressful" ongoing situations. Study participants were asked to rate the level of stress associated with each event, identifying the major life events, which were also stressful life events. Because cross-sectional designs preclude the possibility of determining directionality, it remains unclear whether the event or chronic migraine is primary in the AMPP Study cross sectional analysis. However, the Frequent Headache Epidemiology Study assessed the role of major life events as risk factors for the new onset of chronic daily headache using a case control design. [66] Chronic daily headache and control cases were asked about the same stressful life events as used in the AMPP analysis. Compared with episodic headache controls, chronic daily headache cases had more major life changes in the prior or current year. After adjusting for age, sex, headache type, and year of event, the odds of frequent headaches increased additionally with each antecedent major life event [odds ratio (OR) 1.20 (1.1, 1.3), $P < 0.001$], but not with subsequent events [OR 0.94 (0.8, 1.1), $P < 0.4$]. The specificity of association for events preceding but not following the onset of chronic daily headache supports the possibility of a causal relationship.

Psychiatric Comorbidities as Risk Factors for Migraine Progression

It has been demonstrated that approximately 2.5 percent of individuals with episodic migraine one year progress to chronic migraine the following year. [5] Several studies have examined the role of psychiatric comorbidities as predictors of chronic migraine onset. Researchers examined 6,657 AMPP Study participants with episodic migraine in 2005 and found that 160 (2.4%) developed chronic migraine in 2006 and 144 (2.2%) developed chronic migraine in 2007. [67] Depression was a significant predictor of chronic migraine onset (OR =1.65, 95% CI: 1.12-2.45), after adjusting for sociodemographic variables and headache characteristics. Additionally, there was a depression-dose effect. Relative to study respondents with none or mild depression, those with moderate (OR= 1.77, 95%CI: 1.25- 2.52), moderately-severe (OR= 2.35, 95% CI:1.53-3.62), and severe depression (OR=2.53, 95% CI:1.52-4.21) were at increased risk for the onset of chronic migraine at increasingly higher rates.

A study of 122 adolescent chronic daily headache patients in Taiwan reported that major depression was an independent predictor of persistence of chronic daily headache at two years in multivariate analyses. In univariate analyses panic disorder, social phobia, and obsessive-compulsive disorder were also risk factors. [68] Anxiety was also identified as a risk factor for progression in the AMPP Study. [69] Smitherman and colleagues postulate that anxiety disorders, rather than depression, contribute more to migraine progression, and that possible mechanisms include shared dysfunction of the serotonergic system, medication overuse derived from a lack of appropriate coping behaviors, and inherent ideology that magnifies pain and unpleasant associated features. [70]

Conversely, researchers tested whether reducing headache days from chronic migraine to episodic migraine would improve risk factors and related outcomes. [71] Thirty-two outpatients (age >18 years) with chronic migraine and comorbid depressive disorders were recruited from three outpatient centers. Participants were treated with onabotulinumtoxinA. At 24 weeks, treatment of chronic migraine with onabotulinumtoxinA was associated with reductions in headache and migraine frequency as well as reductions in depression, anxiety, headache-related disability and impact and improvement in health related quality of life. As onabotulinumtoxinA has no known direct effect on mood, the improvements seen may be attributable to improvement in headache. Additional blinded studies with larger samples are necessary to fully explore the results seen in all of these studies.

Treatment of Psychiatric Comorbidities of Migraine

Psychiatric conditions can be treated with pharmacologic and nonpharmacologic treatments. Several empirically supported nonpharmacologic treatments for psychological conditions also have evidence for migraine management including most notably cognitive behavioral therapy (CBT)[72-74] and biobehavioral training (biofeedback, relaxation training, and stress management). [75, 76] These techniques have demonstrated efficacy when learned and practiced correctly, and may be used individually or in conjunction with pharmacological and other interventions. Notably, these techniques are particularly effective for the treatment of migraine in individuals with diagnoses of depression and/or anxiety. [77]

Information and referrals for CBT can be found at www.abct.org, biofeedback information and referrals can be found at www.aapb.org, relaxation exercises and instruction can be found at dawnbuse.com, additional information for patients can be found at www.achenet.org and www.headaches.org.

Psychological Factors in the Medical and Surgical Treatment of Migraine

Medication Adherence

People with migraine are estimated to use two to five times more healthcare services people without migraine, in part because their symptoms are often not well controlled. [78] Medication adherence refers to the pattern of medication-taking necessary to manage headache optimally, or "the extent of agreement between a patient's treatment-related behaviors and a health professional's advice." This definition implies an active role and collaborative involvement in treatment by the patient. Across chronic diseases, a large literature suggests that only 50% of patients are adherent with their medication regimen. [79] People with migraine frequently have difficulty with medication adherence, including filling prescriptions, following medication-related recommendations, and keeping appointments with prescribing providers. [80] Moreover, medication adherence in migraines is of importance for several reasons including prevention of excessive use of both over-the-counter and prescription medications, headache progression and potential drug interaction, decrease in emergency room visits and decreased chronicity of symptoms.

Most adherence research has focused almost exclusively on medications that are used on a fixed schedule, as opposed to medications taken on managing episodic symptoms such as headaches. [16] Optimal use of acute headache medications, such as triptans or non-steroidal anti-inflammatories, is more complex and a higher patient burden than daily medications. A person using acute medication to manage migraine must make in-the-moment decisions about the benefits, cost, and timing of medication on the self-evaluation of the progressing, disabling symptoms of a migraine. [16, 81] Behaviors considered by patients and providers to be required for adherence with acute headache medications including keeping the medication accessible, communicating with the prescribing provider, distinguishing between migraine and non-migraine headaches accurately, optimal choice of medication type, dose, timing, and limiting medication use appropriately to avoid medication overuse headache. [16] Given the high burden on the patient to make these in-the-moment decisions, it is not surprising that patients have difficulty taking acute headache medication optimally. People with migraine frequently choose a non-specific pain medication rather than a migraine-specific medication to treat migraine headaches. [82, 83] Further, between 40-85% of people with migraine wait to take abortive medications until after they are most likely to be effective. [82, 84-87] Additionally, four percent of people with migraine take acute migraine medication more than three days per week, a pattern of medication use associated with medication overuse headache. [87-89]

Socio-economic factors such as gender, stage of life and racial differences have also been shown to influence triptan use among persons with episodic migraines. In the AMPP study, adherence to triptans has been associated with higher education, having health insurance, being female, Caucasian, aged between 40-49 years, and with a household income of over $40,000. [90] Behavioral studies have demonstrated that headache sufferers develop a psychological dependency on their medications because they see them as being indispensable and as the only object that provides them with relief when the headaches disrupt their lives. People with migraine may hold onto the indispensable medication just in case they may need it, contributing to overuse of the medication. [91] With the exception of the AMPP study, most medication adherence studies are cross-sectional, making causal attributions difficult.

Research demonstrates that discontinuation of medications is most correlated with lack of efficacy, and the type of medication often influences the differing patterns of discontinuation. In one multicenter cross-sectional study, people with migraine who discontinued triptans (n = 69) had higher rates of medication overuse, were more likely to have used opioids for headache management and had higher MIDAS and BDI scores. People with migraine who continued triptans (n = 207), however, were more likely to have been given their prescription by a specialist, were more likely to report headache reduction or resolution from the triptan, were also more likely to report greater confidence in their prescribers, feel a greater sense of control over their migraines, and were more educated about their triptan use. [92) In the AMPP study, compared to opioid users for the treatment of migraine headaches, triptan users were less likely to discontinue medication use due to headache-related disability or due to side effects. Opioid users were likely to discontinue medications because of return of migraine pain, concerns regarding drug interactions, and stomach upset. [93]

Rains and colleagues recommended the following strategies to improve adherence: send reminders to patients to encourage them to attend their appointments, simplify and tailor medications to meet patient's specific needs, screen and assess for psychiatric comorbidities, and improve self-efficacy in the management of chronic migraine. [80, 94, 95] Because the most common cause of discontinuation is lack of efficacy, further research on understanding individually targeted therapies is warranted.

Psychological Factors in Surgical Interventions

Surgery is often a threatening experience for most individuals because it creates concerns about one's physical well-being, anticipation of the pain, worries about treatment response and potential risks. [96] As surgical interventions and their costs are on the rise, it has become more important to identify factors that predict optimal surgical outcomes. Early research, exploring the role of socio-demographic factors, clinical variables, anatomic structures, and associated comorbidities, found that these factors did not explain the significant variability in post-operative recovery time. More recently, research has begun to examine the influence of psychological factors in post-surgical outcomes. While a significant impact of psychosocial factors on surgical outcomes have been identified in knee arthroscopies, ACL reconstruction, hip fractures and spine surgeries [97], in refractory headaches research is still in its early stages. Depression and anxiety have been associated with worse outcomes following cardiac surgeries [98, 99]. A review conducted by Rosenberger et al., (2006) attempted to determine whether psychosocial factors demonstrated effectiveness in predicting surgical outcomes while controlling for clinical factors. They examined mood disturbances, attitudes, social support, coping factors, and personality factors. Their conclusions regarding mood were that, 1) negative mood states impacted different aspects of recovery trajectory, 2) specific pre-operative worries were the best predictors of short-term surgical outcomes and patient's ratings of recovery, and 3) depression most-likely predicted long-term pain and functional impairment. However, when clinical factors were added to the predictors, mood disturbance lacked predictive power. Their conclusions regarding attitudinal factors (positive expectations, self-efficacy, patient-perceived control, optimistic outlook and involvement in recovery) revealed that attitudinal factors were predictors of quicker recovery, especially with functional tasks such as activities of daily living. Their conclusions regarding social support revealed significant effects on long-term physical outcome and survival. Other findings revealed that more research was needed to understand the role of coping factors and personality in surgical outcomes. Similar research is needed to understand the influence of these variables in refractory headache disorders.

Neuromodulation in Migraines and Assessment for Treatment

While the mechanism of numerous anti-migraine medications are rooted in neuromodulation, neuromodulation therapy specifically refers to medical non-pharmacologic modulation of neuronal structures that are involved in the detection or transmission of painful stimuli or in the processing of the information in the brain. The neuronal structures involved in migraines are thought to be the cerebral cortex, the brainstem, the trigeminal system as well as the associated vasculature components. [100] Emerging, promising treatments include noninvasive techniques such as transcranial magnetic stimulation and transcranial direct current stimulation, which modulate cortical excitability; invasive procedures such as vagal nerve stimulation, cervical spinal cord stimulation, and occipital nerve stimulation, which modulates inhibitory anti-nonciceptive pathways [101-104].

Most patients start evaluation of their migraines in a primary care setting and advance to a specialist's care when their headaches are refractory to conservative measures. Typically, they are considered for neuromodulation if they have severe chronic headaches lasting longer than 2 years, and conventional medical therapies were tried for more than 3-6 months without success. [105] Initial evaluation covers headache history, medications, alternative therapies, disability status, and visual analog scale rating the headache pain. Careful history taking should help to rule out medication overuse, and thorough diagnostic workup should rule out specific vascular causes via cerebral MRI scan with angiography of the vessels [106].

Psychological evaluation has become an increasingly important component of prescreening for invasive neuromodulation as well as during and after the trial. The role of psychosocial influences on successful outcomes in these therapies is being widely recognized. Extant research on the role of psychiatric illness on the efficacy of spinal cord stimulation consistently found that depression had a negative effect on the success of this modality. [107] Additionally, higher levels of anxiety and catastrophization have also been associated with less favorable outcomes. [108, 109]

Many patients with chronic migraines may not have had a prior contact with mental health providers and maybe unwilling to be evaluated by one. Therefore, referring physicians should preface the encounter with clear reasons for the referral, explaining that this information will assist the physician and the patient to make the most appropriate decision after determining whether the patient will have the best chance of a successful outcome. These evaluations are conducted by a licensed psychologist with expertise in pain management and tend to be both, evaluative and educational in nature. In addition to the clinical interview, an integral part of the assessment is the patient's response to this interactive process as it provides information about their readiness for the procedure. Besides eliciting the illness narrative and treatment history, pain psychologists find it useful to consider a comprehensive history that includes the patient's emotional condition; chemical dependency; character pathology; psychiatric symptoms of depression, anxiety, thought disorder, sleep, cognitive, or sexual impairment; current living situation; current external stressors; childhood and development history. [110] They also ask about the patient's understanding of the technical aspects of the implantable device, surgical procedure, follow-up, and expectations for pain relief, strategies to cope with inadequate pain relief, and relationship with the pain physician. [111] They may find it useful to include significant others or family members as part of the interview to obtain more information.

Numerous red flags are associated with outcomes and include: personality disorders, unstable family and personal relationships, poor vocational adjustment, active litigation, suicidality, homicidality, severe depression, somatoform disorders, alcohol or drug dependency, cognitive deficits, and poor social support [112, 113]. Contrary to this approach, Doleys [114] highlighted the following positive indicators for a successful outcome: general psychological stability, moderate levels of self-confidence and self efficacy, realistic concern regarding illness and proposed therapy, mild depression appropriate to the current circumstances, a sense of optimism, ability to cope with flareup and complications, adequate knowledge about the procedure, adequate social support, history of treatment adherence, ability to follow instructions, appropriate expectations and ability to tolerate paresthesias.

As an objective component of the psychological assessment, patients may be asked to complete screening assessment measures like Beck Depression Inventory, Beck Anxiety Inventory, Minnesota Multiphasic Personality Inventory, Millon Clinical Multiaxial Inventory, and Symptom Check List 90-R, and specific pain screening measures. [110] Through the history gathering, mental status examination, and standardized psychological tests, pain psychologists make recommendations regarding contraindications, whether these contraindications are amenable to change or mitigated by close follow-up, and likelihood that the patient will benefit from the procedure in terms of restored functioning and/or improved quality of life.

Upon completion of the psychological evaluation and recommendations to proceed with the trial, a trial stimulator may be placed percutaneously in the initial period before the consideration for a permanent stimulator. A majority of patients report back either a markedly positive response or that the trial stimulator was not effective at all for their headache; if they do report that they respond well to a neurostimulator, typically all aspects show improvement: decreased medication requirement, increased sense of well-being, and a return to previous activities of daily living [115]. The physician and the patient should discuss in advance the specific goals of the trial and the measures of success important to the patient. If returning to work is the primary goal, a rehabilitation specialist could be invited to be part of the evaluation process. [106]. Two questions, vital to the assessment, arise: First of all, does the patient respond to therapy? Typically, they are not recommended to continue with implantation if their pain is not reduced by more at least 50% during the trial [104]. Secondly, does the patient tolerate the planned modality? The treatment modality should be sufficiently free of adverse effects. In addition, there should be a discussion regarding expectations of the efficacy of treatment modality, possible complications, and the necessary follow-up appointment.

Behavioral Treatments for Migraine

Non-drug approaches to headache management are especially important for patients who have not responded sufficiently to pharmacologic therapies, who prefer a non-drug approach, are pregnant or planning a pregnancy, as well as for those for whom drug therapies are contraindicated. [116] Furthermore, these therapies may be particularly relevant for patients who evidence poor psychological coping or for whom stress is a headache trigger. Mind-body treatments have good evidence of benefit for the management of chronic pain symptoms [117, 118] and have shown roughly comparable benefit to each other with regard to managing headache symptoms [117, 119, 120]. These therapies have been found to be superior to no treatment [76] and roughly comparable to drug therapies with regard to headache management. [121] Relaxation training, thermal biofeedback combined with relaxation training; electromyographic biofeedback; and cognitive behavioral therapy (for prevention) have been designated as Grade A therapies with regard to treatment of migraines. [116] Mind-body approaches require moderate to minimal effort, are palatable to patients, cost effective, and pose little-to-no risk. [122] Hypnosis, biofeedback, and relaxation training can be effectively combined with each other, as well as with other cognitive behavioral and meditative techniques, for pain management [118].

Relaxation Training and Biofeedback

Biofeedback works through bringing biological processes to the awareness of the patient, which provides them with an opportunity for enhanced control over these processes. Specifically, computerized feedback about physiologic processes trains the subject to bring involuntary and other physiologic responses (e.g., peripheral skin temperature, muscle tension, heart rate, etc.) under voluntary, or conscious, control. [123] This happens by "rewarding" the subject via audible tone or visual indicators when he or she successfully achieves the target physiological response (whether of increased peripheral skin temperature, decreased muscle tension, or other markers indicative of enhanced relaxation or decreased arousal; [123] Relaxation training is often paired with biofeedback and further facilitates increased parasympathetic and decreased sympathetic. [121, 123, 124] Relaxation training typically involves one or more of the following: progressive muscle relaxation, meditation (including mindfulness meditation, which will be described in a subsequent section), and autogenic training. [125] The latter usually involves instruction in one or more self-induced sensations such as hand warming or warming other areas of the body, forehead cooling, arm heaviness, and deep, easy breathing. Biofeedback and relaxation exercises are taught in sessions with a trained provider with instructions to continue practice at home [123, 125] and thus emphasizes an active role for patients in managing migraine symptoms. [124]

Several meta-analyses of mind body therapies have found that treatments including biofeedback and autogenic training reduced migraine symptoms considerably over no treatment and comparably to drug therapies. [76, 116, 117, 125] Furthermore, improvement in migraine-related pain associated with biofeedback has been estimated at between 35 and 60%. [124] The benefits of biofeedback extend well past the conclusion of formal treatment. [126] Despite evidence supporting their efficacy, however, and that several approaches (diaphragmatic breathing, progressive muscle relaxation, etc.) can be taught quickly in the physician's office and then practiced at home, mind-body therapies are often underused in the medical setting. [117]

The US Headache Consortium [116] developed guidelines for the use of behavioral and physical treatments for migraines. They concluded that relaxation training, thermal biofeedback combined with relaxation training, electromyographic biofeedback, and cognitive-behavioral therapy are all "somewhat effective" in preventing migraine headaches when compared with controls. The authors concluded that no claims could be made with regard to the superiority of one behavioral treatment over another, but that the above treatments may be considered "Grade A" therapies. Grade A evidence of benefit was determined to be based on multiple well-designed randomized controlled trials (RCTs) revealing a consistent pattern of positive findings. The combination of behavioral and pharmacologic treatments has been associated with even greater effects [126] and received a designation of Grade B by the US Headache Consortium [116]. Grade B evidence of benefit was denoted based on the Consortium's determination that the findings were from randomized clinical trials supporting the recommendation, but the scientific support was not optimal. For instance, either few randomized trials existed, the trials that did exist were somewhat inconsistent, or the trials were not directly relevant to the recommendation.

A White Paper review by Nestoriuc and colleagues [124] found that the greatest treatment gains with regard to migraine management with biofeedback were associated with blood volume pulse biofeedback and EEG biofeedback, also known as neurofeedback. Blood volume pulse involves monitoring arterial blood flow and providing feedback enabling patients to decrease or constrict blood flow. [126] A blood volume pulse sensor is worn on a finger and measures heart rate, provides blood volume pulse amplitude, blood volume pulse waveform, and heart rate variability feedback. This type of biofeedback is less frequently used in clinical practice, however, perhaps because of the increased difficulty of administration and complexity of data interpretation, and thus, the authors did not make a recommendation with regard to its use in the treatment of migraines. With regard to EEG biofeedback, the authors included three studies in their review. EEG biofeedback for migraine typically aims to increase the amplitudes of slow brain wave activity (delta, theta, and alpha) and decrease higher amplitudes of faster brain wave activity (beta). Effects sizes for this modality ranged from small to medium, but the authors concluded that additional well-controlled investigations are needed before this treatment can be recommended for treatment of migraine headaches. [124]

With regard to other biofeedback approaches, an overall medium effect size was found for temperature biofeedback in combination with relaxation and electromyograpic feedback. Small-to-medium effect sizes were reported for electromyograpic feedback and temperature biofeedback alone. Differences between treatments were negligible and benefits were clinically meaningful. Furthermore, it was predicted that migraine patients treated with biofeedback would experience symptom improvements of 56-65% over that of patients in a wait-list control condition; however, biofeedback gains were not reliably higher than gains in a psychological placebo group. Thus, the authors concluded there is strong evidence for biofeedback's efficacy, but that this is comparable to the efficacy of relaxation training.

Biofeedback instruction can be conducted by appropriately trained professionals. Psychologists who are trained to administer biofeedback do not require certification to use biofeedback in clinical practice; however, other health professionals or technicians should be certified to administer this treatment. One resource for locating certified biofeedback providers is the Association for Applied Psychophysiology and Biofeedback (www.aapb.org), and another is the Biofeedback Certification Institute of America (bcia.org). The American Psychological Association (APA.org) and state psychological associations maintain referral databases that can be searched for psychologists who offer biofeedback, stress management, and who work with chronic pain issues.

Cognitive Behavioral Therapy

Cognitive Behavioral Therapy draws from both cognitive and behavioral philosophies, the underlying theory being that both thought and behavior patterns are critical in the development and maintenance of illness. [125] Treatment may incorporate any number of components from each realm and combinations may be tailored to individuals' needs. [127] Cognitive components commonly used in cognitive behavioral therapy include reality testing (examining evidence for and against automatic thoughts), cognitive restructuring (modifying thoughts and reframing situations), and challenging maldaptive core beliefs. Behavioral components include relaxation training, deep-breathing, meditation, self-monitoring, goal-setting, guided imagery, hypnosis and biofeedback. [76, 125, 128-131]

While the specific course may vary, treatment generally begins with assessment and socialization to cognitive behavioral therapy. [130, 132] Monitoring records, commonly pre-prepared forms that solicit particular information from the client, are often employed in the early stages and are used to help the client build awareness of his or her thoughts, emotions and behaviors. A headache diary may ask about the presence or absence of a headache, its severity, medication used, symptoms experienced, and any effects on role performance and sleep. Thought- and behavior-monitoring records ask about factors like situations, thoughts, and emotions that occur. [131]

Therapy may move into a more intensely cognitive phase, in which therapist and client conceptualize patterns that the client's thoughts, emotions and behaviors form and the consequences of those patterns. Once recognized, these patterns can be addressed with cognitive strategies, like questioning the validity of negative automatic thoughts, replacing these thoughts with more productive ones, and reframing situations.

These tools are used to engender in the client feelings of agency, confidence, and calm regarding migraine management and open up possibilities for more adaptive behaviors. [133]

Behavioral strategies may be incorporated simultaneously to help the client actively address situations more adaptively. [133] Tools like relaxation and deep breathing, meditation and guided imagery may be employed to help clients persevere in responding to migraine-related situations in novel ways. [131] More extensive monitoring records may be introduced, often including space to write down possible alternative responses to situations and outcome of enacting those responses. [130, 134, 135].

The US Headache Consortium has labeled the evidence supporting cognitive behavioral therapy for migraine Grade A based on findings across randomized controlled trials. [48] Indeed, meta-analyses report that cognitive behavioral therapy is consistently more effective than control conditions. [76, 125] In one trial, cognitive behavioral therapy reduced headaches by an average of 68% compared with 56% and 20% for biofeedback and control groups respectively. [129] In another study, the number of participants considered to be at least moderate responders was significantly greater in the cognitive behavioral therapy group than in a control group. [44] Cognitive behavioral therapy has been shown to reduce the salient features of migraine. In one study, for example, cognitive behavioral therapy was found to reduce migraine frequency, severity and duration as well as medication use while increasing quality of life. [127] Trials of behavioral migraine management—a program integrating relaxation, biofeedback and stress management—have reported average reductions in migraine headaches of 40-50%, a rate similar to that reported in trials of preventive drug treatment. The combination of preventative drug treatment and behavioral migraine management was even more effective, significantly improving reductions in migraine frequency and related quality of life achieved by an initial 5 week tailored acute drug-treatment. [136]

Cognitive behavioral therapy is time- and cost-effective and can be successfully delivered in the home with minimal therapist contact augmented through the telephone or internet. [128, 137, 138] Additionally, because cognitive behavioral therapy allows for a range of combinations of tools, it can be tailored to individual needs and sensitivities. [132] Nevertheless, a significant drawback is that a large percentage of participants—roughly 40%–70%—may not experience clinically significant reductions in migraine symptoms. [76] Cognitive behavioral therapy may have larger effects, however, on other factors related to quality of life, like disability, anxiety, depression, self-efficacy, isolation and activity engagement. [139] For example, while Thorn and colleagues [44] did not find differences between changes in headache frequency and intensity experienced by cognitive behavioral therapy and wait-list control groups, they reported significant decreases in pain-related catastophizing and anxiety and increases in headache management self-efficacy in the cognitive behavioral therapy group as compared with wait-list controls. [44] Similarly, Sajadinejad, and colleagues reported significant decreases in depression and disability after nine weeks of group cognitive behavioral therapy for migraine. [140]

Resources about cognitive behavioral therapy and referrals for cognitive behavioral therapists can be found through the American Psychological Association (APA.org) and Association for Behavioral and Cognitive Therapies (www.abct.org), as well as through local and regional psychology organizations.

Mindfulness and Acceptance-Based Treatments

A newer generation of "third wave" behavioral interventions have demonstrated efficacy for other chronically painful conditions and offer a promising direction for the development of behavioral treatment for migraine. This burgeoning "third wave" is often distinguished by therapies sharing a mindfulness component. [141] The most commonly used third-wave interventions include mindfulness-based stress reduction (Kabat-Zinn, 1990),[142] mindfulness-based cognitive therapy (Segal, Williams, & Teasdale, 2002)[143] and acceptance and commitment therapy (Hayes, Strosahl, & Wilson, 1999). [144-146]

Among third wave therapies, mindfulness denotes the practice of attending to and refining awareness of private thoughts, feelings and sensations in the present moment, without engaging judgment. [147] The nonjudgmental aspect of these therapies is defined as acceptance, denoting nonjudgmental awareness of and willingness to experience internal thoughts, feelings and sensations without the attempt to alter or fix them. Mindfulness-based stress reduction was developed as a holistic approach for addressing a broad range of health concerns, from chronic illness and pain to psychological disorders and general well being. A rigorous and structured eight-week program, mindfulness-based stress reduction teaches participants self-care from a perspective that combines Eastern, Buddhist principals of compassion and present-moment awareness with traditionally Western ideals of controlling affliction and its impact on life. [148] Still to be studied in migraine, mindfulness-based stress reduction has shown some efficacy in improving physical health in populations with other chronic health conditions, suggesting that the investigation of mindfulness-based stress reduction for migraine would be worthwhile. Meta-analyses looking at the effects of mindfulness-based stress reduction on physical health reveal mixed results, however, indicating a need for more high-quality research. [149-151]

Mindfulness-based cognitive therapy is essentially the combination of cognitive therapy and mindfulness-based stress reduction. [152] Upon discovering mindfulness-based stress reduction, psychologists seeking new ways to help patients avoid depressive relapse realized that mindfulness-based stress reduction utilized a valuable tool that cognitive therapy lacked—non-judgment of the observed thoughts and feelings. Mindfulness-based stress reduction had also already been shown to be effective in the treatment of chronic pain, which was associated with depression. [143] One randomized, controlled pilot study has investigated the effects of mindfulness-based cognitive therapy for headache (including migraine) and found reduced pain-related interference but no difference in headache diary outcomes compared to control conditions. [153] Mindfulness-based cognitive therapy for migraine, therefore, warrants further study.

Acceptance and commitment therapy is a bottom-up, inductive, and process-based approach to behavior therapy [154] Integrating clients' core values with mindfulness and acceptance, acceptance and commitment therapy supports committed action towards valued goals. There are six core processes—acceptance, cognitive defusion (de-coupling thought and fact/identity), being present, self as context (viewing experiences as transient within a stable self that houses them), values, and committed action—and increasing psychological flexibility is their central aim. [155] Acceptance and commitment therapy has demonstrated efficacy to address a range of problems, including psychiatric disorders and management of chronic illness. [141] To date, only two studies have addressed acceptance in migraine: acceptance of pain was related to decreased pain-related disruption in daily life [156] and a brief acceptance and commitment therapy intervention reduced disability and distress compared to a control group. [157] Further research on the role of acceptance in migraine is warranted.

This, although little research has investigated the efficacy of mindfulness and acceptance-based therapies in migraine, these therapies have shown promise in the treatment of chronic pain with effect sizes comparable to cognitive behavioral therapy. [158] Research has indicated that mindfulness-based interventions generally may impart nonspecific (placebo-like) effects that reduce pain and decrease depression in chronic pain patients. [159] A more recent review found specific effects of mindfulness-based interventions for pain, leading to reduced pain intensity. [160] Further investigation of these relationships is needed and should continue to be examined in the context of migraine and related disability.

Hypnosis

Hypnosis represents a change in awareness characterized by increased absorption in or focus on one's inner world, disattention to extraneous stimuli, and a reduction in spontaneous cognition. [161] There is a good deal of overlap between hypnosis, guided imagery, and autogenic training; however, hypnosis goes beyond imagery and relaxation training in that it deliberately fosters dissociation and focuses attention via specific suggestions. [118, 162] Hypnosis decreases EEG-measured beta activity (associated with information processing) and increases EEG-measured alpha activity (associated with enhanced relaxation), which may explain hypnosis' global calming effect on the brain. [122] It has been theorized that both positive rapport between the hypnotherapist and patient as well as receptivity to hypnotic induction and suggestion are facilitated by activation of mirror neurons. [163]

Hypnosis sessions with a trained provider often begin with a formal induction, which is a set of suggestions aimed at deepening one's state of relaxation and inner focus and fostering disattention to external stimuli prior to the presentation of suggestions related to the patient's specific goal. Prior to the end of the session, post-hypnotic suggestions can be given to help the patient remember consciously whatever is helpful and reinforce positive change beyond the duration of the formal hypnosis. [122] "Ego-strengthening" suggestions, which emphasize enhanced patient self-efficacy, as well as future oriented suggestions that instill the expectation of benefit, can instill confidence and decrease anxiety about whether the treatment will be successful. [122] Self-hypnosis recordings may be helpful adjuncts to standard treatment for those who are resistant to or otherwise unable to seek individual hypnotherapy. At-home practice can reinforce suggestions initiated during sessions [162, 164], enhance feelings of self-efficacy, and improve outcomes [118].

Hypnosis satisfies American Psychological Association criteria as an efficacious and specific treatment for chronic pain and has demonstrated efficacy for reducing pain severity, improving pain coping, as well as reducing the psychological distress and insomnia associated with headaches. [162, 164, 165] Self-hypnosis been shown to be beneficial during invasive medical procedures, having more pronounced effects on pain and anxiety reduction, and resulting in improved hemodynamic stability, over standard care or structured attention. [166] Hypnosis has specific effects beyond expectation of benefit or motivation for treatment [122].

Although hypnosis is considered both safe and effective, the American Society of Clinical Hypnosis (ASCH) recommends choosing a health care provider who is properly trained, licensed (e.g., holds a valid license in a health care field, has an academic degree from a regionally accredited institution of higher education, and has had supervised experience in offering their professional services to clients and patients), and certified in clinical hypnotherapy. "Hypnotists" denote lay practitioners who may have little to no formal training, and should not be consulted for hypnotherapy. For more information, or to access referral information to certified providers, visit ASCH.net. Psychologists who offer hypnotherapy and work with chronic pain patients can be located via the referral directories of the American Psychological Association (APA.org) and state psychological associations.

Conclusion

Migraine is a common neurologic condition characterized by episodes of head pain. Migraine can be disabling and burdensome. Migraine can affect all aspects of life (e.g., occupational, academic, social, familiar, and personal) and is most prevalent during one's most productive years of life. Treating migraine requires a comprehensive treatment plan, including potentially acute and preventive pharmacologic treatments, and empirically supported behavioral therapies. [48, 123] Psychological assessment is key to successful treatment of migraine, and can include assessment of migraine-related disability, stress and other psychological risk factors, current coping efforts, and psychiatric comorbidity. Psychological and behavioral variables, including psychiatric comorbidity, have been associated with migraine-related disability, as well as progression from episodic to chronic migraine. Adherence to medical recommendations is essential for the success of any medical intervention, including pharmacological and surgical interventions. Psychological assessment can identify the psychological and behavioral factors associated with adherence, and behavioral interventions often involve enhancing adherence to medical interventions for migraine. Behavioral interventions, particularly biofeedback, relaxation and cognitive-behavioral therapy, have demonstrated efficacy to treat migraine and can be useful adjunctive treatments. This chapter has provided resources to assist medical providers in locating behavioral providers in your area who offer these services, including the American Psychological Association (APA.org), Association for Behavioral and Cognitive Therapies (www.abct.org), Association for Applied Psychophysiology and Biofeedback (www.aapb.org), Biofeedback Certification Institute of America (bcia.org).

References

[1] The International Classification of Headache Disorders, 3rd edition (beta version). *Cephalalgia*, 2013 Jul, 33(9), 629-808. PubMed PMID: 23771276. Epub 2013/06/19. eng.

[2] Lipton, RB; Bigal, ME; Diamond, M; Freitag, F; Reed, ML; Stewart, WF. Migraine prevalence, disease burden, and the need for preventive therapy. *Neurology*, 2007 Jan 30, 68(5), 343-9. PubMed PMID: 17261680. Epub 2007/01/31. eng.

[3] Buse, DC; Loder, EW; Gorman, JA; Stewart, WF; Reed, ML; Fanning, KM; et al. Sex differences in the prevalence, symptoms, and associated features of migraine, probable migraine and other severe headache: results of the American Migraine Prevalence and Prevention (AMPP) Study. *Headache*, 2013 Sep, 53(8), 1278-99. PubMed PMID: 23808666. Epub 2013/07/03. eng.

[4] Buse, DC; Manack, AN; Fanning, KM; Serrano, D; Reed, ML; Turkel, CC; et al. Chronic migraine prevalence, disability, and sociodemographic factors: results from the American Migraine Prevalence and Prevention Study. *Headache*, 2012 Nov-Dec, 52(10), 1456-70. PubMed PMID: 22830411. Epub 2012/07/27. eng.

[5] Bigal, ME; Serrano, D; Buse, D; Scher, A; Stewart WF; Lipton, RB. Acute migraine medications and evolution from episodic to chronic migraine: a longitudinal population-based study. *Headache*, 2008, Sep 48(8), 1157-68. PubMed PMID: 18808500. Epub 2008/09/24. eng.

[6] Lipton, RB; Stewart, WF; Diamond, S; Diamond, ML; Reed, M. Prevalence and burden of migraine in the United States: data from the American Migraine Study II. *Headache*, 2001 Jul-Aug, 41(7), 646-57. PubMed PMID: 11554952. Epub 2001/09/14. eng.

[7] Buse, D; Manack, A; Serrano, D; Reed, M; Varon, S; Turkel, C; et al. Headache impact of chronic and episodic migraine: results from the American Migraine Prevalence and Prevention study. Headache. 2012 Jan, 52(1), 3-17. PubMed PMID: 22106869. Epub 2011/11/24. eng.

[8] Martelletti, P; Birbeck, GL; Katsarava, Z; Jensen, RH; Stovner, LJ; Steiner, TJ. The Global Burden of Disease survey 2010, Lifting The Burden and thinking outside-the-box on headache disorders. *J Headache Pain.* 2013 Dec, 14(1), 13. PubMed PMID: 23565711. Pubmed Central PMCID: Pmc3620501. Epub 2013/04/10. eng.

[9] Leonardi, M; Steiner, TJ; Scher, AT; Lipton, RB. The global burden of migraine: measuring disability in headache disorders with WHO's Classification of Functioning, Disability and Health (ICF). *J Headache Pain.*, 2005 Dec, 6(6), 429-40. PubMed PMID: 16388337. Pubmed Central PMCID: Pmc3452308. Epub 2006/01/03. eng.

[10] Smitherman, TA; Burch, R; Sheikh, H; Loder, E. The prevalence, impact, and treatment of migraine and severe headaches in the United States: a review of statistics from national surveillance studies. *Headache*, 2013 Mar, 53(3), 427-36. PubMed PMID: 23470015. Epub 2013/03/09. eng.

[11] Buse, DC; Bigal, MB; Rupnow, M; Reed, M; Serrano, D; Lipton, RB. Development and validation of the Migraine Interictal Burden Scale (MIBS): a self-administered instrument for measuring the burden of migraine between attacks. *Neurology*, 2007, 67(1), A89.

[12] Brandes, JL. The migraine cycle: patient burden of migraine during and between migraine attacks. *Headache*, 2008 Mar, 48(3), 430-41. PubMed PMID: 18179565. Epub 2008/01/09. eng.

[13] Dowson, A; Jagger, S. The UK migraine patient survey: quality of life and treatment. *Current medical research and opinion.*, 1999, 15(4), 241-53. PubMed PMID: 10640257. Epub 2000/01/20. eng.

[14] Lipton, RB; Bigal, ME; Kolodner, K; Stewart, WF; Liberman, JN; Steiner, TJ. The family impact of migraine: population-based studies in the USA and UK. *Cephalalgia.*, 2003 Jul, 23(6), 429-40. PubMed PMID: 12807522. Epub 2003/06/17. eng.

[15] Young, WB; Park, JE; Tian, IX; Kempner, J. The stigma of migraine. *PloS one.*, 2013, *8*(1), e54074. PubMed PMID: 23342079. Pubmed Central PMCID: Pmc3546922. Epub 2013/01/24. eng.

[16] Seng, EK; Holroyd KA. Optimal use of acute headache medication: a qualitative examination of behaviors and barriers to their performance. *Headache.*, 2013 Oct, 53(9), 1438-50. PubMed PMID: 23808788. Epub 2013/07/03. eng.

[17] Hazard, E; Munakata, J; Bigal, ME; Rupnow, MF; Lipton, RB. The burden of migraine in the United States: current and emerging perspectives on disease management and economic analysis. Value in health: *the journal of the International Society for Pharmacoeconomics and Outcomes Research.* 2009 Jan-Feb, 12(1), 55-64. PubMed PMID: 18671771. Epub 2008/08/02. eng.

[18] Pesa, J; Lage, MJ. The medical costs of migraine and comorbid anxiety and depression. *Headache*, 2004 Jun, 44(6), 562-70. PubMed PMID: 15186300. Epub 2004/06/10. eng.

[19] Natoli, JL; Manack, A; Dean, B; Butler, Q; Turkel, CC; Stovner, L. et al. Global prevalence of chronic migraine: a systematic review. *Cephalalgia*, 2010 May, 30(5), 599-609. PubMed PMID: 19614702. Epub 2009/07/21. eng.

[20] Buse, DC; Manack, A; Serrano, D; Turkel, C; Lipton, RB. Sociodemographic and comorbidity profiles of chronic migraine and episodic migraine sufferers. *Journal of neurology, neurosurgery, and psychiatry.*, 2010 Apr, 81(4), 428-32. PubMed PMID: 20164501. Epub 2010/02/19. eng.

[21] Ruscheweyh, R; Muller, M; Blum, B; Straube, A. Correlation of Headache Frequency and Psychosocial Impairment in Migraine: A Cross-Sectional Study. *Headache*, 2013 Aug 23. PubMed PMID: 23980919. Epub 2013/08/29. Eng.

[22] Serrano, D; Manack, AN; Reed, ML; Buse, DC; Varon, SF; Lipton, RB. Cost and predictors of lost productive time in chronic migraine and episodic migraine: results from the American Migraine Prevalence and Prevention (AMPP) Study. Value in health: *the journal of the International Society for Pharmacoeconomics and Outcomes Research.* 2013 Jan-Feb, 16(1), 31-8. PubMed PMID: 23337213. Epub 2013/01/23. eng.

[23] Turk, DC; Okifuji, A. Psychological factors in chronic pain: evolution and revolution. *Journal of consulting and clinical psychology*, 2002 Jun, 70(3), 678-90. PubMed PMID: 12090376. Epub 2002/07/02. eng.

[24] Buse, DC; Sollars, CM; Steiner, TJ; Jensen, RH; Al Jumah, MA; Lipton, RB. Why HURT? A review of clinical instruments for headache management. *Current pain and headache reports.* 2012 Jun, 16(3), 237-54. PubMed PMID: 22487847. Epub 2012/04/11. eng.

[25] Lipton, RB; Stewart, WF; Sawyer, J; Edmeads, JG. Clinical utility of an instrument assessing migraine disability: the Migraine Disability Assessment (MIDAS) questionnaire. *Headache.*, 2001 Oct, 41(9), 854-61. PubMed PMID: 11703471. Epub 2001/11/13. eng.

[26] Stewart, WF; Lipton, RB; Kolodner, KB; Sawyer, J; Lee, C; Liberman, JN. Validity of the Migraine Disability Assessment (MIDAS) score in comparison to a diary-based

measure in a population sample of migraine sufferers. *Pain.*, 2000 Oct, 88(1), 41-52. PubMed PMID: 11098098. Epub 2000/12/01. eng.

[27] Stewart, WF; Lipton, RB; Kolodner, K; Liberman, J; Sawyer, J. Reliability of the migraine disability assessment score in a population-based sample of headache sufferers. *Cephalalgia.*, 1999, 19, 107-14.

[28] Bjorner, JB; Kosinski, M; Ware, JE. Jr. Calibration of an item pool for assessing the burden of headaches: an application of item response theory to the headache impact test (HIT). Quality of life research: *an international journal of quality of life aspects of treatment, care and rehabilitation.*, 2003 Dec, 12(8), 913-33. PubMed PMID: 14651412. Epub 2003/12/04. eng.

[29] Bjorner, JB; Kosinski, M; Ware, JE. Jr. Using item response theory to calibrate the Headache Impact Test (HIT) to the metric of traditional headache scales. Quality of life research: *An international journal of quality of life aspects of treatment, care and rehabilitation.*, 2003 Dec, 12(8), 981-1002. PubMed PMID: 14651417. Epub 2003/12/04. eng.

[30] Stewart, WF; Lipton, RB; Simon, D; Von Korff, M; Liberman, J. Reliability of an illness severity measure for headache in a population sample of migraine sufferers. *Cephalalgia.*, 1998, 18, 44-51.

[31] Rendas-Baum, R; Bloudek, LM; Maglinte, GA; Varon, SF. The psychometric properties of the Migraine-Specific Quality of Life Questionnaire version 2.1 (MSQ) in chronic migraine patients. Quality of life research: *An international journal of quality of life aspects of treatment, care and rehabilitation.*, 2013 Jun, 22(5), 1123-33. PubMed PMID: 22797868. Pubmed Central PMCID: Pmc3664759. Epub 2012/07/17. eng.

[32] Martin, BC; Pathak, DS; Sharfman, MI; Adelman, JU; Taylor, F; Kwong, WJ; et al. Validity and reliability of the migraine-specific quality of life questionnaire (MSQ Version 2.1). *Headache*, 2000 Mar, 40(3), 204-15. PubMed PMID: 10759923. Epub 2000/04/12. eng.

[33] Martin, B; Pathak, D; Sharfman, M; Adelman, J; Taylor, F; Kwong, W; et al. Validity and reliability of the Migraine-Specific Quality of Life Questionnaire (MSQL Version 2.1). *Headache*, 2000, 40, 204-15.

[34] Ware, JE. Jr., Sherbourne CD. The MOS 36-item short-form health survey (SF-36). I. Conceptual framework and item selection. *Medical care.* 1992 Jun, 30(6), 473-83. PubMed PMID: 1593914. Epub 1992/06/11. eng.

[35] McHorney, CA; Ware, JE. Jr., Raczek AE. The MOS 36-Item Short-Form Health Survey (SF-36): II. Psychometric and clinical tests of validity in measuring physical and mental health constructs. *Medical Care.*, 1993 Mar, 31(3), 247-63. PubMed PMID: 8450681. Epub 1993/03/01. eng.

[36] Ware, JE. Jr; Kosinski, M; Keller, SD. A 12-Item Short-Form Health Survey: construction of scales and preliminary tests of reliability and validity. *Medical care.*, 1996 Mar, 34(3), 220-33. PubMed PMID: 8628042. Epub 1996/03/01. eng.

[37] Ware, JE; Sherbourne, CD. The MOS 36-item Short-Form Health Survey ((SF-36). I. Conceptual frameworks and item selection. *Medical Care.*, 1992, 30, 473-83.

[38] Buse, DC; Rupnow, MF; Lipton, RB. Assessing and managing all aspects of migraine: migraine attacks, migraine-related functional impairment, common comorbidities, and quality of life. *Mayo Clinic proceedings.*, 2009 May, 84(5), 422-35. PubMed PMID: 19411439. Pubmed Central PMCID: Pmc2676125. Epub 2009/05/05. eng.

[39] Tietjen, GE; Brandes, JL; Peterlin, BL; Eloff, A; Dafer, RM; Stein, MR; et al. Childhood maltreatment and migraine (part II). Emotional abuse as a risk factor for headache chronification. *Headache.*, 2010 Jan, 50(1), 32-41. PubMed PMID: 19845781. Epub 2009/10/23. eng.

[40] Waldie, KE. Childhood headache, stress in adolescence, and primary headache in young adulthood: A longitudinal cohort study. Headache: *The Journal of Head and Face Pain.* 2001, 41(1), 1-10.

[41] Winter, AC; Berger, K; Buring, JE; Kurth, T. Associations of socioeconomic status with migraine and non-migraine headache. *Cephalalgia.* 2012 Jan, 32(2), 159-70. PubMed PMID: 22174348. Pubmed Central PMCID: Pmc3266434. Epub 2011/12/17. eng.

[42] Stewart, WF; Roy, J; Lipton, RB. Migraine prevalence, socioeconomic status, and social causation. *Neurology.*, 2013 Sep 10, 81(11), 948-55. PubMed PMID: 23990405. Epub 2013/08/31. eng.

[43] Thorn, BE; Cognitive therapy for chronic pain: a step-by-step guide. New York: The Guilford Press; 2004.

[44] Thorn, BE; Pence, LB; Ward, LC; Kilgo, G; Clements, KL; Cross, TH; et al. A randomized clinical trial of targeted cognitive behavioral treatment to reduce catastrophizing in chronic headache sufferers. The journal of pain: *official journal of the American Pain Society.*, 2007 Dec, 8(12), 938-49. PubMed PMID: 17690017. Epub 2007/08/11.

[45] Holroyd, KA; Drew, JB; Cottrell, CK; Romanek, KM; Heh, V. Impaired functioning and quality of life in severe migraine: The role of catastrophizing and associated symptoms. *Cephalalgia.*, 2007, 27(10), 1156-65.

[46] Rosenstiel, AK; Keefe, FJ. The use of coping strategies in chronic low back pain patients: relationship to patient characteristics and current adjustment. *Pain.*, 1983 Sep, 17(1), 33-44. PubMed PMID: 6226916. Epub 1983/09/01. eng.

[47] Riley, JL. 3rd, Robinson ME. CSQ: five factors or fiction? *The Clinical journal of pain.* 1997 Jun, 13(2), 156-62. PubMed PMID: 9186023. Epub 1997/06/01. eng.

[48] Silberstein, SD. Practice parameter: evidence-based guidelines for migraine headache (an evidence-based review): report of the Quality Standards Subcommittee of the American Academy of Neurology. *Neurology.*, 2000 Sep 26, 55(6), 754-62. PubMed PMID: 10993991. Epub 2000/09/20.

[49] Buse, DC; Silberstein, SD; Manack, AN; Papapetropoulos, S; Lipton, RB. Psychiatric comorbidities of episodic and chronic migraine. *Journal of neurology.* 2013 Aug, 260(8), 1960-9. PubMed PMID: 23132299. Epub 2012/11/08. eng.

[50] Peterlin; BL; Tietjen, G; Meng, S; Lidicker, J; Bigal, M. Post-traumatic stress disorder in episodic and chronic migraine. Headache: *The Journal of Head and Face Pain.*, 2008, 48(4), 517-22.

[51] Breslau, N; Davis, GC. Migraine, physical health and psychiatric disorder: a prospective epidemiologic study in young adults. *Journal of psychiatric research.*, 1993 Apr-Jun, 27(2), 211-21. PubMed PMID: 8366470. Epub 1993/04/01. eng.

[52] Zwart, J-A; Dyb, G; Hagen, K; Ødegård, KJ; Dahl, AA; Bovim, G; et al. Depression and anxiety disorders associated with headache frequency. The Nord-Trøndelag Health Study. *European Journal of Neurology.*, 2003, 10(2), 147-52.

[53] Juang, KD; Wang, SJ; Fuh, JL; Lu, SR; Su, TP. Comorbidity of depressive and anxiety disorders in chronic daily headache and its subtypes. *Headache.*, 2000 Nov-Dec, 40(10), 818-23. PubMed PMID: 11135026. Epub 2001/01/03. eng.

[54] Smitherman, TA; Kolivas, WD; Bailey, JR. Panic disorder and migraine: Comorbidity, mechanisms, and clinical implications. Headache: *The Journal of Head and Face Pain.*, 2013, 53(1), 23-45.

[55] Merikangas, KR; Angst, J; Isler, H. Migraine and psychopathology. Results of the Zurich cohort study of young adults. *Archives of general psychiatry.* 1990 Sep, 47(9), 849-53. PubMed PMID: 2393343. Epub 1990/09/01. eng.

[56] Merikangas, KR; Merikangas, JR; Angst, J. Headache syndromes and psychiatric disorders: association and familial transmission. *Journal of psychiatric research.*, 1993 Apr-Jun, 27(2), 197-210. PubMed PMID: 8366469. Epub 1993/04/01. eng.

[57] Chen, YC; Tang, CH; Ng, K; Wang, SJ. Comorbidity profiles of chronic migraine sufferers in a national database in Taiwan. *J Headache Pain.*, 2012 Jun, 13(4), 311-9. PubMed PMID: 22527034. Pubmed Central PMCID: Pmc3356468. Epub 2012/04/25. eng.

[58] Blumenfeld, AM; Varon, SF; Wilcox, TK; Buse, DC; Kawata, AK; Manack, A; et al. Disability, HRQoL and resource use among chronic and episodic migraineurs: results from the International Burden of Migraine Study (IBMS). *Cephalalgia.*, 2011 Feb, 31(3), 301-15. PubMed PMID: 20813784. Epub 2010/09/04. eng.

[59] Anda, R; Tietjen, G; Schulman, E; Felitti, V, Croft J. Adverse childhood experiences and frequent headaches in adults. *Headache.*, 2010 Oct, 50(9), 1473-81. PubMed PMID: 20958295. Epub 2010/10/21. eng.

[60] Tietjen, GE; Khubchandani, J; Herial, NA; Shah, K. Adverse childhood experiences are associated with migraine and vascular biomarkers. *Headache.* 2012 Jun, 52(6), 920-9. PubMed PMID: 22533684. Epub 2012/04/27. eng.

[61] Golding, JM. Sexual assault history and headache: five general population studies. *The Journal of nervous and mental disease.*, 1999 Oct, 187(10), 624-9. PubMed PMID: 10535656. Epub 1999/10/27. eng.

[62] Tietjen, GE; Brandes, JL; Digre, KB; Baggaley, S; Martin, VT; Recober, A; et al. History of childhood maltreatment is associated with comorbid depression in women with migraine. *Neurology.*, 2007 Sep 4, 69(10), 959-68. PubMed PMID: 17785664. Epub 2007/09/06. eng.

[63] Fuller-Thomson, E. Baker, TM; Brennenstuhl, S. Investigating the association between childhood physical abuse and migraine. *Headache.*, 2010 May, 50(5), 749-60. PubMed PMID: 20236339. Epub 2010/03/20. eng.

[64] Tietjen, GE; Buse, DC; Fanning, KM; Serrano, D; Reed, ML; Lipton, RB. The relationship of childhood maltreatment with migraine and tension-type headache: Results of the American Migraine Prevalence & Prevention (AMPP) Study. *Headache.*, 2012, 52, 910.

[65] Manack, AN; Serrano, D; Turkel, CC; Lipton, RB; Buse, DC. Major life events, stress appraisal, and migraine: results of the American Migraine Prevalence and Prevention (AMPP) study. *Journal of Headache Pain.*, 2013, 14(1), 9. Epub 13 February 21.

[66] Scher, AI; Stewart, WF. Buse, D; Krantz, DS; Lipton RB. Major life changes before and after the onset of chronic daily headache: a population-based study. *Cephalalgia.*, 2008 Aug, 28(8), 868-76. PubMed PMID: 18557980. Epub 2008/06/19. eng.

[67] Ashina, S; Serrano, D; Lipton, RB; Maizels, M; Manack, AN; Turkel, CC; et al. Depression and risk of transformation of episodic to chronic migraine. *J Headache Pain.*, 2012 Nov, 13(8), 615-24. PubMed PMID: 23007859. Pubmed Central PMCID: Pmc3484253. Epub 2012/09/26. eng.

[68] Wang, SJ; Fuh, JL; Lu, SR; Juang, KD. Outcomes and predictors of chronic daily headache in adolescents: a 2-year longitudinal study. *Neurology.*, 2007 Feb 20, 68(8), 591-6. PubMed PMID: 17182975. Epub 2006/12/22. eng.

[69] Ashina, S; Buse, DC; MM; Manack, A; Serrano, D; Turkel, C; et al. Self-reported anxiety as a risk factor for migraine chronification: Results from The American Migraine Prevalence and Prevention (AMPP) study. *Headache.*, 2010, *50*(1), S4.

[70] Smitherman, TA; Penzien, DB; Maizels, M. Anxiety disorders and migraine intractability and progression. *Current pain and headache reports.*, 2008 Jun, 12(3), 224-9. PubMed PMID: 18796274. Epub 2008/09/18. eng.

[71] Boudreau, GP; Grosberg, BM; PJM; Sheftell, FD; Lipton, RB; Buse, DC. Open-label, multicenter study of the efficacy and outcome of onabotulinumtoxin-A treatment in patients with chronic migraine and comorbid depressive disorders. Presented at the 2nd European *Headache and Migraine Trust (EHMTIC) International Congress.*, 2010 Nice(France) October, 28-31.

[72] Beck, AT. Cognitive therapy of depression. New York: *Guilford Press*, 1979, 425 p. p.

[73] Holroyd, KA; Andrasik, FA. cognitive-behavioral approach to recurrent tension and migraine headache. In: Kendall PC, editor. *Advances in cognitive-behavioral research and therapy.* 1. New York: Academic; 1982, p. 275-320.

[74] McCarran, MS; Andrasik, F. Migraine and tension headaches. In: Michelson L, Ascher M, editors. Anxiety and stress disorders: Cognitive-behavioral assessment and treatment NY: Guilford; 1987, p. 465-83.

[75] Nestoriuc, Y; Martin, A. Efficacy of biofeedback for migraine: a meta-analysis. *Pain.*, 2007 Mar, 128(1-2), 111-27. PubMed PMID: 17084028. Epub 2006/11/07. eng.

[76] Andrasik, F. What does the evidence show? Efficacy of behavioural treatments for recurrent headaches in adults. Neurological sciences: *official journal of the Italian Neurological Society and of the Italian Society of Clinical Neurophysiology.*, 2007 May, 28 Suppl 2, S70-7. PubMed PMID: 17508184. Epub 2007/05/18. eng.

[77] Seng, EK; Holroyd, KA. Psychiatric comorbidity and response to preventative therapy in the treatment of severe migraine trial. *Cephalalgia.*, 2012, 32(5), 390-400.

[78] Burns, JW; Kubilus, A; Bruehl, S; Harden, RN; Lofland K. Do changes in cognitive factors influence outcome following multidisciplinary treatment for chronic pain? A cross-lagged panel analysis. *Journal of consulting and clinical psychology.* 2003, 71(1), 81-91.

[79] Dunbar-Jacob, J; Erlen, JA; Schlenk, EA; Ryan, CM; Sereika, SM; Doswell, WM. Adherence in chronic disease. *Annu Rev Nurs Res.*, 2000, 18, 48-90. PubMed PMID: 10918932. eng.

[80] Rains, JC; Lipchik, GL; Penzien, DB. Behavioral facilitation of medical treatment for headache--part I: Review of headache treatment compliance. *Headache.*, 2006 Oct, 46(9), 1387-94. PubMed PMID: 17040335. Epub 2006/10/17. eng.

[81] The fear-avoidance model of chronic pain. Validation and age analysis using structural equation modeling, (2006).

[82] Malik, SN; Hopkins, M; Young, WB; Silberstein, SD. Acute migraine treatment: patterns of use and satisfaction in a clinical population. *Headache.*, 2006 May, 46(5), 773-80. PubMed PMID: 16643580. eng.
[83] Flor, H; Fydrich, T; Turk, DC. Efficacy of multidisciplinary pain treatment centers: A meta-analytic review. *Pain.*, 1992, 49(2), 221-30.
[84] Turk, DC; Rudy, TE. Cognitive factors and persistent pain: A glimpse into Pandora's box. *Cognitive Therapy and Research.* 1992, 16(2), 99-122.
[85] Martin, NJ; Holroyd, KA; Penzien, DB. The Headache-Specific Locus of Control Scale: Adaptation to recurrent headaches. 1990, 30(11), 729-34.
[86] McCracken, LM; Zayfert, C; Gross RT. The Pain Anxiety Symptoms Scale: Development and validation of a scale to measure fear of pain. *Pain.*, 1992, 50(1), 67-73.
[87] Roelofs, J; McCracken, L; Peters, ML; Crombez, G; van Breukelen, G; Vlaeyen, JWS. Psychometric Evaluation of the Pain Anxiety Symptoms Scale (PASS) in Chronic Pain Patients. *J Behav Med.*, 2004, 27(2), 167-83.
[88] McCracken, LM; Dhingra, LA. short version of the Pain Anxiety Symptoms Scale (PASS--20): *Preliminary development and validity. Pain Research & Management.*, 2002, 7(1), 45-50.
[89] Silberstein, S. Practice Parameter: evidence-based guidelines for migraine headache (an evidence-based review). *Neurology.*, 2000, 55(6), 754-62.
[90] Chu, MK; Buse, DC; Bigal, ME; Serrano, D; Lipton, RB. Factors associated with triptan use in episodic migraine: results from the American Migraine Prevalence and Prevention Study. *Headache.*, 2012 Feb, 52(2), 213-23. PubMed PMID: 22413150. Epub 2012/03/14. eng.
[91] Jonsson, P; Jakobsson, A; Hensing, G; Linde, M; Moore, CD; Hedenrud, T. Holding on to the indispensable medication--a grounded theory on medication use from the perspective of persons with medication overuse headache. *J Headache Pain.*, 2013 Dec, 14(1), 43. PubMed PMID: 23697986. Pubmed Central PMCID: Pmc3671143. Epub 2013/05/24. eng.
[92] Wells, RE; Markowitz, SY; Baron, EP; Hentz, JG; Kalidas, K; Mathew, PG; et al. Identifying the Factors Underlying Discontinuation of Triptans. *Headache.*, 2013 Sep 3. PubMed PMID: 24001117. Epub 2013/09/05. Eng.
[93] Holland, PR; Maskrey, MV; Swift, DL; Notley, DC; Robinson, MA; Nagar J; et al. Treatment retention, drug use and social functioning outcomes in those receiving three months versus one month of supervised opioid maintenance treatment. Results from the Super C randomised controlled trial. Addiction (Abingdon, England). 2013 Dec 4. PubMed PMID: 24304349. Epub 2013/12/07. Eng.
[94] Rains, JC; Penzien, DB; Lipchik, GL. Behavioral facilitation of medical treatment of headache: implications of noncompliance and strategies for improving adherence. *Headache.*, 2006 Oct, 46 Suppl 3, S142-3. PubMed PMID: 17034392. Epub 2006/10/13. eng.
[95] Rains, JC; Penzien, DB; Lipchik, GL. Behavioral facilitation of medical treatment for headache--part II: Theoretical models and behavioral strategies for improving adherence. *Headache*, 2006 Oct, 46(9), 1395-403. PubMed PMID: 17040336. Epub 2006/10/17. eng.
[96] Kiecolt-Glaser, JK; Page, GG, Marucha, PT; MacCallum, RC; Glaser, R. Psychological influences on surgical recovery. Perspectives from psychoneuroimmunology. *The*

American psychologist., 1998 Nov, 53(11), 1209-18. PubMed PMID: 9830373. Epub 1998/11/27. eng.

[97] Thorvaldsen, P; Sorenson, E. Psychological vulnerability as a predictor for short-term outcome in lumbar spine surgery. *Acta Neurochirurgica*, 1990, 102(32), 58-60.

[98] Brand, EJN. Patient outcomes following ACL reconstruction: The influence of psychological factors. *Orthopedics.*, 2009, 32(335).

[99] Tully, P; Baker, R; Knight, J. Anxiety and depression as risk factors for mortality after coronary artery bypass surgery. *Journal of Psychosomatic Research.*, 2008, 64, 285-90.

[100] Schoenen, J. The pathophysiology of migraine: *a review based on the literature and on personal contributions. Funct Neurol.*, 1998 Jan-Mar, 13(1), 7-15. PubMed PMID: 9584870. Epub 1998/05/19. eng.

[101] Jenkins, B; Tepper, S. Neurostimulation for primary headache disorders, part 2: Review of central neurostimulators for primary headache, overall therapeutic efficacy, safety, cost, patient selection, and future research in headache neuromodulation. *Headache.*, 2011, 51(9), 1408-18.

[102] Antal, A; Kriener, N; Lang, N; Boros, K; Paulus, W. Cathodal transcranial direct current stimulation of the visual cortex in the prophylactic treatment of migraine. *Cephalalgia*, 2011, 31, 820-8.

[103] Lipton, R; Dodick, D; Silberstein, S; Saper, J; Aurora, S; Pearlman, S; et al. Single-pulse transcranial magnetic stimulation for acute treatment of migraine with aura: a randomised, double-blind, parallel-group, sham- controlled trial. *Lancet Neurology.*, 2010, 9, 373-80.

[104] Caudill, M; Holman, G; Turk, D. Effective ways to manage chronic pain. *Patient Care.*, 1996, 31, 154-66.

[105] Schulman, EA; Peterlin, BL; Lake, AE; 3rd, Lipton, RB; Hanlon, A; Siegel, S; et al. Defining refractory migraine: results of the RHSIS Survey of American Headache Society members. *Headache.*, 2009 Apr, *49*(4), 509-18. PubMed PMID: 19245385. Epub 2009/02/28. eng.

[106] Prager, J; Jacobs, M. Evaluation of patients for implantable pain modalities: medical and behavioral assessment. *The Clinical journal of pain.*, 2001 Sep, 17(3), 206-14. PubMed PMID: 11587110. Epub 2001/10/06. eng.

[107] Burchiel, KJ; Anderson, VC; Wilson, BJ; Denison, DB; Olson, KA; Shatin, D. Prognostic factors of spinal cord stimulation for chronic back and leg pain. *Neurosurgery.*, 1995 Jun, 36(6), 1101-10; discussion 10-1. PubMed PMID: 7643988. Epub 1995/06/01. eng.

[108] Schocket, KG; Gatchel, RJ; Stowell, AW; Deschner, M; Robinson, R; Lou, L; et al. A DEMONSTRATION OF A PRESURGICAL BEHAVIORAL MEDICINE EVALUATION FOR CATEGORIZING PATIENTS FOR IMPLANTABLE THERAPIES: A PRELIMINARY STUDY. Neuromodulation: *journal of the International Neuromodulation Society.*, 2008 Oct 8, 11(4), 237-48. PubMed PMID: 20657728. Pubmed Central PMCID: Pmc2909129. Epub 2008/10/08. Eng.

[109] North, RB; Kidd, DH; Wimberly, RL; Edwin, D. Prognostic value of psychological testing in patients undergoing spinal cord stimulation: a prospective study. *Neurosurgery.*, 1996 Aug, 39(2), 301-10; discussion 10-1. PubMed PMID: 8832667. Epub 1996/08/01. eng.

[110] Doleys, DM; Marino, L; Howell, M; Nicholson, B. Pain management programs in hand therapy: a literature review and appraisal. Journal of hand therapy: *official journal of the American Society of Hand Therapists.*, 1997 Apr-Jun, 10(2), 175-82. PubMed PMID: 9188036. Epub 1997/04/01. eng.

[111] Dumoulin, K; Devulder, J; Castille, F; De Laat, M; Van Bastelaere, M; Rolly, GA. psychoanalytic investigation to improve the success rate of spinal cord stimulation as a treatment for chronic failed back surgery syndrome. *The Clinical journal of pain.*, 1996 Mar, 12(1), 43-9. PubMed PMID: 8722734. Epub 1996/03/01. eng.

[112] Daniel, MS; Long, C; Hutcherson, WL; Hunter, S. Psychological factors and outcome of electrode implantation for chronic pain. *Neurosurgery.*, 1985 Nov, 17(5), 773-7. PubMed PMID: 4069329. Epub 1985/11/01. eng.

[113] Nelson, DV; Novy, DM. Psychological characteristics of reflex sympathetic dystrophy versus myofascial pain syndromes. *Regional anesthesia.*, 1996 May-Jun, 21(3), 202-8. PubMed PMID: 8744661. Epub 1996/05/01. eng.

[114] Doleys, DM. Psychologic evaluation for patients undergoing neuroaugmentative procedures. *Neurosurgery clinics of North America.*, 2003 Jul, 14(3), 409-17. PubMed PMID: 14567142. Epub 2003/10/22. eng.

[115] Reed, K. Peripheral neuromodulation and headaches: history, clinical approach, and considerations on underlying mechanisms. *Current pain and headache reports.*, 2013, 17(1), 305.

[116] Sullivan, MJL; Thorn, B; Haythornthwaite, JA; Keefe, F; Martin, M; Bradley, LA; et al. Theoretical perspectives on the relation between catastrophizing and pain. *The Clinical journal of pain.*, 2001, 17(1), 52-64.

[117] Sierpina, V; Astin, J; Giordano, J. Mind-body therapies for headache. American family physician. 2007, 76, 1518-22.

[118] Donatone, B. Focused suggestion with somatic anchoring technique: rapid self-hypnosis for pain management. *American Journal of Clinical Hypnosis.*, 2013, 55, 325-42.

[119] Penzien, DB; Johnson, C; Carpenter, D. Drug vs. behavioral treatment of migraine: long-acting propranolol vs. home-based self-management training. *Headache.*, 1990, 30, 300.

[120] ter Kuile, M; Spinhoven, P; Linssen, A; Zitman, F; Van Dyck, R; Rooijmans, H. Autogenic training and cognitive self-hypnosis for the treatment of recurrent headaches in three different subject groups. *Pain.*, 1994, 58(3), 331-40.

[121] Holroyd, KA; Penzien, DB. Pharmacological versus non-pharmacological prophylaxis of recurrent migraine headache: A meta-analytic review of clinical trials. *Pain.*, 1990, 42(1), 1-13.

[122] Jensen, MP; Ehde, DM; Gertz, KJ; Stoelb, BL; Dillworth, TM; Hirsh, AT; et al. Effects of self-hypnosis training and cognitive restructuring on daily pain intensity and catastrophizing in individuals with multiple sclerosis and chronic pain. *The International journal of clinical and experimental hypnosis.*, 2011 Jan, 59(1), 45-63. PubMed PMID: 21104484. Epub 2010/11/26. eng.

[123] Buse, DC; Andrasik, F. Behavioral medicine for migraine. *Neurologic clinics.*, 2009 May, 27(2), 445-65. PubMed PMID: 19289225. Epub 2009/03/18. eng.

[124] Nestoriuc, Y; Martin, A; Rief, W; Andrasik, F. Biofeedback treatment for headache disorders: a comprehensive efficacy review. *Applied psychophysiology and*

biofeedback., 2008 Sep, 33(3), 125-40. PubMed PMID: 18726688. Epub 2008/08/30. eng.

[125] Rains, JC; Penzien, DB; McCrory, DC; Gray, RN. Behavioral Headache Treatment: History, Review of the Empirical Literature, and Methodological Critique. *Headache: The Journal of Head and Face Pain.*, 2005, 45(Suppl2), S92-S109.

[126] Andrasik, F. Biofeedback in headache: an overview of approaches and evidence. *Cleveland Clinic journal of medicine.*, 2010 Jul, 77 Suppl 3, S72-6. PubMed PMID: 20622082. Epub 2010/08/07. eng.

[127] Nash, JM; Park, ER; Walker, BB; Gordon, N; Nicholson, RA. Cognitive-Behavioral Group Treatment for Disabling Headache. *Pain Medicine.*, 2004, 5(2), 178-86.

[128] Schafer, AM; Rains, JC; Penzien, DB; Groban, L; Smitherman, TA; Houle, TT. Direct costs of preventive headache treatments: comparison of behavioral and pharmacologic approaches. *Headache.*, 2011 Jun, 51(6), 985-91. PubMed PMID: 21631481. Pubmed Central PMCID: 3303196. Epub 2011/06/03.

[129] Martin, PR; Forsyth, MR; Reece, J. Cognitive-behavioral therapy versus temporal pulse amplitude biofeedback training for recurrent headache. *Behavior Therapy.*, 2007, 38(4), 350-63.

[130] Beck, JS; Beck, JS. Cognitive behavior therapy: basics and beyond. 2nd ed. New York: Guilford Press; 2011, xix, 391 p. p.

[131] Holroyd, KA. Behavioral Management for Migraine Headaches. In: Cottrell CK, editor. A Treatment Program For Controlling Migraines. Ohio: Ohio University; 2000.

[132] Gatchel, RJ; Rollings, KH. Evidence-informed management of chronic low back pain with cognitive behavioral therapy. The spine journal: *official journal of the North American Spine Society.*, 2008 Jan-Feb, 8(1), 40-4. PubMed PMID: 18164452. Pubmed Central PMCID: 3237294. Epub 2008/01/01.

[133] Weeks, RE. Application of behavioral therapies in adult and adolescent patients with chronic migraine. Neurological sciences: *official journal of the Italian Neurological Society and of the Italian Society of Clinical Neurophysiology.*, 2013 May, 34 Suppl 1, S11-7. PubMed PMID: 23695037. Epub 2013/05/25. eng.

[134] Wenzel, A; Brown, GK; Karlin, BE. Cognitive Behavioral Therapy for Depression in Veterans and Military Servicemembers: Therapist Manual. Washington, DC: Department of Veterans Affairs; 2011.

[135] Dubord, G. Part 9. Thought records. Canadian family physician Medecin de famille canadien. 2011 Aug, 57(8), 913-4. PubMed PMID: 21841114. Pubmed Central PMCID: Pmc3155448. Epub 2011/08/16. eng.

[136] Holroyd, KA; Cottrell, CK; O'Donnell, FJ; Cordingley, GE; Drew, JB; Carlson, BW; et al. Effect of preventive (β blocker) treatment, behavioural migraine management, or their combination on outcomes of optimised acute treatment in frequent migraine: Randomised controlled trial. BMJ: *British Medical Journal.*, 2010, 341(7776), 1-12.

[137] Richardson, GM; McGrath, PJ. Cognitive-Behavioral Therapy for Migraine Headaches: A Minimal-Therapist-Contact Approach Versus a Clinic-Based Approach. *Headache: The Journal of Head and Face Pain.*, 1989, 29(6), 352-7.

[138] Holroyd, KA. Assessment and psychological management of recurrent headache disorders. *Journal of consulting and clinical psychology.* 2002, 70(3), 656-77.

[139] Weeks, RE. Behavioral management of headache. *Techniques in Regional Anesthesia & Pain Management.*, 2009, 13(1), 50-7.

[140] Sajadinejad, MS; Mohammadi, N; Taghavi, SMR; Ashgazadeh, N. Therapeutic effects of cognitive-behavioral group therapy on headache disability and depression in patients with migraine and tension headache. [Therapeutic effects of cognitive-behavioral group therapy on headache disability and depression in patients with migraine and tension headache.]. *Iranian Journal of Psychiatry and Clinical Psychology.* 2009, 14(4), 411-8.
[141] Hayes, SC; Strosahl, K; Wilson, KG. Acceptance and commitment therapy: the process and practice of mindful change. 2nd ed. New York: Guilford Press; 2012, xiv, 402 p. p.
[142] Kabat-Zinn, J. University of Massachusetts Medical Center/Worcester. Stress Reduction Clinic. Full catastrophe living: using the wisdom of your body and mind to face stress, pain, and illness. New York, N.Y.: Delacorte Press; 1990, xxi, 453 p. p.
[143] Segal, ZV; Williams, JMG; Teasdale, JD. Mindfulness-based cognitive therapy for depression: a new approach to preventing relapse. New York: Guilford Press; 2002, xiv, 351 p. p.
[144] Hayes, SC; Strosahl, K; Wilson, KG. Acceptance and commitment therapy: an experiential approach to behavior change. New York: Guilford Press; 1999, xvi, 304 p. p.
[145] Hayes, SC. Acceptance and Commitment Therapy, Relational Frame Theory, and the Third Wave of Behavioral and Cognitive Therapies. *Behavior Therapy.*, 2004, 35(4), 639-65.
[146] Brown, LA; Gaudiano, BA; Miller, IW. Investigating the similarities and differences between practitioners of second- and third-wave cognitive-behavioral therapies. *Behavior Modification.*, 2011, 35(2), 187-200.
[147] Kabat-Zinn, J. Mindfulness-based interventions in context: Past, present, and future. Clinical Psychology: *Science and Practice.* 2003, 10(2), 144-56.
[148] Kabat-Zinn, J. Full catastrophe living: using the wisdom of your body and mind to face stress, pain, and illness. Revised and updated edition, Bantam Books trade paperback edition. ed. New York: Bantam Books; 2013, pages cm p.
[149] Grossman, P; Niemann, L; Schmidt, S; Walach, H. Mindfulness-based stress reduction and health benefits: A meta-analysis. *Journal of Psychosomatic Research.* 2004, 57(1), 35-43.
[150] Ledesma, D; Kumano, H. Mindfulness-based stress reduction and cancer: A meta-analysis. *Psycho-Oncology*, 2009, 18(6), 571-9.
[151] Lauche, R; Cramer, H; Dobos, G; Langhorst, J; Schmidt, S. A systematic review and meta-analysis of mindfulness-based stress reduction for the fibromyalgia syndrome. *Journal of Psychosomatic Research.*, 2013, No Pagination Specified.
[152] Williams, JM; Russell, I; Russell, D. Mindfulness-based cognitive therapy: further issues in current evidence and future research. *Journal of consulting and clinical psychology.*, 2008 Jun, *76*(3), 524-9. PubMed PMID: 18540746. Pubmed Central PMCID: Pmc2834575. Epub 2008/06/11. eng.
[153] Day, MA; Thorn, BE; Ward, LC; Rubin, N; Hickman, SD; Scogin, F; et al. Mindfulness-based Cognitive Therapy for the Treatment of Headache Pain: A Pilot Study. *The Clinical journal of pain.*, 2013 Feb, 26. PubMed PMID: 23446085. Epub 2013/03/01. Eng.
[154] Hayes, SC; Levin, ME; Plumb-Vilardaga, J; Villatte, JL; Pistorello, J. Acceptance and commitment therapy and contextual behavioral science: Examining the progress of a distinctive model of behavioral and cognitive therapy. *Behavior Therapy.*, 2013, 44(2), 180-98.

[155] Hayes, SC; Luoma, JB; Bond, FW; Masuda, A; Lillis, J. Acceptance and commitment therapy: Model, processes and outcomes. *Behaviour Research and Therapy.*, 2006, 44(1), 1-25.

[156] Chiros, C; O'Brien, W. Acceptance, appraisals, and coping in relation to migraine headache: an evaluation of interrelationships using daily diary methods. *J Behav Med.*, 2011 2011/08/01, 34(4), 307-20. English.

[157] Mo'tamedi, H; Rezaiemaram, P; Tavallaie, A. The effectiveness of a group-based acceptance and commitment additive therapy on rehabilitation of female outpatients with chronic headache: Preliminary findings reducing 3 dimensions of headache impact. Headache: *The Journal of Head and Face Pain.*, 2012, 52(7), 1106-19.

[158] Veehof, MM; Oskam, M; Schreurs, KMG; Bohlmeijer, ET. Acceptance-based interventions for the treatment of chronic pain: A systematic review and meta-analysis. Pain. *2011*, 152(3), 533-42.

[159] Chiesa, A; Serretti, A. Mindfulness-based interventions for chronic pain: A systematic review of the evidence. *The Journal of Alternative and Complementary Medicine.* 2011, 17(1), 83-93.

[160] Reiner, K; Tibi, L; Lipsitz, JD. Do mindfulness-based interventions reduce pain intensity? A critical review of the literature. *Pain Medicine.*, 2013, 14(2), 230-42.

[161] Oakley, DA; Halligan, PW. Hypnotic suggestion and cognitive neuroscience. *Trends in cognitive sciences.*, 2009 Jun, 13(6), 264-70. PubMed PMID: 19428287. Epub 2009/05/12. eng.

[162] Patterson, DR; Jensen, MP; Wiechman, SA; Sharar, SR; Virtual reality hypnosis for pain associated with recovery from physical trauma. The International journal of clinical and experimental hypnosis. 2010 Jul, 58(3), 288-300. PubMed PMID: 20509069. Pubmed Central PMCID: Pmc2913598. Epub 2010/05/29. eng.

[163] Rossi, EL; Rossi, KL. The neuroscience of observing consciousness & mirror neurons in therapeutic hypnosis. American Journal of Clinical Hypnosis. 2006 April 2006, 48(4), 263-78.

[164] Hammond, DC. Review of the efficacy of clinical hypnosis with headaches and migraines. *The International journal of clinical and experimental hypnosis.*, 2007 Apr, 55(2), 207-19. PubMed PMID: 17365074. Epub 2007/03/17. eng.

[165] Crasilneck, HB. The use of the Crasilneck Bombardment Technique in problems of intractable organic pain. *The American journal of clinical hypnosis.*, 1995 Apr, 37(4), 255-66. PubMed PMID: 7741081. Epub 1995/04/01. eng.

[166] Lang, EV; Benotsch, EG; Fick, LJ; Lutgendorf, S; Berbaum, ML; Berbaum, KS; et al. Adjunctive non-pharmacological analgesia for invasive medical procedures: a randomised trial. *Lancet.*, 2000 Apr 29, 355(9214), 1486-90. PubMed PMID: 10801169. Epub 2000/05/09. eng.

In: Migraine Surgery
Editor: Antonios Mammis

ISBN: 978-1-63321-761-4

Chapter 5

Interventional Treatment of Migraine 1: Botox - Trigger Point Injections

Anthony Sifonios [*] ***and Vanny Le***
Department of Anesthesiology,
Rutgers New Jersey Medical School, Newark, New Jersey, US

Myofascial pain syndrome is a chronic pain disorder characterized by the presence of trigger points (TrPs) within muscles associated with taut bands, muscle spasm, stiffness, limited range of motion, and referred pain. Myofascial TrPs are defined as focally tender points in skeletal muscle, fascia, or both that can consistently reproduce a referred pain pattern upon palpation [1]. Myofascial TrPs are often overlooked when diagnosing and treating headaches.

There have been few and small clinical control trials evaluating myofascial trigger points' role in the production of both chronic tension type headache (CTTH) and migraine headaches (MH). Patients with MH without aura have been shown to have focal cervical and pericranial muscle tenderness with referred pain that reproduce their migraine headache. These pericranial muscles are more tender in migraine patients than in nonheadache controls even when the migraine patients are headache free [1]). In a prospective study evaluating migraine patients with active TrPs of the neck with referral patterns that can mimic migraine, 78 patients underwent electrical pain threshold measurement in skin, subcutis, and muscle in TrPs and referred areas at baseline and after 3, 10, 30, and 60 days after TrP anesthetic injection. Fifty four patients underwent TrP anesthetic injection and 24 patients received no treatment. At baseline, all the patients exhibited below normal thresholds in TrPs and in referred sites representing hyperalgesia. In the TrP injected group, the pain threshold increased progressively indicating a reduction in hyperalgesia and migraine headache. In the untreated group, no changes occurred, thus indicating that cervical and pericranial TrPs

[*] Corresponding author: Anthony Sifonios, M.D. Assistant Professor, Department of Anesthesiology, 90 Bergen Street, Suite 8100, Newark NJ, 07103, sifonian@njms.rutgers.edu.

contribute and enhance MH [3]. There are a number of muscles within the head and neck, in which TrPs can refer pain to the head and hence contribute to chronic tension type headache and migraine headaches [2]. In a study aimed at mapping the referred pain areas of active myofascial TrPs, 13 patients suffering from CTTH were analyzed. It was found that these patients had a mean number of 7 active TrPs. It was found that TrPs in the suboccipital muscles were most prevalent in these patients [2]. TrPs within the trapezius, sternocleido-mastoid, masseter, temporalis, occipitofrontalis, splenius capitus, splenius cervicus, and others have referral patterns that can mimic both migraine and chronic tension type headaches [1].

TrPs of Cervical Muscles

The trapezius muscle is a frequently overlooked source of temporal and cervicogenic headache. TrPs within the upper trapezius muscle often refers pain from the posterolateral aspect of the neck to the posterior ear and ipsilateral temple. TrPs within the lower trapezius muscle tend to radiate to the posterior neck, mastoid process, and scapula [1].

The sternocleidomastoid muscle consists of two heads, the sternal head and the clavicular head. The facial pain referred from trigger points within this muscle is frequently the basis for the diagnoses of atypical facial neuralgia, tension headache, and cervicocephalalgia. TrPs within the sternal head often refers pain to the occiput, the vertex of the head, and periorbitally. TrPs within the clavicular head often refer pain to the forehead and the ipsilateral periauricular area [1].

TrPs in the splenius capitis will refer pain to the vertex of the head. Pain from the splenius cervicis is referred cephalad to the occiput, through the skull to the orbit. TrPs within the upper portion of the semispinalis capitis refer pain in a band like pattern projected above the orbit mimicking a greater occipital neuralgia. TrPs from the mid portion of the muscle is felt over the posterior occiput [1] similar to a lesser occipital neuralgia.

TrPs of Pericranial Muscles

TrPs within the masseter muscle may radiate to the supraorbital area, the maxilla, the mandible and the ear [1]. Identification of TrPs within the masseter muscle is slightly more challenging as an intraoral examination is needed. TrPs within the temporalis muscle can refer pain to the supraorbital area, the maxilla, and the temporomandibular joint. Pain referred from TrPs in the occipitofrontalis muscle radiates over the forehead, to the back of the head through the cranium [1].

Trigger Point Injection Technique

Trigger point injections (TPI) are a fairly safe therapeutic option with few contraindications. TPIs can effectively inactivate TrPs, provide prompt symptomatic relief, and is the gold standard for treatment of TrPs [4]. Once a trigger point has been located, the skin is then cleansed with alcohol or betadine. The clinician then isolates the TrP by pinching the muscle between the thumb and index finger. Using sterile technique, a 25 gauge 1.5 inch needle is then inserted into the trigger point. After negative aspiration for blood or cerebrospinal fluid, an injectate of 3-5 mL of local anesthetic with or without a non-particulate steroid is then injected in a fan-like distribution. The stabilizing fingers apply pressure on either side of the injection site, ensuring adequate tension of the muscle fibers to allow penetration of the trigger point but preventing it from rolling away from the advancing needle and isolating the muscle. The application of pressure may also help to prevent the serious complication of pneumothorax especially with injection of the trapezius muscle [5].

Dry needling (performing a TPI without a local anesthetic) has also been described, and was found to be as effective as a TPI with local anesthetic. Dry needling, however, resulted in more post-injection soreness [1].

Botulinum Toxin

Botulinum toxin or BOTOX® (Allergan, Inc., Irvine, CA) injections have been FDA-approved for preventive treatment in patients with chronic migraines. [6,7] The medication is a neurotoxin derived from the anaerobic bacterium Clostridium botulinum and at this time, only the onabotulinumtoxin A preparation is permitted for patient use. The exact mechanism of action is not clearly understood but the botulinum toxin seems to inhibit craniofacial muscle nociceptive mediators such as substance P, CGRP and glutamate causing a decrease in peripheral mechanical sensitization as well as central sensitization. [8,9] In addition, there is evidence that botulinum toxin A also impedes the expression of ion channels on trigeminovascular neurons which are linked to mechanical pain thereby decreasing hypersensitivity and cutaneous allodynia associated with migraines. [9, 10]

Earlier studies showed conflicting evidence regarding the efficacy of onabotulinumtoxin A and its advantage over established oral medications. Multiple retrospective or open-label trials together with small, double-blinded, randomized trials have shown a beneficial role of onabotulinumtoxin A in reducing migraine attacks. However, these studies were limited by sample size, poorly defined end points and heterogeneous patient populations. [9] Botulinum toxin injections were compared to oral topiramate in two small clinical trials and showed that patients had a similar reduction in headache days with no statistical significance. [7, 11] Other studies compared onabotulinumtoxin A to amitriptyline or to valproate for chronic migraines in a randomized prospective trial and demonstrated that the two outcomes were comparable in reducing the number of pain days. [12, 13] However, the two PREEMPT clinical trials (Phase III Research Evaluating Migraine Prophylaxis Therapy) were large, randomized, double-blinded, prospective studies that investigated the effect of botulinum toxin vs. placebo injections in 31 fixed muscle sites for a total of 155 units. All patients, regardless of headache symptoms, were injected in the procerus, bilateral corrugators, frontalis, temporalis, occipitalis, cervical, paraspinal, and superior trapezius muscles. In the PREEMPT I trial, the authors specifically examined patients with chronic migraines in combination with medication overuse and found that after 24 weeks, patients receiving onabotulinumtoxin A (N=445) vs. placebo (N=459) had fewer headache/migraine episodes, headache/migraine days, and cumulative headache hours while improving quality of life and functioning. [6] In addition, many patients in the onabotulinumtoxin A treated group shifted to no medication overuse for at least 3 to 6 months after the primary endpoint of 24 weeks. [6] The PREEMPT II trial evaluated patients for the full 56-weeks or five 12-week treatment cycles. [14] Patients received either onabotulinumtoxin A for all five treatment cycles or placebo for 2 cycles then onabotulinumtoxin A for 3 cycles. A total of 1384 patients were randomized and 1005 patients (N = 513 onabotulinumtoxin A only, N = 492 placebo/onabotulinumtoxin A) completed all treatment cycles. Similar to the PREEMPT I results, the PREEMPT II study showed that onabotulinumtoxin A was safe and effective as a long-term treatment decreasing the frequency of migraine and headache days per month, migraine/headache episodes, and cumulative headache hours compared to placebo. [6, 14, 15] It also had a positive impact on the Headache Impact Test (HIT)-6 score and Migraine-Specific Quality of Life Questionnaire score. More patients had a significant response of >50% reduction from baseline in frequency of headache days when botulinum toxin injections were initiated earlier, i.e., in the 5 cycle onabotulinumtoxin A group. (14]

The common botulinum toxin injection sites are the glabellar, frontal, temporal and occipital regions. The muscles involved are the procerus, corrugator, frontalis, temporalis, occipitalis, splenius capitus, suboccipital, posterior cervical paraspinal and the trapezius muscles. The injections can be injected at fixed sites bilaterally, specifically at the sites of pain or tenderness or a combination of both techniques. [9] The fixed-site approach may be more beneficial in patients with migraines while the follow-the-pain approach is appropriate for tension-type headaches. Using the follow-the-pain approach may have the detrimental effects of a poor cosmetic outcome and triggering the pain to shift to the unaffected side. [9] Although the doses have varied, 5 units are typically injected at each site every 3 months. [16]

Adverse effects related to onabotulinumtoxin A range in mild to moderate severity and resolve without sequelae. The most commonly reported side effects include mild fatigue, nausea, difficulty concentrating or with memory, and mood swings. Nausea is the most significant adverse effect seen in 59.1% of patients on onabotulinumtoxin A as compared to 27.3% in patients taking topiramate. [11] Botulinum toxin injections are better tolerated than amitriptyline with a significantly higher incidence of weight gain, somnolence, dry mouth, and constipation in patients taking amitriptyline. [12] Other side effects include blepharoptosis, muscle weakness, neck pain, neck stiffness, paresthesias and skin tightness. [13]

Although botulinum toxin is expensive, the long term benefit of reducing daily pain medications, such as triptans, and increasing quality-adjusted life years, may make the injections a cost-effective treatment. [7, 17]

Conclusion

Myofascial pain syndromes that originate from trigger points are one of the most frequent causes of headaches. Myofascial TrPs within cervical and pericranial muscles can contribute and refer pain in patterns resembling migraine and chronic tension type headache helping to explain why some patients may be resistant to medication management. A thorough history and physical examination of both cervical and pericranial muscle anatomy may help in diagnosing myofascial pain syndrome as a cause of the headache. When myofascial TrPs are found to be the cause or a contributing factor of headache, patients may benefit from TrP injections. If Trp injections are beneficial but temporary, injection with botulinum toxin may be a beneficial and cost-effective treatment.

References

[1] Simons, D. G., Travell, J. & Simons, L. S. (1999). Travell and Simons' Myofascial Pain and Dysfunction: the Trigger Point Manual, second ed., Vol. 1 Williams & Wilkins, Baltimore.

[2] Fernandez-de-las Penas, C., Ge, H., Alonso-Blanco, C. Gonzalez-Iglesias, J. & Arendt-Nielsen, L. (2010). Referred pain areas of active myofascial trigger points in head, neck, and shoulder muscles, in chronic tension type headache. *Journal of Bodywork & Movement Therapies*, *14*, 391-396.

[3] Giamberardino, M. A., Tafuri, E., Savini, A., Fabrizio, A. Affaitati, G., Lerza, R., Di Ianni, L. Lapenna, D. & Mezzetti, A. (2007). Contribution of Myofascial Trigger Points to Migraine Symptoms. *J. of Pain*, Vol *8*, No 11, 869-878.

[4] Giamberardino, M. A., Affaitati, G., Fabrizio, A. & Costantini, R. (2011). Myofascial pain syndromes and their evaluation. *Best Practice & Research Clinical Rheumatology*, *25*, 185-198.

[5] Alvarez, D. J. & Rockwell, P. G. (2002). Trigger points: Diagnosis and Management. *Am Fam Physician*, *65* (4), 653-661.

[6] Silberstein, S. D. et al. (2013). OnaboltulinumtoxinA for treatment of chronic migraine: PREEMPT 24-week pooled subgroup analysis of patients who had acute headache medication overuse at baseline. *Journal of Neurological*, *331*, 48-56.

[7] Evans, Randolph W. A (2013). rational approach to the management of chronic migraine. *Headache*, *53*, 168-176.

[8] Gazerani, P. et al. (2010). Botulinum neurotoxin type A (BoNTA) decreases the mechanical sensitivity of nociceptors and inhibits neurogenic vasodilation in a craniofacial muscle targeted for migraine prophylaxis. *Pain*, *151*, 606-616.

[9] Dodick, D. et al. (2004). Botulinum neurotoxin for the treatment of migraine and other primary headache disorders. *Clinics in Dermatology*, *22*, 76-81

[10] Burstein, R. et al. (2014). Selective inhibition of meningeal nociceptors by botulinum neurotoxin type A: Therapeutic implications for migraine and other pains. *Cephalagia*, *0*(0), 1-17.

[11] Cady, R. K. et al. (2011). A multi-center double-blind pilot comparison of onabotulinumtonxinA and topiramate for the prophylactic treatment of chronic migraine. *Headache*, *51*, 21-32.

[12] Magalhaes, E. et al. (2010). Botulinum toxin type A versus amitriptyline for the treatment of chronic daily migraine. *Clinical Neurology and Neurosurgery*, 112, 463-466.

[13] Jackson, J., Kuriyama, A. & Hayashino, Y. (2012). Botulinum Toxin A for prophylactic treatment of migraine and tension headaches in adults: A meta-analysis. *JAMA*, *307* (16), 1736-1745.

[14] Aurora, S. K. et al. (2014). OnabotulinumtoxinA for chronic migraine: efficacy, safety, and tolerability in patients who received all five treatment cycles in the PREEMPT clinical program. *Acta Neurol Scand*, *129*, 61-70.
[15] Carod-Artal, F. (2014). Tackling chronic migraine: Current Perspectives. *Journal of Pain Research*, *7*, 185-194.
[16] Shulman, E. & McGeeney, B. E. (2013). Current concepts in refractory migraine. *Current treatment options in neurology*, *15*, 40-55.
[17] Batty, A., Hansen, R. & Bloudek, L. et al. (2013). The cost-effectiveness of onabotulinumtoxin A for the prophylaxis of headache in adults with chronic migraine in the UK. *Journal of Medical Economics*, *16* (7), 877-887.

In: Migraine Surgery
Editor: Antonios Mammis
ISBN: 978-1-63321-761-4

Chapter 6

Interventional Treatment of Migraine 2: Nerve Blocks

Sam Nia, Antonio Gonzalez-Fiol and Anthony Sifonios
Department of Anesthesiology,
Rutgers New Jersey Medical School, Newark, New Jersey, US

Abstract

Peripheral nerve blocks have traditionally been used to diagnose and treat certain kinds of head pain. They can be quickly and relatively simple to perform in the outpatient setting. These blocks are typically performed with local anesthetics alone, although a combination of local anesthetic and steroid can also be used. The analgesic effects of these peripheral nerve blocks may be transient, however, if the pain relief from the diagnostic block is significantly decreased by more than 50%, radiofrequency ablation of these peripheral nerves can be performed for longer duration of relief.

Keywords: Nerve blocks, Migraine, Headache, Greater Occipital Nerve block, Occipital neuralgia, Cervicogenic headache, Hemicrania continua, Posttraumatic headache, Lesser Occipital nerve block, Trigeminal nerve block, Supraorbital nerve block, Sphenopalatine Ganglion block, Pterygopalatine ganglion block, Gasserian ganglion

Greater Occipital Nerve Block

GON Block Rationale

The most commonly blocked peripheral nerve for the treatment of headaches is the greater occipital nerve (GON). [1, 2] This, and other nerves have been targeted for blockade in an effort to treat headaches for decades. [3] There is sound justification for the injection of local anesthetic and anti-inflammatory agents around the greater occipital nerve as its proximity to the confluence of sensory input to the trigeminal nucleus caudalis (TNC) from both the cervical and trigeminal fibers has been considered a major factor in its contribution to headache discomfort and, by blocking it, the alleviation of this discomfort. [3] Studies using animal models have provided evidence that, when the GON is stimulated, the TNC shows an increase in metabolic activity. [3] Along with evidence from other studies, these findings support the thinking that cervical and trigeminal inputs converge at the level TNC. [3] Furthermore, evidence suggest that humans with GON blockade may experience pain relief in skin areas beyond the innervation of the GON [2], as these data propose that GON stimulation facilitates C2 neuronal response to dural stimulation. [3] Additionally, evidence exists that the analgesic effects peripheral nerve blocks for headache relief far outlast the anesthetic effects of the drugs used, providing even more rationale to consider a centrally mediated cause of headache relief secondary to peripheral nerve block. [2]

Headache Types Treated by GON

GON blockade for the relief of distinct headache types has been investigated in several clinical studies, however the data demonstrate a noticeable paucity of controlled studies. [3] The two most common headache types treated by GON are occipital neuralgia and cervigocenic headache (CEH). [4] In the case of occipital neuralgia, studies exist which demonstrate the success of this technique. [4] CEH has a unique relationship to GON blockade as a positive response to GON blockade is a diagnostic criterion for CEH, which should not only provide pain relief for the regions supplied by the nerve blocked, but also in areas beyond the innervation of the peripheral nerves being injected. [5, 6] A host of other studies exist which demonstrate the efficacy of GON blockade on CEH for not only diagnosis, but also treatment. [3, 6, 7, 8] Blocking the GON has also been shown by a case report to be efficacious in the treatment of trigeminal neuralgia. [7] Post dural puncture headache has also been successfully treated in part by GON blockade. [7] GON block has shown some promise for contributing to the treatment of hemicrania continua, another headache type. [8, 9] Migraine, a headache type that much of the population has the misfortune of being familiar with, has been shown to be successfully treated with GON even in the refractory state [6, 7, 8]. Posttraumatic headache has also been treated successfully with GON. [7] Another headache type, which commonly maligns much of the population, the tension type headache, has been demonstrated, in studies to be treatable, in part, by GON block. [3, 6] Cluster headache is another headache type, which has been shown by several case studies as well as a randomized trial to be successfully treated by GON block. [3, 7, 8]

GON Technique

There is a wide discrepancy between practitioners when it comes to exactly where to inject and which agents to inject for the GON block, as there is no standardized protocol for GON block. [3, 5, 8] There seems to be consensus that shows that most practitioners will tend to use a local anesthetic (generally Lidocaine 1% or 2% or bupivicaine 0.25% or 0.5%) with or without a corticosteroid (Triamcinolone 20mg or Methylprednisolone 80mg). [1, 3, 4, 8]

According to Ashekaazi, et al., as well as others, the evidence for corticosteroid for use in GON block is lacking. [3, 5, 8]

Other technical aspects of the GON block in terms of anatomical landmarks are relatively straightforward which proves this a simple procedure, which can easily and safely be done in an office setting. [3, 8] Injection requires the use of a small gauge needle (typically 23gauge) inserted 3.5 cm infero-lateral to the occipital protuberance. [3] Being careful to aspirate, in order to avoid intravascular injection in the relatively blood-vessel-rich scalp, 2-4ml of local anesthetic with or without steroid is injected. [1, 3]

Lesser Occipital Nerve Block

Headache Types Treated by LON

Similar to the GON, the lesser occipital nerve block (LON) has been used to treat a variety of headache types. [7] Some practitioners support the use of LON in the treatment of CEH as well as post-dural puncture headache (PDPH). [1, 7] There are, however, published accounts that espouse that there is no evidence to support the use of LON block in the treatment of headache disorders. [4]

LON Technique

Different practitioners use different techniques when it comes to the agents and volumes utilized in LON block administration, which is similar to GON block. (1, 3-5, 8)

The location of LON block injection is generally performed by imagining a line drawn from the occipital protuberance to the mastoid process and injecting ⅔ of the way laterally to the occipital protuberance. [1, 4]

Trigeminal Nerve Blocks

The trigeminal nerve, or cranial nerve five (CNV) has been implicated in the cause of various headache types and as a result, blockade of this nerve and its branches has been targeted for headache relief. [7] Blockade of the supratrochlear nerve (STN), the terminal branch of the frontal nerve, the longest branch of the ophthalmic division of CNV [1] has been implicated in the relief of supraorbital neuralgia [7]. as well as its diagnosis [4]; this is due to the anatomic location of where the STN courses, making it prone to traumatic injury. [1, 4]

No consensus exists as to the exact dosage and agents to be used in this block, however, Injection of local anesthetic agents for blockade of this nerve involves the administration of these drugs via a small gauge needle, being careful to aspirate to avoid vascular structures in the area just above the eyebrow over the medial border. [4]

The auriculotemporal nerve (ATN) is a branch of the mandibular portion of CNV is responsible for sensation over the ear and temporalis muscle. [4] Published works claim that some patients derive benefit from blockade of this nerve despite a lack of data supporting its use. [4]

Injection of local anesthetic agents for blockade of this nerve involves the administration of these drugs via a small gauge needle, being careful to aspirate to avoid vascular structures in the location just anterior to the ear or superior to the posterior portion of the zygoma. [4]

Supraorbital Nerve Blocks

The Supraorbital Nerve (SON) is the larger of the terminal branches of the frontal nerve. [1] This nerve innervates the upper eyelid and conjunctiva as well as the skin of the scalp. This nerve is also responsible for innervation of the supraorbital sweat glands. [1] Blockade of this nerve has been implicated in the treatment of hemicrania continua. [9] Blockade of the SON has also been implicated in the cause of supraorbital neuralgia. [7] as well as its diagnosis [4]; this is due to the anatomic location of where the SON courses, making it prone to traumatic injury. [1, 4] Other headache types that have been successfully treated with SON block have been shown to include TTH, CEH, and Migraine headache types. [6, 7]

Technique

Despite the fact that no consensus exists as to the exact anesthetic agents and their volumes to utilize in the blockade of the SON [1,7], Injection of the SON should be done in the area immediately above the supraorbital notch. [1] Injections should be done in a fanlike manner to ensure adequate infiltration of anesthetic agents for nerve branch coverage.

Sphenopalatine Ganglion Block

The sphenopalatine ganglion (SPG) or pterygopalatine ganglion lies in the pterygopalatine fossa (PPF), posterior to the middle nasal turbinate. [10, 11] This ganglion contains sensory, motor and autonomic components. This complex autonomic and sensory relation in the ganglion has being implicated in the pathophysiology of headaches, particularly, cluster headaches. [12, 13]

Hence, the sphenopalatine ganglion has gain acceptance for the treatment of acute migraines and acute and chronic cluster headaches. [10-16]

This block can be performed using one of three approaches: Intranasal, Transoral (Greater Palatine Foramen approach) or Infrazygomatic arch (Lateral infratemporal).

The Intranasal Approach

This is the easiest and least invasive technique. It is performed by using a cotton-tipped applicator filled with lidocaine 4% directed towards the posterior aspect of the middle nasal turbinate. [10] This technique is easy to perform, but the variability of absorption of the local anesthetic and anatomy might limit the efficacy or predictability of the block. [10, 17] This has prompt to the modification of the technique by using new delivery devices as in the case of Candido et al. and Windsor et al. [11], or performing the block with transnasal endoscopic assistance. [18]

Felisati et al. [18] describes a transnasal endoscopic technique to approach the PPF via the lateral nasal wall, and in this way perform a SPG block using a 20G needle and a mixture of local anesthetics and steroids. They performed 20 SPG blocks, during the years of 2002 to 2005, for patients suffering cluster headaches refractory to pharmacotherapy. His group reports eight patients [8] with complete (yet temporary) relief and three [3] additional patients with partial relief. That is, eleven out of the twenty patients (55%) benefited from the block. Pipolo et al. [19] was able to reproduce similar results with 15 patients (years 2008-2009) using a similar endoscopic transnasal technique with a success rate of 60%. These studies support the use of the SPG block for the treatment of cluster headaches unresponsive to pharmacotherapy.

Although the aforementioned modification seems promising for patients suffering from headaches (particularly those who do not respond well to pharmacotherapy), there is paucity of studies performed using randomized controlled trials and with a higher number of patients. Besides, the use of local anesthetics to perform this block offers the patients a temporary relief at most. Hence, radiofrequency might offer prolonged relief of symptoms for patients that showed improvement with the SPG block. [10, 12, 15]

The Transoral (Greater Palatine Foramen Approach) Approach

This approach provides the most direct route to the SPG, but also the most difficult to perform and with the greatest risk of complications. [10] The technique is performed by directing a curved needle through the greater palatine foramen to gain access to the superior aspect of the PPF. [10] Because of the increase risk of complications many physicians avoid this technique.

The Infrazygomatic Arch (Lateral Infratemporal) Approach

This technique is the most commonly reserved for neurolysis [10, 12] of the SPG after a successful diagnostic test, i.e., an intranasal SPG block. This technique can be performed blindly or with fluoroscopic aid. [10, 12] Patients are placed in the supine position and the PPF is localized with C-arm fluoroscopic guidance. A line is drawn over the PPF and the intersection between this line and the inferior zygomatic arch is used as the entry site of the needle. [12, 15] After local anesthesia infiltration the SPG is confirmed by electrical stimulation [15] and the radio frequency ablation (RFA) is performed. Sanders et al. [15] performed RF lesions of the SPG on 66 patients suffering from episodic [56] or chronic [10] cluster headaches. From the group with episodic cluster headaches 34 patients experienced complete relief, 14 partial relief and 8 patients had no relief. From the group with chronic CH 3 patients experienced complete relief, 3 partial relief and 4 no relief. The results from both groups were statistically significant. Narouze et al. [12] were able to demonstrate a decrease on the mean attack intensity, mean attack frequency and pain disability index on seven [7] out of fifteen [15] patients with chronic CH. Hence, RF lesioning might be an alternative for those patients suffering CH that do not respond to pharmacotherapy and have responded well to less invasive SPG blocks.

Gasserian Ganglion

The Gasserian Ganglion, or Trigeminal Ganglion is a sensory ganglion of the trigeminal nerve, which occupies a cavity known as Meckel's Cave, or Trigeminal Cave near the apex of the petrous part of the temporal bone. [20]

Evidence exists supporting the use of Gasserian Ganglion ablation for the treatment of headache. In the case of the rare and debilitating type of headache known as the severe, unremitting cluster headache, clinical evidence has been put forth by Pieper, et al. suggesting that the ablation of this nerve ganglion provides long term relief of associated headache symptoms. [21]

Ablation of neural tissue renders it unable to conduct electrical impulses, and as a result stops the propagation of signals. The principle behind injecting local anesthetic agents is predicated on the same principle as it eliminates neural signaling through the manipulated tissue. It stands to reason, therefore, that the results obtained by nerve blockade are expected to be the same, albeit more short-term than those of full nerve ablation.

Technique

This nerve block injection is performed when the patient is supine. Local skin anesthesia is obtained at the corner of the mouth ipsilateral to the Gasserian Ganglion targeted. A 13cm 20-gauge Hinck needle is inserted at the corner of the mouth and is aimed at the auditory meatus travelling perpendicular to a midposition pupil. After needle contact with the skull base is achieved, the tip is withdrawn several millimeters and carefully advanced posteriorly to the foramen ovale.

After needle entry to the foramen ovale is achieved, it is then aspirated making sure that there is free flow of CSF and no blood present. The needle position should be confirmed by radiography before local anesthetic agents are injected. Common medications injected include 1% lidocaine for diagnostic blockade or 0.5% bupivicaine for therapeutic blocks. It must be kept in mind that there can be variability in the size of Meckel's Cave and as a result, care must be taken to not inject a large volume of anesthetic agent that a small Meckel's Cave cannot accommodate. Doing so may cause nerve compression, injury and could result in further neuralgia symptomatology. [20]

Conclusion

Headaches can be very debilitating, sometimes dwindling our ability to perform even the simplest of the activities of daily living. Nerve blocks are part of the resources that physicians in the field of pain management can use to help patients with migraines and other types of headaches. It is important for patients seeking help for their headaches to have an interdisciplinary team that can offer the patient the different alternatives and treatments available for their particular headache. Neurologist and or neurosurgeons should take in consideration the use of these nerve blocks particularly when pharmacologic treatments have failed, particularly as a step before surgery. Although, in some cases, surgery is unavoidable, since some of the aforementioned blocks can provide transitory relief.

References

[1] Blumenfeld, A; Ashkenazi, A; Napchan, U; Bender, SD; Klein, BC; Berliner, R; et al. Expert Consensus Recommendations for the Performance of Peripheral Nerve Blocks for Headaches – A Narrative Review. *Headache*, 2013, 53(3), 437–46.

[2] Robbins, MS; Blumenfeld, A. Peripheral Nerve Blocks for Headaches. americanheadachesocietyorg

[3] Ashkenazi, A; Levin, M. Greater occipital nerve block for migraine and other headaches: Is it useful? Curr Pain Headache Rep. *Current Science Inc*, 2007, 11(3), 231–5.

[4] Levin, M. Nerve blocks in the treatment of headache. Neurotherapeutics. *Springer-Verlag*, 2010 Apr, 7(2), 197–203.

[5] Bogduk, N. Role of anesthesiologic blockade in headache management. *Curr Pain Headache Rep.*, 2004 Oct, 8(5), 399–403.

[6] Ashkenazi, A; SILBERSTEIN, S. Headache management for the pain specialist. *Regional Anesthesia and Pain Medicine*, 2004 Oct, 29(5), 462–75.

[7] Ashkenazi, A; Blumenfeld, A; Napchan, U; Narouze, S; Grosberg, B; Nett, R; et al. Peripheral nerve blocks and trigger point injections in headache management - a systematic review and suggestions for future research. Headache. *Blackwell Publishing Inc*, 2010 Jun, 50(6), 943–52.

[8] Young, WB. Blocking the Greater Occipital Nerve: Utility in Headache Management. Curr Pain Headache Rep. *Current Science Inc*, 2010, 14(5), 404–8.

[9] Guerrero, ÁL; Herrero-Velázquez, S; Peñas, ML; Mulero, P; Pedraza, MI; Cortijo, E; et al. Peripheral nerve blocks: a therapeutic alternative for hemicrania continua. *Cephalalgia*. SAGE Publications, 2012 Apr, 32(6), 505–8.

[10] Piagkou, M; Demesticha, T; Troupis, T; Vlasis, K; Skandalakis, P; Makri, A; et al. The pterygopalatine ganglion and its role in various pain syndromes: from anatomy to clinical practice. *Pain Practice*. Blackwell Publishing Ltd., 2012 Jun, 12(5), 399–412.

[11] Windsor, RE; Jahnke, S. Sphenopalatine ganglion blockade: a review and proposed modification of the transnasal technique. *Pain Physician*. 2004.

[12] Narouze, S; Kapural, L; Casanova, J; Mekhail, N. Sphenopalatine ganglion radiofrequency ablation for the management of chronic cluster headache. *Headache.* Blackwell Publishing Inc, 2009 Apr, 49(4), 571–7.

[13] Schoenen, J; Jensen, RH; Lantéri-Minet, M; Láinez, MJ; Gaul, C; Goodman, AM; et al. Stimulation of the sphenopalatine ganglion (SPG) for cluster headache treatment. Pathway CH-1: A randomized, sham-controlled study. *Cephalalgia.* SAGE Publications, 2013 Jul 1, 33(10), 816–30.

[14] Candido, KD; Massey, ST; Sauer, R; Darabad, RR; Knezevic, NN. A novel revision to the classical transnasal topical sphenopalatine ganglion block for the treatment of headache and facial pain. *Pain Physician.,* 2013 Nov, 16(6), E769–78.

[15] Sanders, M; Zuurmond, WW. Efficacy of sphenopalatine ganglion blockade in 66 patients suffering from cluster headache: a 12- to 70-month follow-up evaluation. *J Neurosurg.* 1997 Dec, 87(6), 876–80.

[16] Tepper, SJ; Rezai, A; Narouze, S; Steiner, C; Mohajer, P; Ansarinia, M. Acute Treatment of Intractable Migraine With Sphenopalatine Ganglion Electrical Stimulation. *Headache.* Blackwell Publishing Inc, 2009, 49(7), 983–9.

[17] Cohen, S; Trnovski, S; Zada, Y. A new interest in an old remedy for headache and backache for our obstetric patients: a sphenopalatine ganglion block. *Anaesthesia.* Blackwell Publishing Ltd, 2001, 56(6), 606–7.

[18] Felisati, G; Arnone, F; Lozza, P; Leone, M; Curone, M; Bussone, G. Sphenopalatine endoscopic ganglion block: *a revision of a traditional technique for cluster headach*e. Laryngoscope. John Wiley & Sons, Inc, 2006 Aug, 116(8), 1447–50.

[19] Pipolo, C; Bussone, G; Leone, M; Lozza, P; Felisati, G. Sphenopalatine endoscopic ganglion block in cluster headache: a reevaluation of the procedure after 5 years. *Neurol Sci. Springer Milan*, 2010, 31(1), 197–9.

[20] Waldman, S. (2007) *Pain Management.* Philadelphia, PA: Saunders.

[21] Pieper, D; Dickerson, J; Hassenbusch, SJ. Percutaneous retrogasserian glycerol rhizolysis for treatment of chronic intractable cluster headaches: long-term results. *Neurosurgery*, 2000 Feb, 46(2), 363-70.

In: Migraine Surgery
Editor: Antonios Mammis

ISBN: 978-1-63321-761-4

Chapter 7

Decompression Procedures

Adam M. Feintisch, Edward S. Lee and Mark S. Granick *
Division of Plastic Surgery, Department of Surgery,
Rutgers New Jersey Medical School Newark, New Jersey, US

Introduction

Since man first experienced migraine headaches, there have been surgical attempts to relieve the associated pain and misery. As early as 7,000 BCE and as recently as the 17th century, "letting evil spirits escape" through trephination of the calvarium has been documented. [1-3] However, as one could imagine, few fortunate souls survived such procedures.

Within the United States, migraine headaches represent a huge economic burden, costing $14-16 billion annually. [4,5] Although the prevalence and distribution of migraine headaches has remained relatively stable over the last 15 years migraine-associated disability remains pervasive and substantial. [6-10]. Approximately 10% of the worldwide population is affected annually, and an estimated 35 million Americans suffer from this disease. [11,12] There is also a significant prevalence within the pediatric population, affecting 5% of young children and 10% of adolescents. [13]

Although there have been major advances in pharmacologic therapy, patients must wait for rescue medications to take effect and many continue to experience poor quality of life despite aggressive medication regimens. [14] Moreover, many of the available preventive and abortive medications have side effects that may lead to treatment discontinuation. Potential adverse effects range from weight gain and cognitive impairment to gastrointestinal disturbances (i.e.: gastric ulcers, gastrointestinal bleeding, nausea, vomiting) and medication overuse headaches. Although the medical management of migraines has seen significant progress, a large subset of patients remains refractory to current therapeutic standards of care. [15] Migraineurs who either fail medical therapy or are not candidates for medical management may benefit from surgical management.

*Corresponding author: Mark S. Granick, M.D. mgranickmd@njms.rutgers.edu Office: 973-972-9383, 973-972-5377.

Table 1. Migraine headache diagnostic criteria

Migraine without aura	
A	At least 5 attacks fulfilling criteria B-D
B	Headache attacks lasting 4-72 hours (untreated or unsuccessfully treated)
C	Headache has at least 2 of the following characteristics: 1. Unilateral location 2. Pulsating quality 3. Moderate or severe pain intensity 4. Aggravation by or causing avoidance of routine physical activity (e.g., walking or climbing stairs)
D	During headache at least 1 of the following: 1. Nausea and/or vomiting 2. Photophobia and phonophobia
E	Not attributed to another disorder
(Adapted from International Headache Society website: hyyp://ihs-classification.org)	

Migraine with aura	
A	At least 2 attacks fulfilling criteria B-D
B	Aura consisting of at least 1 of the following, but no motor weakness: 1. Fully reversible visual symptoms including positive features (e.g., flickering lights, spots or lines) and/or negative features (e.g., loss of vision) 2. Fully reversible sensory symptoms including positive features (e.g., pins and needles) and/or negative features (e.g., numbness) 3. Fully reversible dysphasic speech disturbance
C	At least 2 of the following: 1. Homonymous visual symptoms and/or unilateral sensory symptoms 2. At least 1 aura symptom develops gradually over ≥5 minutes and/or different aura symptoms occur in succession over ≥5 minutes
D	Headache fulfilling criteria B-D for migraine without aura begins during the aura or follows aura within 60 minutes
E	Not attributed to another disorder
(Adapted from International Headache Society website: hyyp://ihs-classification.org)	

Recently, a variety of surgical procedures for the relief of migraine headaches have been suggested and are actively being researched. Interventions have included cauterization, cryotherapy or ligation of the superficial vessels of the scalp, removal of possible sites of muscle or fascial nerve entrapment, neurectomies, osteotomies, intranasal ablative procedures and even repair of certain congenital heart defects. Most of the current focus for surgical intervention, however, has been on the deactivation of extracranial trigger sites of migraine headache. We will discuss the techniques and outcomes for trigger site decompression, neurectomy, and arterial ligation.

Trigger Site Decompression

Over the past decade, there has been a flurry of interest in the surgical deactivation of extracranial trigger sites for treatment of migraine headaches. Although migraine headaches were initially thought to be a primary disorder of the cerebral vasculature, a more contemporary view is that migraines are a primary neurogenic disorder. Current surgical treatment focuses on the role of the distal trigeminal nerve in the pathogenesis of migraines. Although the exact mechanisms are unclear, it has been demonstrated that stimulation of this cranial nerve, whether through muscle contraction, compression, or irritation of perinasal sinus linings, results in the release of neuropeptides such as substance P, neurokinin A and calcitonin gene-related peptide. [16,17] These proinflammatory neuropeptides produce a localized sterile meningitis and likely play a crucial role in migraine headache development. [18-21]

Currently, migraine surgery can be performed at four common trigger sites: frontal, temporal, intranasal and occipital. This method was first introduced by Dr. Bahman Guyuron who after performing corrugator supercilii muscle resection in patients undergoing forehead rejuvenation procedures noticed that a significant number of his patients had experienced alleviation of their migraine headaches. [22] In conjunction with reports of the efficacy of botulinum toxin in migraine treatment, further support was generated in the peripheral theory of migraine triggers. [23]

Patient Selection

The success of migraine surgery depends upon appropriate patient selection. Establishing a diagnosis of migraine headaches requires careful examination by a neurologist and a conformation to the diagnostic criteria set forth by the International Headache Society (Table 1]. [24] Patients may have additional headache disorders (i.e.: cluster headaches, tension-type headaches, cervicogenic headaches), and must be selected appropriately. More serious causes of headaches must be excluded and patients must display a history of migraine headaches not amenable to traditional medical treatment and demonstrate an acceptable surgical risk. After a careful history of symptoms and physical exam suggest a potential trigger site, a variety of validated questionnaires are used to collect baseline data of migraine characteristics. Migraine-associated pain has been described to originate from a variety of locations, mainly the forehead, temple and occiput. Septonasal triggers are suggested through a history of retroocular pain and supported by intranasal exam and CT scans showing septal deviation with turbinate enlargement. [21] Patients are then ready for trigger site identification via botulinum toxin type A trial injections or local anesthetic nerve blocks. A proposed algorithm for the stepwise identification of migraine trigger sites by botulinum toxin injection and for progression to surgical intervention are detailed in Figures 1 and 2. [21] Surgical intervention should be considered for each trigger site that yields either sustained migraine elimination or a significant improvement for at least 4 consecutive weeks, which Guyuron and colleagues have defined as at least 50 percent reduction in intensity and/or frequency of migraines from baseline. [21, 25-30]

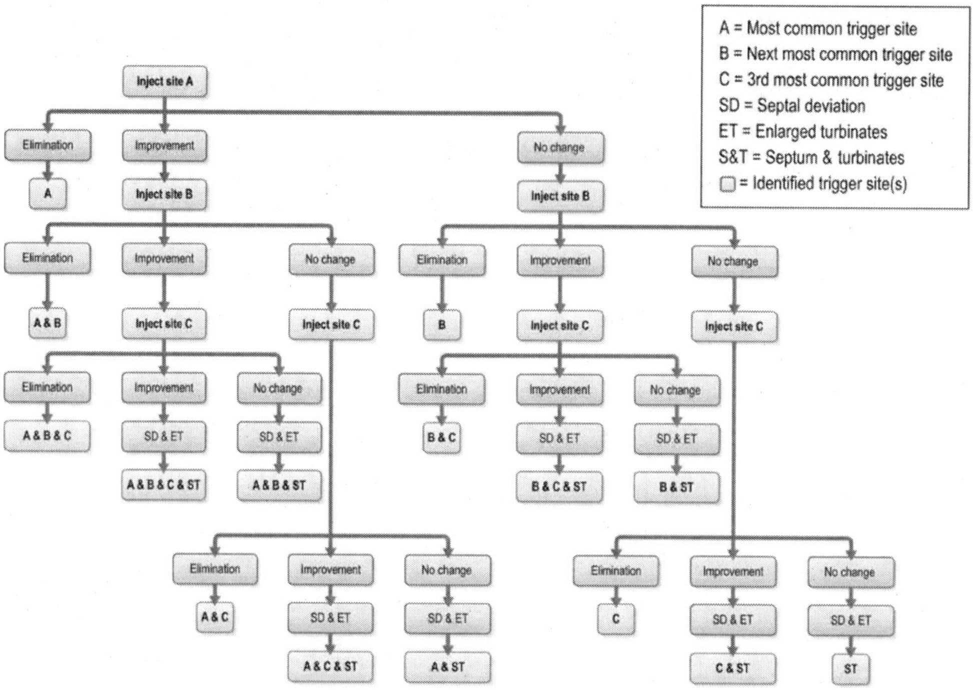

Figure 1. Algorithm for identification of migraine headache trigger sites by botulinum toxin injection. (From Kung, TA, Guyuron, B, Cederna, PS. Migraine Surgery: A Plastic Surgery Solution for Refractory Migraine Headache. Plast Reconstr Surg 2011;127(1):181-189).

Botulinum toxin has been FDA-approved for the treatment of chronic migraine headaches. Although efficacious, the toxins effects are temporary and have an inherent risk of potential adverse events. Side effects may include injection-site pain, blepharoptosis, diplopia and significant muscle atrophy (i.e.: temporal hourglass deformity). [21,31,71] A more permanent solution than chemical denervation would be preferable. Therefore, botulinum toxin injections may be beneficial in determining which patients would benefit from surgical peripheral nerve decompression. Guyuron has described use of botulinum toxin injections as a diagnostic modality in his preoperative patient selection. The botulinum toxin is injected at one trigger site per visit, starting with the most severe and common site based on the patients constellation of symptoms. Injections are performed 1 month apart, if necessary, until all trigger sites are confirmed. [25,26] This enables a maximum of up to three injections so that the involvement of each of the 4 common trigger sites can be confirmed. Such a lengthy diagnostic period (up to 3 months) is not ideal. Not only is surgical intervention delayed until diagnosis is confirmed, however surgery must also be postponed until the effects of the botulinum toxin have subsided as muscle atrophy has been noted to complicate surgical resection. [25]

Recently, in a study of 335 patients, Liu and colleagues showed no statistical difference in overall surgical outcome whether patients were diagnosed using botulinum toxin injections or a constellation of symptoms. [25] In patients diagnosed using Botox versus a constellation of symptoms, 84 versus 80 percent experienced a ≥50 percent reduction in migraine index, with 36 versus 32 percent experiencing complete elimination of migraine headaches, respectively. With no statistical difference regardless of trigger site evaluated, the authors concluded that testing with botulinum toxin type A with stepwise injections is not always necessary for the localization of migraine trigger sites as surgical outcomes are not significantly improved. Instead, trigger sites can be reliably identified through physical exam, symptomatic history and use of computed tomographic scans when necessary (i.e.: evaluation of paranasal sinuses). However, for those surgeons with limited experience in diagnosing trigger sites, the use of Botox or nerve blocks may still be helpful.

Trigger Sites

Trigger site surgery consists of either nerve resection or the excision of muscles, fascia and/or vessels believed to irritate the terminal branches of the trigeminal nerve supplying specific areas of the head and neck associated with migraine pain. The exact operation varies depending on the trigger site involved. Surgical procedures have been developed at all 4 trigger sites: frontal, temporal, occipital, and intranasal. Details of the surgeries have been documented in previously published reports. [21, 22, 26-28, 30, 32, 33] The procedures are performed under general endotracheal tube anesthesia in an ambulatory care setting. They take an average of 1 hour to complete.

Frontal

The peripheral theory of migraine headaches identifies the frontal trigger site as responsible for a large proportion of migraines due to compression and irritation of the supratrochlear and supraorbital nerves [34-36]. Compression occurs as the nerves pass through the glabellar muscle group, including the corrugator supercilii, depressor supercilii and procerus muscles. [35, 37-43] Surgical intervention in this area involves complete resection of these glabellar muscles encasing the involved nerves. [22] This can be accomplished either via a transpalpebral or endoscopic approach (Figure 3). For those who also suffer from temporal trigger sites in conjunction with a frontal trigger, the endoscopic approach can accomplish decompression of these two sites simultaneously. [21, 39, 40, 44, 45] Fat from the upper eyelid can be used to fill the defect after muscle resection and to shield the nerve from further irritation. [33]

Temporal

As the second most likely trigger site, temporal migraine headaches are presumed to be secondary to inflammation of the zygomaticotemporal branch of the trigeminal nerve. [37] Previous anatomical work has indicated nerve activation through contraction of the temporalis muscles. [37, 43] There is also most likely a contribution from adjacent vessels leading to additional irritation. [30, 37] To treat migraines located at this trigger site, approximately 2-3 cm of the zygomaticotemporal branch of the trigeminal nerve is avulsed endoscopically as it passes through the substance of the temporalis muscle. [21, 33]

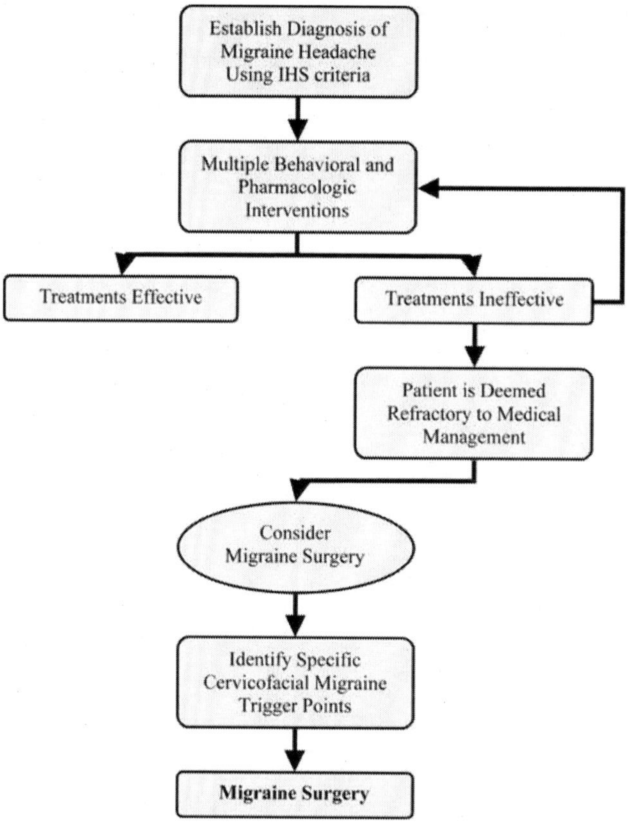

Figure 2. Practice of migraine surgery for patients with refractory migraine headache. IHS, International Headache Society. (From Kung, TA, Guyuron, B, Cederna, PS. Migraine Surgery: A Plastic Surgery Solution for Refractory Migraine Headache. Plast Reconstr Surg 2011;127(1):181-189).

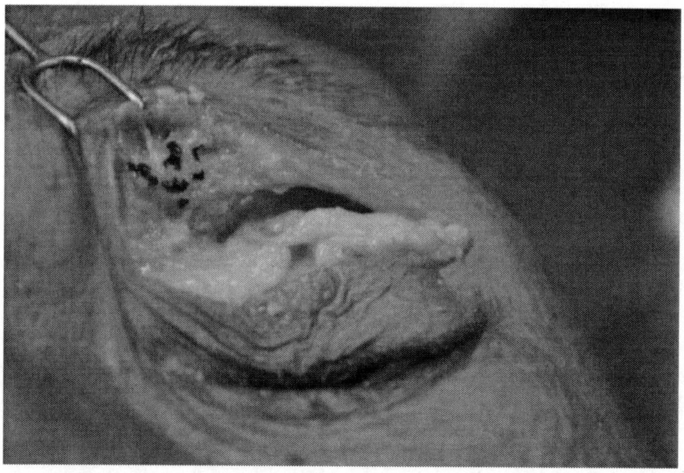

Figure 3. Transpalpebral view of the supraorbital branch of the trigeminal nerve with its accompanying vascular supply.

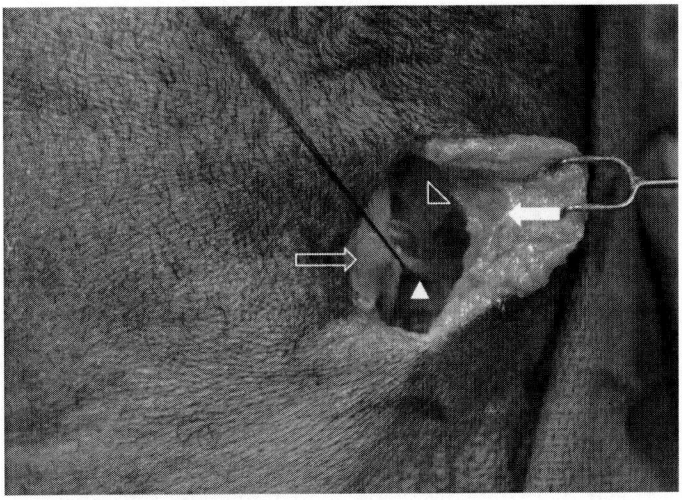

Figure 4. Occipital nerve anatomy identified at surgical decompression. Midline raphe (line arrow), trapezius fascia (solid arrow), occipital nerve – retracted (solid arrowhead), semispinalis muscle fibers (line arrowhead).

Occipital

Occipital headaches may be triggered by irritation of the occipital nerve at a number of identified compression points including the semispinalis capitis muscle and the occipital artery. [36, 46-48] This mechanical entrapment has been shown in numerous studies to be the impetus for nerve irritation. [36-48] Although there has been some suggestion that excision of the occipital artery may be of some benefit, more recent publications have discredited primary arterial inflammation as a mechanism of occipital neuralgia, with studies showing lowered operative success with occipital arterial ligation. [49-53] Relief of occipital neuralgia has been shown to occur with removal of a segment of the semispinalis capitis muscle medial to the greater occipital nerve approximately 1 cm wide and 2.5 cm long, followed by insertion of a subcutaneous flap between the nerve and the muscle to avoid nerve impingement (Figure 4). [21, 33, 54,55].

Septonasal

When diagnostic botulinum toxin type A injections into the previously described trigger sites do not provide adequate relief and symptoms indicate a septonasal trigger, surgical intervention in this area must be considered. [25,33] Termed exploding migraine headaches, these septonasal headaches are resistant to the effects of Botox as they originate in the deeper trigeminal nerve branches within the lining of the turbinates, septum and sinuses. [28,56] Septonasal migraines may involve a variety of intranasal abnormalities including septal deviation, spur-turbinate contact, concha bullosa, septa bullosa and Haller cells. [33,57,58] These anatomic variations are appreciable through a combination of a thorough history, physical exam, and computed tomography. They are thought to irritate the peripheral trigeminal afferents via friction between intranasal structures leading to neuropeptide release and subsequent reduction in migraine threshold initiation. [25, 28, 33, 58-60] Surgical treatment includes septoplasty and turbinectomy in an effort to eliminate contact points and decompress any concha or septa bullosa. [21, 30, 33, 57, 59-61]

Additional Sites

Aside from the abovementioned trigger sites, less common points of nerve irritation have been implicated in the evolution of peripheral migraine headaches. [29] These include the auriculotemporal nerve and lesser and third occipital nerves and their compression via the superficial temporal artery and surrounding investing fascia/muscle, respectively. [62-64] Although surgical approaches have been suggested, detailed anatomical studies have been cadaveric in nature and there remains a paucity of literature consistent with randomized controlled trials (RCTs) to support surgical decompression.

Evidence

Despite promising results, skepticism surrounding decompression procedures continues and widespread acceptance remains hindered by select case studies and few RCTs. In his initial report in 2000, Guyuron et al. showed retrospectively that 79.5 percent of 39 patients identified through questionnaires experienced elimination or improvement in their migraine headaches after forehead rejuvenation surgery. [22] Since then, two published RCTs, both performed by Dr. Guyuron's group, have substantiated this claim. [26,30] In the first prospective study, patients underwent surgical resection of the corrugate supercilii muscles alone or in conjunction with transection of the zygomaticotemporal branch of the trigeminal nerve with soft tissue repositioning to prevent nerve recoaptation. The study showed a 95.5 percent improvement in migraine headaches; 45.5 percent noting complete elimination and 50 percent with significant improvement, as defined previously. Patients experienced a significant reduction in migraine intensity and frequency over an average follow-up of 347 days however this study was non-blinded and did not have a control group. [26] Subsequently, in 2005, the same institution presented another prospective study involving 89 patients who underwent surgical decompression of one to four trigger sites after diagnosis via botulinum toxin injections. At 1-year follow up, complete elimination or significant improvement of migraine headaches were seen in 35 and 57 percent of patients, respectively, equating to a 92 percent benefit of surgery in the treatment group. Also seen was a significant improvement in average migraine headache frequency, intensity, duration and migraine headache index for the treatment group compared with the control group. Interestingly, 15.8 percent in the control group noted headache improvement after 1-year follow up, however no control patients reported migraine elimination. [30]

Additional studies have supported the peripheral theory of nerve compression. Poggi et al. showed in their 2007 retrospective review that 16.7 percent of patients experienced complete elimination of migraines with 72.2 percent experiencing $\geq$ 50 percent improvement. [27] The majority of patients completely discontinued or significantly reduced their medication requirements, and about 60 percent saw decreased frequency, duration and intensity in their migraines. Interestingly, although nearly all patients experienced migraine relief initially, some experienced return of their migraines by 6 months, as central forehead sensation returned. All, however, still continued to relate improved quality of life than prior to surgical intervention. [27] This study was limited, however, by its retrospective nature, low power, inherent selection as well as patient memory bias. Similar outcomes were seen by Dirnberger and Becker who in a prospective study of 60 patients saw a gradual return of headaches between 4 and 6 months postoperatively. Although overall headache quality was improved from baseline, initial success rates of 86.7 percent at 1 month dropped to 68.3 percent of patients experiencing migraine improvement or elimination by 6 months. This was in contrast to the sustained results seen in Guyuron et al. initial studies. Additionally, those with milder forms of migraines had a better chance at surgical success (almost 90 percent), however this was not deemed to be statistically significant. [32]

Although many of these studies offer validity to the peripheral theory of migraine headaches and to surgical decompression of the involved nerves, limitations remain including differences in definitions of migraine improvement, lack of controls and small sample sizes. In response to the criticism of a possible placebo effect, in 2009 Guyuron and colleagues published a randomized, placebo-controlled trial. [28] In this study 49 of 75 patients underwent surgical deactivation of frontal, temporal and occipital trigger sites while the remaining 26 patients in the control group received sham surgery consisting of exposure of the involved areas through similar incisions, however the integrity of the associated muscles and nerves were maintained. Overall, 83.7 percent in the surgery group reported significant improvement at 1 year compared with 57.7 percent in the sham surgery group. Migraine headache elimination was seen in 57.1 percent of those who underwent actual decompression versus 3.8 percent (one of 26 patients) in those who underwent the sham operation. The relatively high incidence of symptomatic improvement seen in the sham surgery group was attributed to a combination of placebo effect and the potential for altered neurosensory function secondary to the actual incision and tissue undermining performed. Additionally, it was suggested that an even higher rate of surgical success might have been achieved if more than the proposed principal trigger site was addressed as this predominant site was not necessarily the sole migraine origin. [28, 65]

A five-year outcome analysis of the 2005 study showed strong evidence to support surgical intervention of one or more trigger sites in the reduction and possible elimination of migraine headaches. [29] Of their initial 89 patients, 79 completed the 5-year follow up requirements. Since the time of the initial surgery, 10 patients underwent surgical deactivation of additional trigger sites and were therefore not included in the analysis. Based on the criteria of a ≥50 percent improvement in headache frequency, duration and intensity, 88 percent of patients maintained an overall improvement with 29 percent experiencing complete elimination. A 90 percent surgical success was seen when the 10 patients who underwent additional decompression were included lending support that most patients have more than one trigger point. [29, 66]. Surgical complications were reported to be low, with few patients experiencing itching, hair thinning, hyper- or hyposensitivity along the course of the supraorbital or supratrochlear nerves, or mild occipital stiffness or weakness. Overall, reports from Guyuron et al. have demonstrated that between 83 and 92 percent of patients experienced positive outcomes at 1 year with almost a 90 success maintained at 5 years. Improvement in surgical outcomes have been noted to occur in patients who are older at the time of migraine onset, have a higher rate of visual symptoms, who undergo surgery at the frontal or temporal sites and those who are deactivated at all four operative sites simultaneously. [61] Surgical failures have been shown to be attributable to factors such as increased intraoperative bleeding and surgery on only 1-2 trigger sites. [61]

Significant cost savings have also been suggested to occur with surgical deactivation of migraine trigger sites, despite the initial high costs associated with the surgery itself. Faber et al. showed that at 5 years postoperatively, a total median cost reduction of $3950 per patient was observed. [67] Patients were shown to spend significantly less time and money on migraine treatments, including drug therapy and alternative treatment modalities. They were also shown to experience an increase in work days and overall productivity, possibly improving indirect costs associated with employers, patients and their families.

Arterial Surgery

There have been numerous studies suggesting involvement of the trigeminovasacular system in the pathogenesis of migraine-associated pain. Specifically, involvement of the terminal branches of the external carotid artery, including the superficial temporal artery (STA) and its frontal branch, as well as the occipital artery, have been implicated. Release of neuropeptides and vasodilatation are largely thought to be responsible, however, there remains considerable controversy as to whether the vascular component of pain arises from intracranial vessels, extracranial vessels or both. [68]

Initially described by Abu al-Qasim Al-Zahrawi (936-1013 AD), arterial surgery for the treatment of migraines was largely pioneered in the 1940s by Harold Wolff and colleagues. Their research supported the vascular theory of migraine development and believed distention of the terminal branches of the external carotid artery were responsible for the symptoms of pain and hyperesthesia. [69-71] There have, however, been numerous attempts to discredit Wolff's vascular theory, and until recently, arterial surgery had largely been forgotten as a therapeutic option. Elliot Shevel, a headache specialist in South Africa, has been largely responsible for a renewed interest in minimally invasive arterial surgery.

Patient Selection

Minimally invasive arterial surgery should only be considered in those patients with presumed extracranial vascular pain. Patients who experience relief by direct digital pressure over a terminal external carotid arterial branch, or through the use of a tension band around the head, may benefit from surgical cauterization or ligation of the relevant artery. [72,73] Similarly, surgery may be indicated in patients who experience pain relief with use of vasoconstrictive medications (i.e.: triptans, ergots). Surgery should only be considered in those who have not responded to conventional drug therapy, who are unable to tolerate pharmacotherapy due to side effects or drug interactions, or those who do not wish to be on permanent medication. Minimally invasive arterial surgery has had promising results in select patients with severely compromised quality of life, and in particular, those who do not experience relief from pharmacotherapy. [74] In addition to pain relief, Shevel also demonstrated enhanced quality of life and improved migraine associated symptoms such as aura, photophobia, phonophobia, nausea and vomiting. [74]

Surgical Technique

The vessels found most frequently to be associated with pain are the main trunk of the STA, the frontal branch of the STA, occipital artery and posterior auricular artery. In Shevel's description, an ultrasonic doppler was used to identify each vessel of interest. Following identification of the vessel, a small 1-2 cm incision was made directly over the vessel. The vessel was then ligated. Numerous anatomical descriptions of the abovementioned arteries have been previously published and ought to prove useful should arterial ligation surgery be considered as a theraputic intervention. [75-79].

Arterial Surgery Results

To date, there have been no randomized controlled trials involving arterial ligation, excision or cauterization for the treatment of migraine headaches. Although intriguing, Dr. Shevel's results have not been duplicated by others. While the potential for therapeutic applicability may be valid, currently there remains a paucity of data to support the use of arterial surgery within the migraine treatment algorithm. There remains a need for future research.

Barriers and the Future

There is significant interest and growing support within the plastic surgery community for the treatment of migraine headaches through surgical intervention. Unfortunately, several barriers to offering this treatment exist and have prevented widespread practice. Such barriers include lack of knowledge of the disease and treatment process, minimal familiarity with surgical techniques as well as difficulty in public relations and patient referrals. Increased referrals by neurologists of suitable patients and enhanced familiarity with the disorder of migraines, surgical techniques and available supportive literature may motivate more plastic surgeons to perform migraine surgery. [80] It is therefore our job as informed physicians to not only educate our patients, but more importantly our colleagues in order to provide additional options in the armamentarium against migraine headaches.

Reported patient outcomes after surgical intervention for migraine headaches have ignited intense interest in these procedures. With high levels of patient satisfaction and results showing near complete to total resolution of migraines in select patient groups, this is an exciting time for migraineurs and the field of Plastic Surgery. The majority of available research suggests a significant potential benefit from nerve decompression of trigger sites for migraine headache relief. Currently, however, there remains insufficient evidence to recommend or establish standards of care. The need for more placebo-controlled randomized clinical trials by additional research groups to uphold or challenge the current published literature is apparent.

Lastly, although it has been suggested that other types of headaches (i.e.: tension-type) may also be triggered by trigeminal nerve irritation, a mechanism of action is less established for headaches other than migraines. Therefore, although intriguing, the potential for a surgical benefit through similar treatment techniques cannot be recommended until published studies have evaluated such interventions for non-migraine headaches.

References

[1] Miller, Neil. (2005). Walsh and Hoyt's clinical neuro-ophthalmology: 6th Edition. Philadelphia, PA: Lippincott Williams & Wilkins. p1275.

[2] Colen, C, B. & Colen, R. E. (2008). Operative Dictation: Neurosurgery. Green Pointe Woods, MI: Colen Publishing, LLC. p1.

[3] Daniel, B. T. (2010). Migraine: The History of Migraine. Bloomington, IN: AuthorHouse. p.101.

[4] Hu, X. H., Markson, L. E., Lipton, R. B. et al. (1999). Burden of migraine in the United States: Disability and economic costs. *Arch Intern Med*, *159*, 813-818.

[5] Goldberg, L. D. (2005). The cost of migraine and its treatment. *Am J Manag Care*, *11*(2 Suppl), S62–S67

[6] Stewart, W. F., Shechter, A. & Rasmussen, B. K. (1994). Migraine prevalence: A review of population-based studies. *Neurology*, *44*(Suppl 4), S17-S23.

[7] Lipton, R. B., Stewart, W. F. Diamond, S. et al. (2001). Prevalence and burden of migraine in the United States: Data from the American Migraine Study II. *Headache*, *41*, 646-657.

[8] Patel, N. V., Bigal, M. E., Kolodner, K. B., et al. (2004). Prevalence and impact of migraine and probable migraine in a health plan. *Neurology*, *63*, 1432-1438.

[9] Lipton, R. B., Bigal, M. E., Diamond, M., et al. (2007). Migraine prevalence, disease burden, and the need for preventive therapy. *Neurology*, *68*, 343-349.

[10] Rasmussen, B. K., Jensen, R., Schroll, M. & Olesen, J. (1992). "Interrelations between migraine and tension-type headache in the general population". *Arch Neurol.*, *49*(9), 914–8.

[11] Jensen, R. & Stovner, L. J. (2008). "Epidemiology and comorbidity of headache". *The Lancet Neurology*, *7* (4), 354–361.

[12] Bigal, M. E. & Lipton, R. B. (2009). The epidemiology, burden, and comorbidities of migraine. *Neurol Clin.*, *41*, 646-657.

[13] Hämäläinen, M. L. (2006). Migraine in children and adolescents: A guide to drug treatment. *CNS Drugs*, *20*, 813-820

[14] Solomon, G. D., Skobieranda, F. G. & Gragg, L. A. (1993). "Quality of life and well-being of headache patients: measurement by the medical outcomes study instrument.". *Headache*, *33* (7), 351–8.

[15] D'Amico, D., Leone, M., Grazzi, L. & Bussone, G. (2008). When should "chronic migraine" patients be considered "refractory" to pharmacological prophylaxis? *Neurol Sci.*, *29*, S55-58.

[16] Moskowitz, M. A. (1984). The neurobiology of vascular head pain. *Ann Neurol.*, *16*, 157.
[17] Goetz, C. & Pappert, E. (1999). *Textbook of Clinical Neurology.* Philadelphia: Saunders.
[18] Spierings, E. L. (2003). Pathogenesis of the migraine attack. *Clin J Pain.*, *19*, 255-262
[19] Fusco, M., D'Andrea, G., Miccichè, F., Stecca, A., Bernardini, D. & Cananzi, A. L.(2003). Neurogenic inflammation in primary headaches. *Neurol Sci.*, *24*, S61-64
[20] Aoki, K. R. (2003). Evidence for antinociceptive activity of botulinum toxin type A in pain management. *Headache*, *43*, S9-15.
[21] Kung, T. A., Guyuron, B. & Cederna, P. S. (2011). Migraine surgery: a plastic surgery solution for refractory migraine headache. *Plast Reconstr Surg.*, Jan, *127*(1), 181-9.
[22] Guyuron, B., Varghai, A., Michelow, B. J., Thomas, T. & Davis, J. (2000). Corrugator supercilii muscle resection and migraine headaches. *Plast Reconstr Surg.*, *106*, 429–434; discussion 435–436.
[23] Janis, J. E., Dhanik, A. & Howard, J. H. (2011). Validation of the peripheral trigger point theory of migraine headaches: single-surgeon experience using botulinum toxin and surgical decompression. *Plast Reconstr Surg.*, Jul, *128*(1), 123-31.
[24] Headache Classification Subcommittee of the International Headache Society. *International Classification of Headache Disorders, 2nd Ed. Cephalalgia, 24* (Suppl. 1). 2004. Available at: http://ihs-classification.org/downloads/mixed/Watermarked ShortForm%20ICHD-II.pdf. Accessed Dec 29, 2013.
[25] Liu, M. T., Armijo, B. S. & Guyuron, B. (2012). A comparison of outcome of surgical treatment of migraine headaches using a constellation of symptoms versus botulinum toxin type A to identify the trigger sites. *Plast Reconstr Surg.* Feb, *129*(2), 413-9.
[26] Guyuron, B., Tucker, T. & Davis, J. (2002). Surgical treatment of migraine headaches. *Plast Reconstr Surg.*, 109, 2183–2189.
[27] Poggi, J. T., Grizzell, B. E. & Helmer, S. D. (2008). Confirmation of surgical decompression to relieve migraine headaches. *Plast Reconstr Surg.*, *122*, 115–122.
[28] Guyuron, B., Reed, D., Kriegler, J. S., Davis, J., Pashmini, N. & Amini, S. (2009). A placebo-controlled surgical trial of the treatment of migraine headaches. *Plast Reconstr Surg.*, *124*, 461–468.
[29] Guyuron, B., Kriegler, J. S. Davis, J. & Amini, S. B. (2009). Five year outcome of surgical treatment of migraine headaches. *Plast Reconstr Surg.*, *124*, 11.
[30] Guyuron, B., Kriegler, J. S., Davis, J. & Amini, SB. (2005). Comprehensive surgical treatment of migraine headaches. *Plast Reconstr Surg.*, *115*, 1–9.
[31] Aurora, S. (2006). Botulinum toxin type A for the treatment of migraine. *Expert Opin Pharmacother.*, *7*, 1085-95.
[32] Dirnberger, F. & Becker, K. (2004). Surgical treatment of migraine headaches by corrugator muscle resection. *Plast Reconstr Surg.*, *114*, 652–657.
[33] Guyuron, B. & Totonchi, A. (2013). Surgical management of migraine headaches. In: Rodriguez, ED, Losee JE, eds. Plastic Surgery, 3rd Edition, Volume 3: Craniofacial, *Head and Neck Surgery and Pediatric Plastic Surgery*. Saunders/Elsevier, 491-499.
[34] Sjaastad, O., Stolt-Nielsen, A., Pareja, J. A., Fredriksen, T. A. & Vincent, M. (1999). Supraorbital neuralgia. On the clinical manifestations and a possible therapeutic approach. *Headache*, Mar, *39*(3), 204-12.

[35] Chepla, K. J., Oh, E. & Guyuron, B. (2012). Clinical outcomes following supraorbital foraminotomy for treatment of frontal migraine headache. *Plast Reconstr Surg.*, Apr, *129*(4), 656e-62e.

[36] Mosser, S. W., Guyuron, B., Janis, J. E. & Rohrich, R. J. (2004). The anatomy of the greater occipital nerve: Implications for the etiology of migraine headaches. *Plast Reconstr Surg.*, 113, 693–697.

[37] Totonchi, A., Pashmini, N. & Guyuron, B. (2005). The zygomaticotemporal branch of the trigeminal nerve: An anatomical study. *Plast Reconstr Surg.*, 115, 273–277.

[38] Janis, J. E., Ghavami, A., Lemmon, J. A., Leedy, J. E. & Guyuron, B. (2008). The anatomy of the corrugator supercilii muscle: Part II. Supraorbital nerve branching patterns. *Plast Reconstr Surg.*, 121, 233–240.

[39] Liu, M. T., Chim, H. & Guyuron, B. (2012). Outcome comparison of endoscopic and transpalpebral decompression for treatment of frontal migraine headaches. *Plast Reconstr Surg.*, May, *129*(5), 1113-9.

[40] Amirlak, B. (2012). Discussion: outcome comparison of endoscopic and transpalpebral decompression for treatment of frontal migraine headaches. *Plast Reconstr Surg.*, May; *129*(5), 1120-2.

[41] Janis, J. E., Hatef, D. A., Hagan, R., Schaub, T., Liu, J. H., Thakar, H., Bolden, K. M., Heller, J. B. & Kurkjian, T. J. (2013). Anatomy of the supratrochlear nerve: implications for the surgical treatment of migraine headaches. *Plast Reconstr Surg.*, Apr, *131*(4), 743-50.

[42] Fallucco, M., Janis, J. E. & Hagan, R. R. (2012). The anatomical morphology of the supraorbital notch: clinical relevance to the surgical treatment of migraine headaches. *Plast Reconstr Surg.*, Dec, *130*(6), 1227-33.

[43] Janis, J. E., Hatef, D. A., Thakar, H., Reece, E. M., Theivagt, C. & Guyuron, B. (2010). The zygomaticotemporal branch of the trigeminal nerve: Part II. Anatomic variations. *Plast Reconstr Surg.*, *126*, 435–442.

[44] Guyuron, B. (2001).Corrugator supercilii resection through blepharoplasty incision. *Plast. Reconstr. Surg.*, 107, 604.

[45] Janis, J. E., Ghavami, A., Lemmon, J. A., Leedy, J. E. & Guyuron, B. (2007). Anatomy of the corrugator supercilii muscle: Part I. Corrugator topography. *Plast Reconstr Surg.*, *120*, 1647–1653.

[46] Janis, J. E., Hatef, D. A., Ducic, I., et al. (2010). The anatomy of the greater occipital nerve: Part II. Compression point topography. *Plast Reconstr Surg.*, 126, 1563–1572.

[47] Ducic, I., Moriarty, M. & Al-Attar, A. (2009). Anatomical variations of the occipital nerves: Implications for the treatment of chronic headaches. *Plast Reconstr Surg.*, *123*, 859–863.

[48] Janis, J. E., Hatef, D. A., Reece, E. M., McCluskey, P. D., Schaub, T. A. & Guyuron, B. (2010). Neurovascular compression of the greater occipital nerve: Implications for migraine headaches. *Plast Reconstr Surg.*, 126, 1996–2001.

[49] Cornely, C., Fischer, M., Ingianni, G. & Isenmann, S. (2011). Greater occipital nerve neuralgia caused by pathological arterial contact: treatment by surgical decompression. *Headache*, Apr, *51*(4), 609-12.

[50] Ducic, I., Felder, J. M., 3rd, & Janis, J. E. Occipital artery vasculitis not identified as a mechanism of occipital neuralgia-related chronic migraine headaches. *Plast Reconstr Surg.*, Oct, *128*(4), 908-12.

[51] Guyuron, B. (2011). Discussion. Occipital artery vasculitis not identified as a mechanism of occipital neuralgia-related chronic migraine headaches. *Plast Reconstr Surg*. Oct, *128*(4), 913-4.

[52] Dellon, A. L. (2011). Discussion. Occipital artery vasculitis not identified as a mechanism of occipital neuralgia-related chronic migraine headaches. *Plast Reconstr Surg.*, Oct, *128*(4), 915-7.

[53] Chmielewski, L., Liu, M. T. & Guyuron, B. (2013). The role of occipital artery resection in the surgical treatment of occipital migraine headaches. *Plast Reconstr Surg.*, Mar, *131*(3), 351e-6e.

[54] Li, F., Ma, Y., Zou, J., Li, Y., Wang, B., Huang, H., Wang, Q. & Li, L. (2012). Microsurgical decompression for greater occipital neuralgia. *Turk Neurosurg.*, *22*(4), 427-9.

[55] Ducic, I., Hartmann, E. C. & Larson, E. E. (2009). Indications and outcomes for surgical treatment of patients with chronic migraine headaches caused by occipital neuralgia. *Plast Reconstr Surg*. 2009, *123*, 1453–1461.

[56] Jakubowski, M., McAllister, P. J., Bajwa, Z. H., Ward, T. N., Smith, P. & Burstein, R. (2006). Exploding vs. imploding headache in migraine prophylaxis with botulinum toxin A. *Pain.*, *125*, 286-295.

[57] Welge-Luessen, A., Hauser, R., Schmid, N., Kappos, L. & Probst, R. (2003). Endonasal surgery for contact point headaches: A 10-year longitudinal study. *Laryngoscope*, *113*, 2151–2156.

[58] Behin, F., Lipton, R. B. & Bigal, M. (2006). Migraine and intranasal contact point headache: Is there any connection? *Curr Pain Headache Rep.*, *10*, 312–315.

[59] Behin, F., Behin, B., Bigal, M. E. & Lipton, R. B. (2004). Surgical treatment of patients with refractory migraine headaches and intranasal contact points. *Cephalalgia*, *25*, 439–443.

[60] Behin, F., Behin, B., Behin, D. & Baredes, S. (2005). Surgical management of contact point headaches. *Headache*, *45*, 204-210.

[61] Larson, K., Lee, M., Davis, J. & Guyuron, B. (2011). Factors contributing to migraine headache surgery failure and success. *Plast Reconstr Surg*. Nov, *128*(5), 1069-75.

[62] Janis, J. E., Hatef, D. A., Ducic, I., et al. (2010). Anatomy of the auriculotemporal nerve: Variations in its relationship to the superficial temporal artery and implications for the treatment of migraine headaches. *Plast Reconstr Surg.*, *125*, 1422–1428.

[63] Chim, H., Okada, H. C., Brown, M. S., Alleyne, B., Liu, M. T., Zwiebel, S. & Guyuron, B. (2012). The auriculotemporal nerve in etiology of migraine headaches: compression points and anatomical variations. *Plast Reconstr Surg.*, Aug, *130*(2), 336-41.

[64] Dash, K. S., Janis, J. E. & Guyuron, B. (2005). The lesser and third occipital nerves and migraine headaches. *Plast Reconstr Surg.*, *115*, 1752–1758.

[65] Janis, J. E. (2009). Discussion. A placebo-controlled surgical trial of the treatment of migraine headaches. *Plast Reconstr Surg.*, Aug, *124*(2), 469-70.

[66] Janis, J. E. (2011). Discussion. Five-year outcome of surgical treatment of migraine headaches. *Plast Reconstr Surg.*, Feb, *127*(2), 609-10.

[67] Faber, C., Garcia, R. M., Davis, J. & Guyuron, B. (2012). A socioeconomic analysis of surgical treatment of migraine headaches. *Plast Reconstr Surg.*, Apr, *129*(4), 871-7.

[68] Olesen, J., Diener, H. C., Husstedt, I. W., Goadsby, P. J., Hall, D., Meier, U., Pollentier, S. & Lesko, L. M. (2004). Calcitonin Gene-Related Peptide Receptor Antagonist BIBN

4096 BS for the Acute Treatment of Migraine. *N Engl J Med.*, March, *350*(11), 1104-1110.

[69] Tunis, M. M. & Wolff, H. G. (1953). Studies on headache: long-term observations of the reactivity of the cranial arteries in subjects with vascular headache of the migraine. *Arch. Neurol. Psychiatry.*, *75*, 551.

[70] Wolff, H. G. & Tunis, M. M. (1952). Analysis of cranial artery pressure waves in patients with vascular headaches of the migraine type. *Trans. Assoc. Am. Physicians.* *65*, 240.

[71] Guyuron, B., Rose, K., Kriegler, J. S. & Tucker, T. (2004). Hourglass deformity after botulinum toxin type A injection. *Headache*, *44*, 262-264.

[72] Zanchin, G., Maggioni, F., Granella, F., Rossi, P., Falco, L. & Manzoni, G. C. (2001). Self-administered pain-relieving maneuvers in primary headaches. *Cephalalgia.* Sept, *21*(7), 718-726.

[73] Cianchetti, C., Serci, M. C., Pisano, T. & Ledda, M. G. (2010). Compression of Superficial Temporal Arteries by a Handmade Device: A Simple Way to Block or Attenuate Migraine Attacks in Children and Adolescents. *Jour Child Neurology.* Jan, *25*(1), 67-70.

[74] Shevel, Elliot. (2007). Vascular surgery for chronic migraine. *Therapy.*, *4*(4), 451-456

[75] Pinar, Y. A. & Govsa, F. (2006). Anatomy of the superficial temporal artery and its branches: its importance for surgery. *Surg Radiol Anat*, *28*, 248-253.

[76] McKinnon, B. J., Wall, M. P & Karakla, D. W. (1999). The Vascular Anatomy and Angiosome of the Posterior Auricular Artery: A Cadaver Study. *Arch Facial Plast Surg.*, *1*(2), 101-104.

[77] Whetzel, T. P. & Mathes, S. J. (1992). Arterial anatomy of the face: an analysis of vascular territories and perforating cutaneous vessels. *Plast Reconstr Surg*, *89*(4), 591-603.

[78] Alvernia, J. E., Fraser, K. & Lanzino, G. (2006). The occipital artery: a microanatomical study. *Neurosurgery*, *58*(1), 114-22.

[79] Marques, S. R., Itezerote, A. M., Saviolo, M. R., De Angelis, M. A. & Prates, J. C. (2002). Anatomical Variations of the Occipital Artery: Relate of Two Cases. *Rev. Chil. Anat.*, *20*(2), 193-19

[80] Kung, T. A., Pannucci, C. J., Chamberlain, J. L. & Cederna, P. S. (2012). Migraine surgery practice patterns and attitudes. *Plast Reconstr Surg.*, Mar, *129*(3), 623-8.

In: Migraine Surgery
Editor: Antonios Mammis

ISBN: 978-1-63321-761-4

Chapter 8

Neuromodulation Therapies for Headache

Antonios Mammis[1*] and Nitin Agarwal[1,2]
[1]Department of Neurological Surgery,
Rutgers New Jersey Medical School, Newark, New Jersey, US
[2]Department of Neurological Surgery,
University of Pittsburgh Medical Center, Pittsburgh, Pennsylvania, US

Introduction

Neuromodulation for headache and craniofacial pain has been an evolving process over the past few decades. Early interest in neurostimulation for these conditions, focused on deep brain targets. In 1973, Hosobuchi, Adams, and Rutkin described the use of thalamic stimulation to treat facial anesthesia dolorosa. [1] Mazars and Pull, in 1976, described intermittent stimulation of the ventroposterolateral nucleus of the thalamus (nVPL) to treat intractable headache. [2] Recent trends have shifted focus from central to peripheral targets.

In 1997, Goadsby reported that stimulation of the greater occipital nerve (GON) in cats resulted in increased metabolic activity of the trigeminal nucleus caudalis and cervical dorsal horn. [3] These were among the first experiments to implicate the role of the GON in modulating the trigeminal system. In 1999, Weiner reported that stimulation of the greater occipital nerves can alleviate pain associated with occipital neuralgia. [4] Subsequently, the utility of occipital nerve stimulation (ONS) in treating occipital neuralgia became firmly established. In 2004, Goadsby reported that occipital nerve stimulation was efficacious in treating chronic migraine, sparking further interest in utilizing peripheral neurostimulation (PNS) in a number of headache and craniofacial pain syndromes. [5-10] More recently,

* Corresponding author: Antonios Mammis, M.D., Assistant Professor, Neurological Surgery, Director, Functional and Restorative Neurosurgery, Director, Center for Neuromodulation, Director, Rutgers Center for Headache, Orofacial, and Neuropathic Pain, Rutgers New Jersey Medical School, 90 Bergen Street, Suite 8100, Newark NJ 07103, Tel: 973-972-4836, Fax: 973-972-2333, Email: antonios.mammis@rutgers.edu.

alternatives to ONS have been explored such as the use of high cervical epidural neurostimulation for cluster headaches. [11]

A variety of occipital headache or pain syndromes may be effectively treated with ONS or alternatively with cervical spinal cord stimulation (SCS). This chapter reviews patient selection, pathophysiology, surgical technique, device programming, and potential complications associated with ONS and SCS, as minimally invasive therapeutic strategies.

Patient Selection

Migraine affects an estimated 12% of the population of the United States. Of those who suffer from migraines, about 70% are women. Approximately 3-13% of migraine patients progress to chronic migraine. [7] These patients report that they have headache pain more than 15 days per month. Of those who cope with headaches, approximately 5% suffer from daily headaches (transformed migraine, chronic daily headaches). Moreover, 1–2% may be poorly responsive to medical treatment modalities. Attempted continuity of medical management may lead to hopelessness, despair, activity restrictions, and narcotic dependence. Ultimately, patients that have failed medical management and have headache pain refractory to preventative medications are candidates for ONS or SCS trials.

Occipital Nerve Stimulation

Neuromodulation refers to alteration of electrical or chemical activity of a peripheral nerve, the spinal cord, or the brain for the relief of pain through the processes of inhibition, stimulation, modification, or other forms of regulation. ONS is a form of neuromodulation, which is reversible, adjustable, and may be individualized to a patient's specific therapeutic needs. While the mechanisms of action for the pain relief, obtained from an ONS, are incompletely understood, the following are thought to play some role: subcutaneous electrical conduction, dermatomal stimulation, myotomal stimulation, sympathetic stimulation, local blood flow alteration, peripheral nerve stimulation, peripheral or central neurochemical mechanisms, and the trigeminovascular system or trigeminocervical tract. Ultimately, peripheral neurostimulation may exert its effect by multiple mechanisms, which may differ in the various headache and pain syndromes. [12]

Electromodulation has been suggested to reduce blood flow to areas of pain as well as abnormal excitation of the peripheral pain fibers. Therefore, the central sensitization of the trigeminal sensory nerve pathways is prevented, while the descending system at the level of the dorsal horn may be modulated. [7, 13] However, a more likely mechanism of action of ONS is described by Pain Gate Theory. Described initially by Melzack and Wall in 1965, the pain gate theory describes the enhancement of inhibitory actions of the local circuit neurons in the dorsal horn on the central transmission cells. Stimulation yields activation of large myelinated afferents, which "close the pain gate" in the substantia gelatinosa, by enhancing the inhibitory actions of local circuit neurons in the dorsal horn on central transmission cells. Continuous firing of unmyelinated and small myelinated afferents usually maintain pain states. With a proportionately greater increase in the activation of large myelinated afferents, the physician and the patient's family members may be able to "close the gate" and stop pain transmission via presynaptic inhibition.

Utilizing ONS, Schwedt et al. have demonstrated that 60% of patients treated for various chronic headache syndromes have experienced a 30% reduction in headache frequency and severity. [14] Additionally, Popeney and Aló reported that 85% of patients with transformed migraine showed over a 50% reduction in frequency or severity of the headache following neurostimulation. [8] Multiple studies have also explored the treatment of occipital neuralgia with ONS, including one by Slavin et al. that described benefits in 70% of the patients treated for occipital neuralgia. [10] Whiplash related headaches, traumatic nerve injuries, or cluster headaches may also be treated with ONS after failed attempts with just medical management.

Surgical Technique

When medical management proves to be insufficient, occipital nerve stimulation may be pursued. The patient may be positioned laterally or prone, based on the location of the skin incision. For the trial, a percutaneous lead is introduced under fluoroscopic guidance, and with the patient under sedation. The entry point should be approximately 1 cm superior to the tip of the mastoid process, and the trajectory is towards the tip of the odontoid process. Trajectories superior to this are oftentimes used and are well tolerated as well. The electrode should be placed in the superficial aspect of the subcutaneous fat. Care should be taken to not place the lead in the dermis, nor too close to the fascia. The leads are secured to the skin with a 2-0 nylon drain stitch. The leads are then inserted into the trialing cable, and programming commences. Stimulation is applied using a temporary radiofrequency (RF) transmitter to various select electrode combinations; this enables the patient to report the stimulation location, intensity, and overall sensation. Most patients have reported an immediate stimulation in the selected occipital nerve distribution with 1 to 4 volts with midrange pulse widths and frequencies. The trial period is typically 4 to 7 days, and patients are encouraged to maintain a headache or pain diary. Trial success is defined as greater than 50% improvement in pain on the visual analog scale, or significant reduction in headache days, or improvement in quality of life.

Upon a successful trial of neurostimulation, permanent implantation may be considered. Permanent implantation is performed under general anesthesia. The patient is positioned supine with the head turned towards the left. A retroauricular incision is made on the right side and dissection is carried down to the retromastoid fascia. A small pocket is made within the subcutaneous tissues immediately lateral to the incision to accept a loop of electrode created following placement and tunneling in order to prevent electrode migration. An additional stab incision is made in the midline. A Tuohy needle is curved to conform to the transverse posterior cervical curvature (bevel concave). The needle is passed, without further dissection, transversely in the subcutaneous space across the base of the affected grater and/or lesser occipital nerves, from the midline stab incision towards to left side. A lead is introduced and the needle is withdrawn. Care should be taken to not stab through the skin. The needle is then placed from the retromastoid incision to the midline incision, and the wire is placed through the needle. Upon withdrawing the needle, the lead is tunneled to the retromastoid incision. The lead is then anchored to the retromasoid fascia with silk stitches. The needle is then introduced from the retromastoid incision to the midline, and the ipsilateral lead is introduced. This lead is also anchored to the retromasoid fascia. A subclavicular subcutaneous pocket is then prepared, and the leads are tunneled from the retromastoid incision to the pocket. The leads are then inserted into the pulse generator, and the pulse generator placed in the pocket. The pulse generator may be a primary cell or rechargeable.

Device Programming

Programming of occipital nerve stimulators differs significantly from spinal cord stimulator (SCS) programming. In ONS programming, a wider array of electrodes is used, in order to increase the likelihood of stimulating the terminal branches of the occipital nerves. Furthermore, we have found that patients often times prefer higher pulse widths, as compared to SCS. The frequency is typically lower than SCS. Unlike in SCS, paresthesia coverage is not necessary for pain relief. We have found that adequate headache relief is achieved in locations where there is not paresthesia spread.

Complications

While the placement of an occipital nerve stimulator is a relatively safe procedure, postoperative complications, may occur. [15] In a retrospective analysis by Schwedt et al., 60% of patients undergoing ONS for chronic headache required lead revision within 1 year. [14] Several complications have been reported following ONS, including the following: lead migration, infection, wound erosion, device failure, muscle spasms, and pain. [16, 17] Most commonly, lead migration is associated with ONS. [16, 18] Often lead migration may require surgical intervention. Schwedt et al. demonstrated lead migration rates of 33% after 6 months, 60% after 2 years, and 100% after 3 years. [14] Corrective surgery may be performed using a distal to proximal lead revision technique. As previously described, this technique is designed to efficiently and safely adjust lead position via both lead depth and lead tip location. [19] Moreover the revision technique may be carried out without a need for replacement of individual components or modification of the entire system. Gofeld described a technique of retrograde lead insertion after lead migration of an occipital neurostimulator. [20]

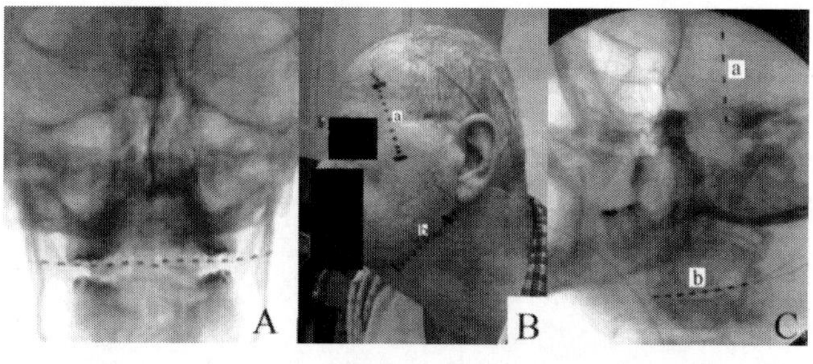

Figure 1. Intraoperative anterior-posterior (AP) radiograph demonstrating bilateral placement of octrode neurostimulator arrays (A). This patient is a 58-year old male who developed left V1 and V3 distribution pain, after a brainstem infarct. Trigeminal branch stimulation trial leads were placed in V1 (a) and V3 (b) regions, corresponding to the painful areas (B). Intraoperative lateral radiograph of the same patient demonstrating final position of the implanted V1 (a) and V3 (b) region leads (C).

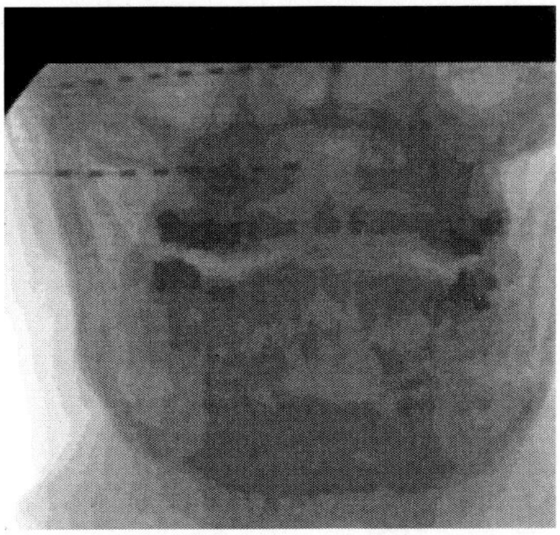

Figure 2. Intraoperative AP radiograph demonstrating stacked occipital percutaneous trial leads, in a patient with hemicrania continua.

Though complications of ONS exist, preventative measures may help to reduce the incidence of complications, such as infection and lead migration. Preoperative patient selection criteria are very important. Since placement of an occipital nerve stimulator is an elective surgery, physicians have an opportunity to ensure patients are medically optimized prior to any surgical operation. In addition, surgeons should consider swabbing all candidates to rule out Methicillin-resistant *Staphylococcus aureus* (MRSA) colonization. Should MRSA colonization be a concern, preoperative antibiotic treatment should be employed prior to implantation. During surgery, sterile surgical technique may help to reduce the incidence of infection. Surgeons should anchor leads to the fascia at the retromastoid incision to prevent lead migration. Postoperatively, local pain at the incision or stimulator sites often may be observed. In addition, ONS induced paresthesia in the area of the greater occipital nerve are typically experienced by all patients; the intensity of this paresthesia may vary with position of the patient's head and neck. [21]

Spinal Cord Stimulation

First described by Shealy, SCS has been used for decades for neurogenic pain. [22] More recently, high cervical SCS has been advocated for the treatment of headache and facial pain as well. One theory postulates the involvement of the trigeminocervical system – the anatomic overlap of the trigeminal and occipital afferent systems at the C2 spinal cord level. These afferents have been cited to converge on second order nociceptors in the spinal trigeminal nucleus. As such, trigeminal afferent pathways, and thereby primary headache disorders, may be controlled at the C2 level. Interestingly, Ward and Levin report a case of persistent headaches developing in a patient subsequent to the placement of a spinal cord stimulator in the upper cervical spine. Repositioning of the stimulator lower in the cervical spine ended the headaches. [23] Given that trigeminal afferent pathways may be controlled at the C2 level, neuromodulation of the cervical spinal cord has been purported for control of headache and facial pain. While both high cervical SCS and ONS are thought to activate the trigeminocervical complex, evidence of any differences is yet to be explicated. [24]

Surgical Technique

Implantation of electrodes for spinal cord stimulation (SCS) has been previously described. [11] Briefly, after local anesthesia, the spinal epidural space is accessed with a 14-G Tuohy needle at the level of T2-T3 under fluoroscopic guidance in two planes. The SCS electrode is then introduced and directed cranially to the upper cervical region. Cessation of movement due to the electrode abutting the inferior margin of the occipital bone indicates the final position. Following a testing phase of variable length, an impulse generator is then implanted under general anesthesia.

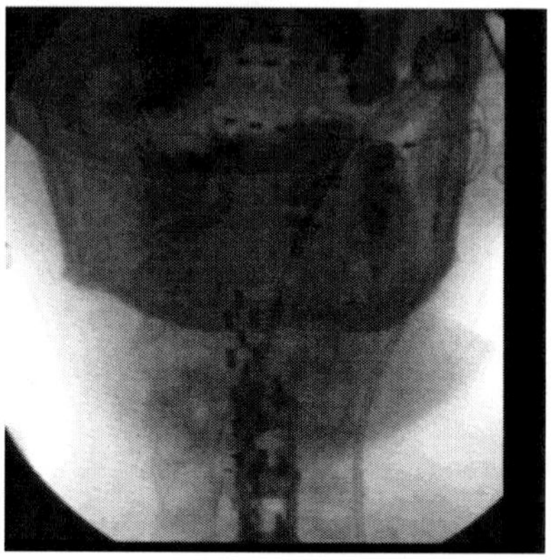

Figure 3. AP radiograph demonstrating implanted stacked occipital leads and a cervical paddle electrode, in a patient with chronic migraine and complex regional pain syndrome of the right upper extremity.

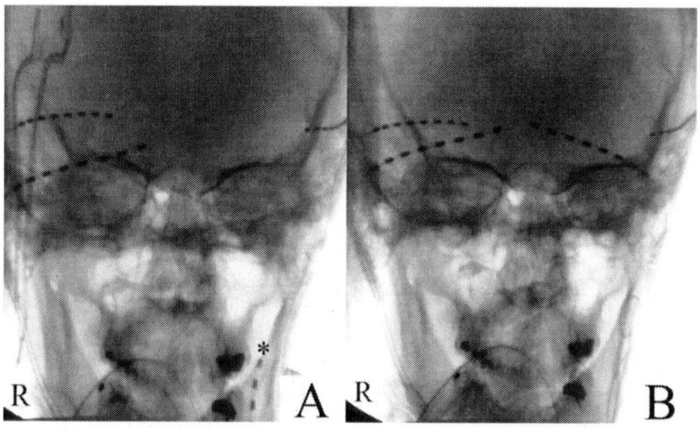

Figure 4. Intraoperative AP radiograph demonstrating migration of left occipital lead (*), in a patient with migraine headaches (A). The left occipital lead was then replaced, during revision surgery (B).

Complications

SCS has already been shown to be safe and effective for variety of chronic pain syndromes affecting the trunk and limbs. [11, 25, 26] While permanent neurological deficit is the most detrimental risk of SCS, of perhaps greater concern are the more frequent device-related complications including: electrode dislocation, lead breakage, and pulse generator battery degeneration. [27] Rates of revision operations due to these device-related complications are reportedly higher for SCS than those for ONS. [24, 28, 29] To date, the sample size of patients treated with high cervical SCS is still small to definitively assess the complication rate.

Conclusion

Neuromodulation therapies offer an efficacious, programmable, and reversible means of treating intractable migraine headache. SCS is a time-tested technique that potentially has a higher efficacy than ONS. However, given its less invasive nature and fewer device-related complications, ONS may be considered a first-line therapy; however, both ONS and SCS are safe and efficacious treatments for a variety of headache disorders. Should medical therapy fail, patients may benefit from and should be educated on neuromodulation therapies. The exact mechanism of action for peripheral neurostimulation is not known, but most likely its effects are due to multiple mechanisms. While complications like lead migration do arise, perioperative preventative measures may help to reduce the incidence of such complication. Should complications like lead migration arise, novel approaches to corrective surgery have been thoroughly described in the literature.

References

[1] Hosobuchi, Y; Adams, JE; Rutkin, B. Chronic thalamic stimulation for the control of facial anesthesia dolorosa. *Archives of neurology*. 1973, 29(3), 158-61. Epub 1973/09/01.

[2] Mazars, G; Pull, H. [Neurosurgical treatment of headaches]. Minerva medica. 1976, 67(31), 2020-2. Epub 1976/06/23. Il trattamento neurochirurgico delle cefalee.

[3] Goadsby, PJ; Knight, YE; Hoskin, KL. Stimulation of the greater occipital nerve increases metabolic activity in the trigeminal nucleus caudalis and cervical dorsal horn of the cat. *Pain*. 1997, 73(1), 23-8. Epub 1997/12/31.

[4] Weiner, RL; Reed, KL. Peripheral neurostimulation for control of intractable occipital neuralgia. *Neuromodulation: journal of the International Neuromodulation Society*. 1999, 2(3), 217-21. Epub 1999/07/01.

[5] Johnstone, CS; Sundaraj, R. Occipital nerve stimulation for the treatment of occipital neuralgia-eight case studies. *Neuromodulation: journal of the International Neuromodulation Society*. 2006, 9(1), 41-7. Epub 2006/01/01.

[6] Kapural, L; Mekhail, N; Hayek, SM; Stanton-Hicks, M; Malak, O. Occipital nerve electrical stimulation via the midline approach and subcutaneous surgical leads for treatment of severe occipital neuralgia: a pilot study. *Anesthesia and analgesia*. 2005, 101(1), 171-4, table of contents. Epub 2005/06/25.

[7] Matharu, MS; Bartsch, T; Ward, N; Frackowiak, RS; Weiner, R; Goadsby, PJ. Central neuromodulation in chronic migraine patients with suboccipital stimulators: a PET study. *Brain: a journal of neurology*. 2004, 127(Pt 1), 220-30. Epub 2003/11/11.

[8] Popeney, CA; Alo, KM. Peripheral neurostimulation for the treatment of chronic, disabling transformed migraine. *Headache*. 2003, 43(4), 369-75. Epub 2003/03/27.
[9] Rodrigo-Royo, MD; Azcona, JM; Quero, J; Lorente, MC; Acin, P; Azcona, J. Peripheral neurostimulation in the management of cervicogenic headache: four case reports. *Neuromodulation: journal of the International Neuromodulation Society*. 2005, 8(4), 241-8. Epub 2005/10/01.
[10] Slavin, KV; Nersesyan, H; Wess, C. Peripheral neurostimulation for treatment of intractable occipital neuralgia. *Neurosurgery*. 2006, 58(1), 112-9, discussion -9. Epub 2005/12/31.
[11] Wolter, T; Kaube, H; Mohadjer, M. High cervical epidural neurostimulation for cluster headache: case report and review of the literature. *Cephalalgia: an international journal of headache*. 2008, 28(10), 1091-4.
[12] Lambru, G; Matharu, MS. Occipital nerve stimulation in primary headache syndromes. *Therapeutic advances in neurological disorders*. 2012, 5(1), 57-67. Epub 2012/01/26.
[13] Bahra, A; Matharu, MS; Buchel, C; Frackowiak, RS; Goadsby, PJ. Brainstem activation specific to migraine headache. *Lancet*. 2001, 357(9261), 1016-7. Epub 2001/04/11.
[14] Schwedt, TJ; Dodick, DW; Hentz, J; Trentman, TL; Zimmerman, RS. Occipital nerve stimulation for chronic headache--long-term safety and efficacy. *Cephalalgia: an international journal of headache*. 2007, 27(2), 153-7. Epub 2007/01/30.
[15] Mammis, A; Sinclair, GL; 3rd; Mogilner, AY. Peripheral neuromodulation for headache and craniofacial pain: indications, outcomes, and complications from a single center. *Clinical neurosurgery*. 2012, 59, 114-8. Epub 2012/09/25.
[16] Trentman, TL; Zimmerman, RS; Dodick, DW. Occipital nerve stimulation: technical and surgical aspects of implantation. *Progress in neurological surgery*. 2011, 24, 96-108. Epub 2011/03/23.
[17] Falowski, S; Wang, D; Sabesan, A; Sharan, A. Occipital nerve stimulator systems: review of complications and surgical techniques. *Neuromodulation: journal of the International Neuromodulation Society*. 2010, 13(2), 121-5. Epub 2010/04/01.
[18] Trentman, TL; Zimmerman, RS. Occipital nerve stimulation: technical and surgical aspects of implantation. *Headache*. 2008, 48(2), 319-27. Epub 2008/02/01.
[19] Mammis, A; Mogilner, AY. A technique of distal to proximal revision of peripheral neurostimulator leads: technical note. *Stereotactic and functional neurosurgery*. 2011, 89(2), 65-9. Epub 2011/02/05.
[20] Gofeld, M. Anchoring of suboccipital lead: case report and technical note. *Pain practice: the official journal of World Institute of Pain*. 2004, 4(4), 307-9. Epub 2006/12/19.
[21] Magis, D; Schoenen, J. Occipital nerve stimulation for intractable chronic cluster headache: new hope for a dreadful disease? Acta neurologica Belgica. 2011, 111(1), 18-21. Epub 2011/04/23.
[22] Shealy, CN; Mortimer, JT; Reswick, JB. Electrical inhibition of pain by stimulation of the dorsal columns: preliminary clinical report. *Anesthesia and analgesia*. 1967, 46(4), 489-91.
[23] Ward, TN; Levin, M. Case reports: headache caused by a spinal cord stimulator in the upper cervical spine. *Headache*. 2000, 40(8), 689-91.
[24] Wolter, T; Kaube, H. Spinal cord stimulation in cluster headache. *Current pain and headache reports*. 2013, 17(5), 324.

[25] Cameron, T. Safety and efficacy of spinal cord stimulation for the treatment of chronic pain: a 20-year literature review. *Journal of neurosurgery*. 2004, 100(3 Suppl Spine), 254-67.

[26] Deer, TR; Skaribas, IM; Haider, N; Salmon, J; Kim, C; Nelson, C; et al. Effectiveness of Cervical Spinal Cord Stimulation for the Management of Chronic Pain. *Neuromodulation: journal of the International Neuromodulation Society*. 2013.

[27] Wolter, T; Kiemen, A; Kaube, H. High cervical spinal cord stimulation for chronic cluster headache. *Cephalalgia: an international journal of headache*. 2011, 31(11), 1170-80.

[28] Burns, B; Watkins, L; Goadsby, PJ. Treatment of medically intractable cluster headache by occipital nerve stimulation: long-term follow-up of eight patients. *Lancet*. 2007, 369(9567), 1099-106.

[29] Fontaine, D; Christophe, Sol, J; Raoul, S; Fabre, N; Geraud, G; Magne, C; et al. Treatment of refractory chronic cluster headache by chronic occipital nerve stimulation. *Cephalalgia: an international journal of headache*. 2011, 31(10), 1101-5.

In: Migraine Surgery
Editor: Antonios Mammis

ISBN: 978-1-63321-761-4

Chapter 9

Patient Selection and Complication Avoidance in Occipital Nerve Stimulation

Nrupen Baxi and Alon Mogilner*
Center for Neuromodulation, Department of Neurosurgery,
New York University Langone Medical Center, New York, NY

Introduction

Chronic migraines affect nearly 2-3% of the world's population. [1] With the development of the International Classification of Headaches Disorders, the definition and criteria for the primary headache disorders were formalized. A chronic migraine was defined as a "headache" occurring 15 or more days a month for more than 3 months which has migrainous features at least 8 days of the month. [2] As described earlier, chronic migraines sufferers can have poor quality of lives from the impact of their disease. It can also lead to productivity losses, increased health care utilization, and is often accompanied by other comorbid conditions such as arthritis, chronic pain, anxiety, depression, hypertension, and obesity. [1]

Chronic migraines can remain refractory to treatment even with the advent of newer pharmacological agents. The refractory nature of these headaches has led clinicians to consider interventional procedures as alternative therapies. Greater occipital nerve blocks which can diagnose and treat occipital neuralgia, were also found to be effective in the treatment of chronic migraines with the effects lasting beyond the half-life of the local anesthetic agents used. [3] This effect sparked interest in utilizing both ablative and decompressive procedures on the occipital nerves to treat chronic migraines. These

* Corresponding author: Alon Y. Mogilner, M.D., Ph.D., Center for Neuromodulation, Department of Neurosurgery New York University Langone Medical Center, 530 First Avenue, Suite 8S, New York, NY 10016, Phone: (212) 263-2607, Email: alon.mogilner@nyumc.org.

procedures have had success in treating chronic migraines but have been complicated by the development of de-afferent neuropathic pain in the area of the initial sensory deficit. This pain often develops in a delayed fashion and can be very difficult to treat. [4]

This led to the development of nondestructive neuromodulation treatment strategies. The hope was that by utilizing electrical stimulation of the peripheral occipital nerve fibers, the delayed failure and neuropathic pain syndromes could be avoided. Current occipital stimulation is performed by utilizing and modifying existing spinal cord stimulation technology in an off-label manner. This peripheral stimulation is thought to reduce pain through two proposed mechanisms.

One mechanism is thought to act via the gate-theory mechanism of pain to reduce nociceptive inputs. Another proposed mechanism is that stimulation directly modulates the trigeminocervical complex in the brainstem which reduces meningeal vasodilation and thus reduces the frequency and intensity of migraines. This speculated activity has been seen on functional PET imaging obtained from the initial cohort of occipital stimulation patients by Matharu et al. [3]. These same neuromodulation treatment strategies have been applied to other headache disorders such as cluster headaches and hemicrania continua where the trigeminocervical complex is also thought to play a pathologic role. [4]

Clinical Trials

Early cohorts of patients with occipital neurostimulation had remarkable initial successes in small published series with nearly 80-95% of patients reporting > 50% reduction in pain and decreased medication usage. [5] The positive results seen in small series encouraged the undertaking of larger, industry sponsored double-blinded randomized clinical trials to test the true efficacy of occipital stimulation and to help gain FDA approval for the technology in the United States (Table 1). The first such trial was the ONSTIM (Occipital Nerve Stimulation for the Treatment of Intractable Chronic Migraines) performed by Saper et al. They found that 39% of patients with adjustable stimulation had at least a 50% reduction in headache days / month or at least a 3 point reduction in pain intensity scores when compared to medical management. Of note sham stimulation or fixed stimulation had 6% of patients experience a 50% reduction as well, however this was not noted to statistically significant. The surgical arm did have a 71% total adverse event rate with a 24% lead migration rate and a 14% device infection rate. [6] In another randomized clinical trial performed by Silberstein et al. with sponsorship from St. Jude Medical, there was no statistically significant difference in responders who had a 50% reduction in their mean pain intensity scores between active stimulation and the sham stimulation groups. [7] This discrepancy between the early case series and the randomized clinical trials raises the point whether a 50% reduction in pain intensity scores is too strict of a primary endpoint. When the pain intensity reduction threshold was dropped to 30%, there was a statistically significant difference between the active stimulation and the sham stimulation groups. The study also found statistically significant differences in pain, headache days, and migraine-related disability. [7] The PRISM trial allowed researchers to trial patients prior to implanting the device however the primary endpoint of a statistically significant reduction in migraine days / month was not achieved. Patients with a successful trial did however obtain a reduction of an average of 8.8 days /

month with active or sham stimulation when compared to trial failures. An inherent issue in all neurostimulation devices is the difficulty in blinding patient when the therapy is paresthesia producing. Currently these studies have given the FDA pause in approving occipital stimulation devices for chronic migraines. Further research is ongoing to determine the optimal endpoints for these trials and whether complications can be reduced with better technology.

Patient Selection

The randomized clinical trials and the smaller earlier series of patients with occipital stimulation have helped guide clinicians on which patients are likely to benefit from occipital neurostimulation for chronic migraines [8-13]. Appropriate candidates should meet the International Classification of Headaches Disorders (ICHD) criteria for chronic migraines. These criteria include: headaches occurring 15 days or more per month which have migrainous features on at least 8 days of the month for at least 3 months. [14] Ideally, patients would have an established diagnosis with a stable headache pattern for 6 months. Working in conjunction with a qualified headache specialist is essential to ensuring that all medical therapeutic options have been attempted prior to considering medical therapy. If ultimately the patient is unable to tolerate the medications which provide relief, it may then be reasonable to consider occipital stimulation. A headache specialist may provide important feedback regarding medication overuse headaches (MOH) which may present in addition to chronic migraines. MOH usually requires discontinuation of the medications which are overused. [14] MOH has been implicated in cases where occipital neurostimulation has failed to improve migraines. [15]

Posteriorly located headaches with spread limited only up to vertex tend to respond best to occipital stimulation. Occipital stimulation is less likely to provide long-term relief for headaches that emanate from the frontal region; although the addition of frontal leads to a previously existing occipital system may be beneficial. Alternatively, frontal (supraorbital) lead placement, rather than occipital placement, may be an appropriate first intervention. Patients with prior destructive lesions to the occipital nerve such as occipital neurectomy or high cervical nerve root section also fare poorly as paresthesias cannot be generated secondary to permanent anesthesia. Initially, it was thought that a positive response to an occipital nerve block was a prerequisite for success with ONS, but later studies have shown this not to be the case, in that ONS has been shown to be successful in patients without previously successful occipital nerve blocks. As for all surgical procedures, patients should also be in medically stable to undergo the procedure, which is usually performed either under general anesthesia or intravenous sedation. At the current time, patients with a need for MRI scanning are not candidates for any peripheral neurostimulator implant, as the devices have not been proven to be MRI compatible. This is true even for the recently introduced MRI-compatible spinal cord stimulation hardware, which despite being the exact same hardware as used in PNS has not been proven to be compatible with MRI. As with all neurostimulation technology, microwave diathermy cannot be performed.

A thorough pain psychological or psychiatric evaluation should be performed to assess for any underlying untreated depression or anxiety which may be contributing an affective component to the headache, as well as to rule out patients with secondary gain, drug addiction, or other conditions which portend a poor outcome. The informed consent discussion should include a detailed explanation of the risks of the procedure, as well as the possibility of further revision surgeries, given the high rate of revision surgeries seen in the larger clinical trials. It is also important for the patient to have reasonable expectations for the outcome of the procedure. Almost all clinical studies have shown that patients can continue to have headache and migrainous symptoms of varying intensity certain days of the month, and that success may not mean freedom from headaches or migrainous symptoms. [15]

A trial of occipital neurostimulation remains an effective way to screen patients who would be candidates for permanent implantation. The PRISM trial demonstrated that patients who had trials of occipital neurostimulation where paresthesias were tolerated and in the appropriate areas of pain had higher reductions of migraine days per month. [13] On the other hand, it has also been speculated that full effect of neuromodulation on the trigeminocervical complex may take up to 6 months and that trialing for a week or so may in the end eliminate patients who would benefit in the long-term. [16]

Complication Avoidance Strategies

Both the large randomized clinical trials and the earlier smaller case series have shown significant rates of complications and adverse events.

Table 1. Initial Case Series Reporting Positive Results with Occipital Neurostimulation

Authors	# of Patients	Positive Results %	Complication Rate
Weiner and Reed[8]	13	12/13 (92.3%)	18 Months to 6 Year Follow-Up
Popeney and Alo[9]	25	22/25 (88.0%)	50% Reduction in Number of Headache Days / Month
Oh et al. [10]	20	16/20 (80%)	95% Satisfaction
Slavin et al. [11]	10	7/10 (70%)	60-90% Reduction in Pain
Levy[4]	45	37/45 (83%)	92% Satisfaction Rate
Mammis et al. [12]	21	19/21 (90%)	Migraine Subseries Extracted
Industry Trials			
Saper et al. [6] (Medtronic) ONSTIM	75	39% Adjustable Stim + 6% Sham Stim	Complications: 24% Lead Migration and 14% infection
Silberstein et al. [7] (St. Jude)	157	No significant difference at 50% improvement in sham vs. control groups. Positive result seen at 30% improvement	Doubled Blinded Randomized Clinical Trial
PRISM Trial[13]	139	8.8 migraine days / month reduction for all comers with implanted devices compared to 0.7 migraines days / month reduction in failed trial patients	Patients trialed and then randomized after implant
OPTIMISE Trial	Ongoing		

Infection

Infection rates from the largest clinical trial to date, by Silberstein et al. ranged from 2.8% to 3.7% in the control and active stimulation groups. [7] As It it has been convincingly demonstrated that the most common cause of surgical-site-infections (SSI) is the patient's own skin flora, reduction of SSIs begins with appropriate identification of potential pathogens. Infections caused by Methicillin-Resistant Staphylococcus aureus (MRSA) have, in recent years, dramatically increased, and MRSA has been found on the skin of individuals with no history of hospitalization or infection. [17]

In our institution, all patients are tested for colonization of MRSA, and, more recently, Methicillin-sensitive s. aureus (MSSA). They are then prophylactically treated in an attempt to reduce the bacterial load on the skin prior to surgery, and are given prophylactic perioperative vancomycin, rather than cephalosporins.

Once a device has found be infected, it can difficult to save the device hardware and often all the hardware must be explanted. Falowski et al. showed a 17.9% rate of infection of which 14.3% were treated solely with oral antibiotics and did not require explantation. Skin erosions over the leads are also often a precursor to infection, or a manifestation of indolent skin infections. 3.7% of patients in a series in the randomized clinical trial by Silberstein et al. had skin erosion over the site. All of these cases were managed with removal and/or revision of the lead. It may be tempting, particularly when therapy has been dramatically effective, to attempt hardware salvage by partial hardware removal or revision. Unfortunately, our experience suggests that, particularly in the case of erosion through the skin, this will just prolong the inevitable and complete hardware removal up front, followed by replacement at a later date, is the most appropriate therapy.

Similarly, impeding wound erosions at the lead tip are revised prophylactically, and can be done via a distal to proximal approach, sparing the need for opening the generator pocket. [18]

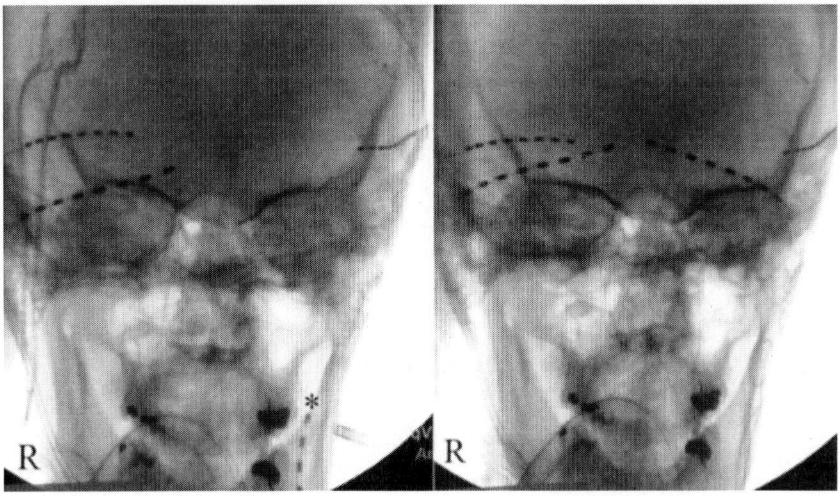

Figure 1.

Lead Migration or Malfunction

The other main complications involve device related issues such lead migration or fracture. Earlier experience with occipital stimulation during the ONSTIM trial demonstrated lead migration rates of 24%. [19] Various strategies have been advocated to reduce lead migrations with positive results in some retrospective series. Falowski et al. reported that by utilizing an additional strain relief loop with a separate incision, the lead migration rate dropped to 10% revision rate versus a 62% revision rate in the group without one. Current ongoing randomized trials utilize standardized strain relief loop and anchors in hopes of reducing complication rates. Use of fluoroscopy in the operating room or postoperative x-rays will help establish the final position of the leads and enable comparisons at a later date to assess for migration (Figure 1).

IPG Related Issues

Lastly, IPG related issues were another significant source of complications and adverse events. In the randomized control trial by Silberstein et al. the incidence was reported at 21.5%. [7] This is a problem not uncommon to permanently implanted neurostimulators including deep brain or spinal cord stimulation systems. Pain in IPG pocket or incision was one of the most commonly reported complaints in both randomized clinical trials and cases series. This can be difficult to rectify as revision surgery may create a new area of pain and focus for the patient's attention. Falowski et al. noted an incidence of 14.3% IPG related pain, of which nearly half required a revision to relocate the generator to a different site. They noted that an abdominal location, though technically more challenging at the time of initial implantation, had fewer rates of IPG pain complaints and revisions. [20] Extensive discussions with the patients at the time of implantation as to the ideal site can be helpful. Flipping of IPGs can lead to difficulty recharging and can place undue torque and stress on the leads themselves. This usually requires surgical revision to ensure that orientation of the device is corrected.

As with any new procedure, one would expect a decrease in complication rate with surgeon experience. Sharan et al. have in fact demonstrated this in a subanalysis of patients in the St. Jude Migraine study. [21] Surgeons with a higher number of PNS implants had a lower incidence of hardware-related adverse events including lead migration, infection and pain, as well as a lower incidence of additional surgeries.

Conclusion

Chronic migraines affect near 2-3% of the population and can be severely disabling. It has a large societal impact in terms of lost productivity and high utilization of health care resources. Occipital neurostimulation offers an additional treatment option for those refractory to treatment. In small initial case series, results were largely positive with nearly 80-90% patients having nearly 50% reduction in their migraine intensity. This success was more measured in larger, randomized clinical trials. All three major industry trials raised important issues. The Medtronic ONSTIM trial had high rates of complications including lead migrations, infection, and IPG complaints. The subsequent randomized clinical trials have had significant improvements in disability and migraine free days, but failed to reach their primary endpoints of 50% improvement in pain. One thing consistently noted in these trials is the high complication rate. As surgeons have more experience and hardware is specially developed for this purpose as opposed to being adapted from spinal cord stimulation, the complications rates may fall. Ongoing clinical trials will hopefully further elucidate the subset of patients who would benefit from this therapy and reduce failure and explantation rates.

References

[1] Carod-Artal, FJ. Tackling chronic migraine: current perspectives. *Journal of pain research*, 2014, 7, 185-94.

[2] Lipton, RB; Bigal, ME; Steiner, TJ; Silberstein, SD; Olesen, J. Classification of primary headaches. *Neurology*, 2004, 63, 427-35.

[3] Matharu, MS; Bartsch, T; Ward, N; Frackowiak, RS; Weiner, R; Goadsby, PJ. Central neuromodulation in chronic migraine patients with suboccipital stimulators: a PET study. *Brain*, 2004, 127, 220-30.

[4] Ellens, DJ; Levy, RM. Peripheral neuromodulation for migraine headache. *Progress in neurological surgery*, 2011, 24, 109-17.

[5] Tavanaiepour, D; Levy, RM., Peripheral neuromodulation for treatment of chronic migraine headache. *Neurosurgery clinics of North America*, 2014, 25, 11-4.

[6] Saper, JR; Dodick, DW; Silberstein, SD; McCarville, S; Sun, M; Goadsby, PJ. Occipital nerve stimulation for the treatment of intractable chronic migraine headache: ONSTIM feasibility study. *Cephalalgia: an international journal of headache*, 2011, 31, 271-85.

[7] Silberstein, SD; Dodick, DW; Saper, J; et al. Safety and efficacy of peripheral nerve stimulation of the occipital nerves for the management of chronic migraine: Results from a randomized, multicenter, double-blinded, controlled study. *Cephalalgia*, 2012, 32, 1165-79.

[8] Weiner, RL; Reed, KL. Peripheral neurostimulation for control of intractable occipital neuralgia. *Neuromodulation: Technology at the Neural Interface*, 1999, 2, 217-21.

[9] Popeney, CA; Aló, KM. Peripheral neurostimulation for the treatment of chronic, disabling transformed migraine. *Headache: The Journal of Head and Face Pain*, 2003, 43, 369-75.

[10] Oh, MY; Ortega, J; Bellotte, JB; Whiting, DM; Aló, K. Peripheral Nerve Stimulation for the Treatment of Occipital Neuralgia and Transformed Migraine Using a C1-2-3 Subcutaneous Paddle Style Electrode: A Technical Report. *Neuromodulation: Technology at the Neural Interface*, 2004, 7, 103-12.

[11] Slavin, KV; Colpan, ME; Munawar, N; Wess, C; Nersesyan, H. Trigeminal and occipital peripheral nerve stimulation for craniofacial pain: a single-institution experience and review of the literature. *Neurosurg Focus*, 2006, 21, E5.

[12] Mammis, A; Sinclair, III GL; Mogilner, Ay. Chapter 16-Ronald Tasker Award-Peripheral Neuromodulation for Headache and Craniofacial Pain: Indications, Outcomes, and Complications From a Single Center. *Clinical Neurosurgery*, 2012, 59, 114.
[13] Lipton, R; Goadsby, P; Cady, R; et al. PRISM study: occipital nerve stimulation for treatment-refractory migraine. *Cephalalgia: an international journal of headache*, 2009: Wiley-Blackwell Publishing, Inc Commerce Place, 350 Main St, Malden 02148, MA USA. p. 30-.
[14] Society, HCCotIH. The international classification of headache disorders, (beta version). *Cephalalgia: an international journal of headache*, 2013, 33, 629-808.
[15] Goadsby, PJ; Sprenger, T. Current practice and future directions in the prevention and acute management of migraine. *Lancet neurology*, 2010, 9, 285-98.
[16] Proietti Cecchini, A; Grazzi, L. Emerging therapies for chronic migraine. *Current pain and headache reports*, 2014, 18, 408.
[17] Pofahl, WE; Goettler, CE; Ramsey, KM; Cochran, MK; Nobles, DL; Rotondo, MF. Active Surveillance Screening of MRSA and Eradication of the Carrier State Decreases Surgical-Site Infections Caused by MRSA. *Journal of the American College of Surgeons*, 2009, 208, 981-6.
[18] Mammis, A; Mogilner, AY. A technique of distal to proximal revision of peripheral neurostimulator leads: technical note. *Stereotact Funct Neurosurg*, 2011, 89, 65-9.
[19] Saper, JR; Dodick, DW; Silberstein, SD; McCarville, S; Sun, M; Goadsby, PJ. Occipital nerve stimulation for the treatment of intractable chronic migraine headache: ONSTIM feasibility study. *Cephalalgia: an international journal of headache*, 2011, 31, 271-85.
[20] Falowski, S; Wang, D; Sabesan, A; Sharan, A. Occipital nerve stimulator systems: review of complications and surgical techniques. *Neuromodulation: journal of the International Neuromodulation Society*, 2010, 13, 121-5.
[21] Sharan, A; Huh, B; Narouze, S; et al. Impact of Surgeon's Experience in Performing Peripheral Nerve Stimulation Implant Procedures on Treatment Efficacy and Safety. *North American Neuromodulation Society Annual Meeting*, 2013, Las Vegas, NV.

In: Migraine Surgery
Editor: Antonios Mammis

ISBN: 978-1-63321-761-4

Chapter 10

Deep Brain Stimulation for Refractory Headache Disorders

Saurabh Sinha and Shabbar F. Danish*
Division of Neurosurgery,
Rutgers Robert Wood Johnson Medical School,
New Brunswick, New Jersey, US

Introduction

Intracranial surgical interventions for refractory headache that has failed trials of multiple medical therapies are predicated on understanding underlying pathophysiologic pathways. Though utilization of intracranial interventions for refractory headache has only recently emerged, two neurosurgical interventions for chronic pain, deep brain stimulation (DBS) and cingulotomy, have been theorized and utilized in some form since the 1960s [1, 2]. Despite a decrease in the use of these procedures in the 1980s and 1990s, there has been a recent resurgence in DBS for refractory headache that follows a refinement in understanding how pain is processed in the brain. The objective of this chapter is to discuss the current understanding of pain pathways in the brain, to assess anatomic and physiologic targets for neurosurgical intervention arising from these studies, to discuss current applications of DBS to chronic cluster headache, and to assess future directions, particularly in regards to an application of DBS for refractory migraine.

Pain Pathways

An understanding of the pathophysiology of headache in the context of intracranial intervention depends in large part on an appreciation of central pain pathways. Though

* Corresponding author: Shabbar F. Danish, M.D., Email: shabbar.danish@rutgers.edu, Phone: 732-235-6678.

different types of headaches manifest differently, there are still pathophysiologic similarities. These similarities can be utilized for neurosurgical lesioning procedures, which depend on targets with sensible physiologic underpinnings.

Pain pathways, which ascend in increasing complexity through the brain, are all inititated by a primary source or insult. These initial insults may be vascular, neuroendocrine, or musculoskeletal in origin [3]. Primary vascular disturbances are signaled by nociceptive fibers that surround intracranial vessels (including those of dura, pia, and venous sinuses) in a plexus that ultimately responds to changes like vasodilation and inflammation [4]. Hormonal flux may be seen in cluster headache, a disorder which has been demonstrated to involve changes in hormones of the hypothalamic-pituitary axis [3]. Though this primary mechanism may be different for different headache disorders, as this information ascends, there exists some overlap in pathways.

Whatever the initial cause of the pain, the ultimate production of the intracranial sensation of that pain necessitates sending afferent fibers to the trigeminocervical complex (TCC), which is comprised of the spinal trigeminal nucleus (SpVC) in the pons, extending down to dorsal horns of C2 and C3 of the cervical spinal cord [3]. In fact, the occipital nerve, which is targeted in the peripheral neuromodulatory technique known as occipital nerve stimulation (ONS), also projects central afferents to the trigeminocervical complex [5]. (ONS is discussed elsewhere in this book as a treatment modality for chronic migraine.) The TCC is, thus, the way station for all intracranial pain processing (Figure 1), and serves an overlapping mechanistic unit that ties together all forms of headache [3].

The TCC routes the trigeminothalamic tract to the thalamus and the trigeminohypothalamic tract to the hypothalamus, both of importance in further discussion in this chapter. Interestingly, triptan medications modulate activity at the trigeminocervical complex for part of their abortive effect on migraines, underscoring the involvement of TCC in pain processing [3].

The brainstem forms reciprocal connections with the TCC (Figure 1). Specific regions of involvement within the brainstem include the ventrolateral periaqueductal grey (vlPAG) and rostral ventromedial medulla (RVM), which receive ascending projections from the TCC and also send efferent projections back to the TCC and also to diencephalic structures such as the hypothalamus and thalamus to further modulate pain processing [3]. These brainstem structures have been demonstrated to affect TCC function. The vlPAG-RVM brainstem pathway has already been demonstrated to be involved in endogenous, opioid-mediated pain modulation, but has also been shown to inhibit nociceptive transmission within the TCC [5]. Moreover, it displays state-dependent activation based on the wake-sleep cycle and is involved in the control of sensory, autonomic, and motor processes via the spinal cord [6]. Given the fact that vlPAG-RVM pathway of the brainstem connects to the TCC pain center, these findings suggest the connection of pain regulation to homeostatic processes such as sleep and hunger [6]. Taken with recent hypotheses that the brainstem serves as a "migraine generator" [5, 6], there exists a connection within neural circuits between common migraine triggers (such as sleep deprivation and hunger) and pain pathways. The "dysfunctional brainstem" angle of migraine pathophysiology is supported by recent neuroimaging analysis as well. Moulton and colleagues recently used functional MRI (fMRI) to assess differences in interictal pain processing in patients with migraine vs. healthy controls, and found that the nucleus cuneiformis of the brainstem was abnormally hypoactive in patients with migraine, a region of the brain demonstrated to have a role in pain modulation [7]. This finding suggests a dysfunctional node within the regulatory pathway of pain in migraine, and a potential target for a neurosurgical intervention, as discussed later.

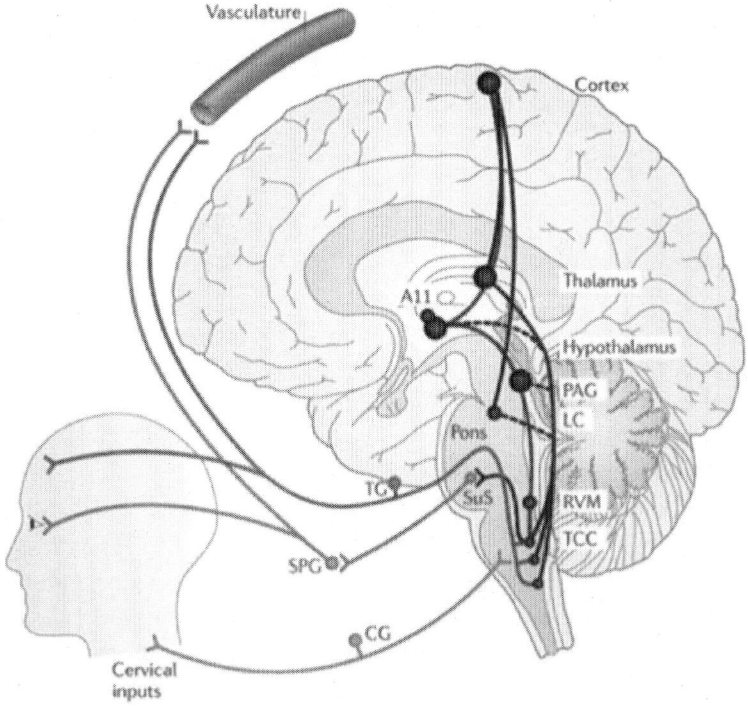

Figure 1. Any source of intracranial pain proceeds through similar central pain pathways. As highlighted here for migraine by Akerman and colleagues, sensory afferents from vasculature, skin, and cervical inputs, synapse at the trigeminocervical complex (TCC). The TCC also has reciprocal connections to the ventrolateral periaqueductal grey (vlPAG) and the rostral ventromedial medulla (RVM) in the brainstem, which functions in pain modulation and integration of other inputs, like the circadian rhythm, hunger, and somatic sensory processes routed from the spinal cord. The TCC then sends afferent signals to specific nuclei within the thalamus, which have demonstrated activity in headache disorders. Thalamic nuclei then send afferents to specific regions of the cortex, including somatosensory cortex, anterior cingulate cortex, and prefrontal cortex.

Moving rostrally in the pain pathway, the trigeminothalamic tract carries somatosensory information (in this case, information about pain) to specific nuclei within the thalamus: ventroposteromedial, posterior, and intralaminar nuclei [8]. Activation of the thalamus is indeed seen in headache disorders, including cluster headache and short-lasting unilateral neuralgiform headache with conjunctival injection and tearing (SUNCT), both of which will be discussed later as refractory headache disorders targeted by neurosurgical intervention [9].

Past the thalamic nuclei, ascending fibers target multiple higher areas, including the somatosensory cortex, anterior cingulate cortex, and prefrontal cortex, with additional projections to the insular cortex, frontal lobes, and basal ganglia. Positron emission tomography (PET) imaging demonstrates activation of many of these cortical areas during acute migraine and cluster headache [9]. Taken with the findings of a brainstem "generator" for migraine and the involvement of the TCC and other nodes in the ascending circuit for both cluster headache and migraine, it is evident that headache utilizes these major cetral pain pathways in the brain. Understanding these pathways and their relevant nodes has been an evolving process over decades resulting in new therapeutic targets for refractory headache disorders, as will be discussed later in this chapter.

Targeting Pain Pathways with Lesioning Procedures

Though the cenral pathways of pain as described above have only recently been elucidated, the involvement of specific regions of the brain like the periaqueductal gray has been known since the 1970s [10, 11]. Based on the knowledge of specific anatomical regions involved in pain, lesioning and neurostimulation procedures for chronic pain have been undertaken for decades. In fact, deep brain stimulation (DBS), a form of neurosurgically-mediated electrical stimulation that we will describe in more detail later, was initially developed for the treatment of chronic pain. As noted above, the PAG was identified as a theoretical target through rodent experiments in the 1970s, and this was followed by PAG DBS initially by Richardson and Akil in 1977 followed by Hosobuchi and colleagues in 1977 [1]. Though none of the patients in whom DBS was utilized was suffering from chronic pain secondary to a refractory headache disorder, there were varying other etiologies, including chronic low back and leg pain from disc herniations, thalamic pain syndrome from brainstem lesions, cancer, and paraplegia. These procedures were efficacious in addressing patients' pain over the long-term, but a decline in DBS usage with the advent of better pharmacological options and an inability to prove efficacy through clinical trials shifted the focus away from DBS for the management of chronic pain [1].

Bilateral anterior cingulotomy is another lesioning procedure that began in the 1950s as a surgical option for refractory psychiatric disease, but was used for chronic pain first in 1962 by Foltz and White [2]. Briefly, cingulotomy is a neurosurgical procedure that involves electrode-mediated thermoablation of a targeted region of the anterior cingulate cortex. As mentioned previously, the anterior cingulate cortex is one of the higher targets of pain pathways after the thalamus. It is located in the ventromedial frontal cortex and has been ascribed a number of functions, including executive function, behavioral control, and monitoring of emotional salience of stimuli [12]. Because of its function in these higher order cognitive and emotional processes, the anterior cingulate cortex appears to be involved in the processing of pain at an affective or cognitive level. Bilateral anterior cingulotomy for chronic, refractory non-cancer pain was assessed in a long-term study in 1999 by Wilkinson and colleagues, who sent questionnaires to patients receiving the procedure from 1979-1996 for chronic pain secondary to failed back syndrome, ischemic leg pain, phantom limb pain, postoperative neck pain, and atypical facial pain [2]. They found that over half of the patients reported relief from pain symptoms, with both psychosocial improvements and decreased need for pain medication. Interestingly, it is the affective component of pain that appears to be affected by cingulotomy; that is, after the surgery, the patients appeared to be less fixated on their pain and even regained some lost functionality [2]. Given the involvement of the anterior cingulate cortex, as previously mentioned, in cognitive and emotional functions, it is logical that cingulotomy appears to affect pain at this higher-order level and, moreover, that this observation was absent in DBS of PAG, and that cingulotomy continues to be utilized for the treatment of psychiatric diseases such as obsessive-compulsive disorder and major depressive disorder.

Though a basic understanding of the aforementioned pain pathways, which are involved in pathologic processes as disparate as chronic low back pain and refractory headache, were utilized to first form a theoretical construct that justified the attempted use of DBS and cingulotomy for pain, absent from these studies were patients with refractory headache disorders. In fact, there has been a general dearth of reported intracranial interventions for refractory headache until recently. A likely reason is that the clinical trials assessing DBS for chronic pain compelled by new FDA regulations in the late 1980s were insufficiently designed to prove benefit, granting DBS only an off-label indication for chronic pain [1]. However, with improvement of DBS technique coupled with refined understanding of pathophysiologic pathways, DBS has been tested in multiple case series for the trigeminal autonomic cephalgias (TAC), a family of headache disorders including and related to cluster headache. Before describing the application of DBS to TACs, let us now discuss DBS in more depth.

Deep Brain Stimulation

Before discussing pathways, targets, and results of DBS for the TACs, it is imperative to understand both the disease entity and the intervention in further detail. Deep brain stimulation (DBS) is a functional neurosurgical technique that has been used primarily in movement disorders such as Parkinson's disease and essential tremor since the early 1990s (though, as described above, it was originally intended to treat chronic pain). The underlying principle of DBS is the application of high-frequency electrical stimulation to specific subcortical targets to affect symptomatic relief [13]. This electrical stimulation is achieved through the placement of electrodes into these identified targets and subsequent modulation of electrical signal. Much research has been performed investigating the underlying mechanism of DBS. While still not fully understood, hypotheses include activation and inhibition of targets and disruption of abnormal circuitry [14, 15].

There are three components in the DBS framework: the electrode, the neurostimulator, and the extension (which connects the former two) [16] (Figure 2). The operative technique to set up these components involves two procedures typically performed in staged sessions, although this can be and is performed in a single sitting as well. The first is intracranial placement of electrodes (also known as leads) into targeted regions in the brain. These can be placed unilaterally or bilaterally depending on what is being treated. Before the procedure, targets are located and mapped out using MR- or CT-based image guidance. Trajectory for insertion of the electrode (or electrodes) is determined, and placement proceeds through a small burr hole in the skull. The second procedure is placement of a battery-powered neurostimulator that provides stimulation to the electrode or electrodes via the extension, ultimately affecting neurophysiological change in the brain [16]. In subsequent appointments, the neurostimulator is programmed by a neurologist, skilled technician, or nurse (with changes in parameters such as voltage, pulse width, and frequency) in order to maximize symptom relief while minimizing adverse effects.

Risks of DBS (Table 1), both intra- and post-operatively, include the standard surgical risk of infection, which can occur up to 12 months after surgery [17], insertional or subcortical hemorrhage in 1% of patients, and hardware malfunction rate of $\leq$ 5% due to electrode fractures [18]. Also reported are seizures, DVT/PE, CSF leak, and complications from anesthesia [19]. Moreover, unique sets of neurological side effects based on location of the electrode may be expected. Programming sessions are utilized to find the right set of parameters on an individualized basis to minimize these side effects. As with any surgery, the patient should be informed of the risk of these complications when discussing the surgical option. Furthermore, with DBS, changes in body image must be explicitly discussed with the patient. Specifically, patients will have two quarter-sized bumps on either side of the skull, a scar three inches from the neurostimulator, and an inch long scar behind the ear, which are changes that warrant frank discussion [19].

Before being considered for surgery, patients must be examined by a multidisciplinary team to receive a formal diagnosis and must have failed multiple trials of medical options (which are discussed elsewhere in this book). In choosing appropriate patients for surgical therapy, it is particularly necessary to understand the poor surgical candidate. Poor candidates for surgical intervention for refractory headache include those with standard contraindications to surgery (such as high cardiopulmonary risk and thromboembolic propensity), patients with coagulopathies, and patients with an inability to undergo MRI [20]. A properly screened and selected surgical candidate is important for maximizing success of the intervention for the patient.

Table 1. Risks/Complications of DBS Surgery

Infection – may necessitate device explantation
Post-operative complications: DVT/PE, pneumonia, wound infection, MI
Subcortical hemorrhage
Stroke and neurological deficits
Seizure
CSF leak
Skin erosion
Memory loss, confusion
Personality change
Coma
Death
Anesthesia complications
Pneumocephalus

Note: Deep brain stimulation is a surgical procedure that carries corresponding surgical risk. The likelihood of complications is less than 10%, with very serious complications ranging from 1-4%. (Adapted from Watson et al., 2007.).

DBS for Trigeminal Autonomic Cephalgias

The best-studied refractory headache disorders treated with DBS are the trigeminal autonomic cephalgias (TAC). TACs constitute a group of rare disorders characterized by paroxysmal sensory hyperactivation in the trigeminal distribution associated with parasympathetic activation. Subtypes of TAC include cluster headache, short-lasting, unilateral, neuralgiform headaches with conjunctival tearing and injection (SUNCT), and paroxysmal hemicrania [20]. The reason that the application of DBS to TACs is the best characterized of the refractory headache disorders is that the associated pathologic pathways in the brain have been studied well, lending to better identification of targets for DBS, as discussed later.

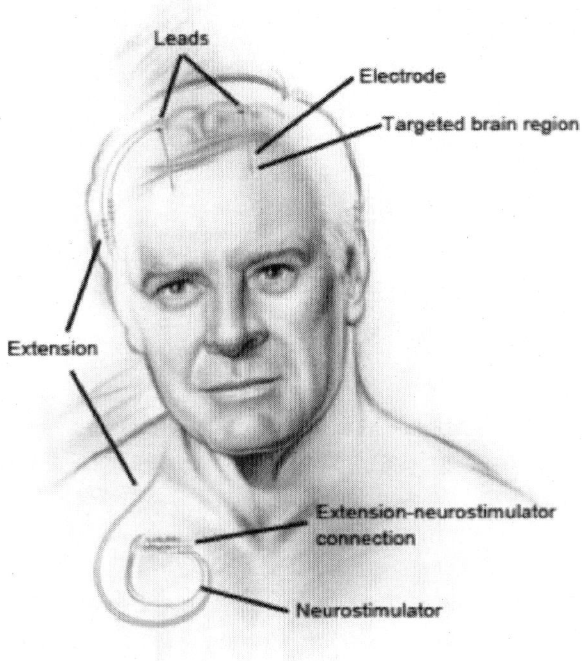

Figure 2. The main components of deep brain stimulation are highlighted here. Typically, the components are surgically implanted in staged sessions, although this can be accomplished in a single sitting as well. (Courtesy of Medtronic, adapted from Watson et al., 2007.).

The study of pain pathways involved in the pathogenesis of TACs is facilitated by their predictable onset, termed circadian recurrence [21]. Neuroimaging, including positron emission topography (PET) studies and functional MRI (fMRI), has been used to analyze activation patterns in the brains of these patients. Posterior hypothalamic neuronal activation has been consistently observed during attacks of cluster headaches, SUNCT, and paroxysmal hemicrania [21], consistent with the previous discussion about the role of the trigeminohypothalamic tract in processing pain. This is demonstrated in Figure 3, where the PET scan of a patient suffering from TAC shows activation of the posterior hypothalamus during an acute attack. Studies in rats have demonstrated that the trigeminal nerve and posterior hypothalamus exhibit reciprocal connections, suggesting a role of the hypothalamus in processing and modulating pain in the trigeminal distribution [14, 22]. Taken together, these findings suggest an elegant pathophysiologic model for the TACs centering on dysregulation of pain modulation. As previously mentioned, for intracranial functional neurosurgical interventions, it is necessary to define a target with demonstrated physiological underpinnings. The posterior hypothalamus, with a further contributory role of the nearby diencephalic-mesencephalic junction [23], has thus emerged as a target for DBS for TACs.

With a target established through these studies, the first hypothalamic DBS procedure for CCH was performed in 2001. Since then, over 50 patients have undergone the procedure, making CCH the best-studied type of refractory headache treated with DBS [20]. In discussing the results of DBS for CCH here, we keep in mind the goal of defining targets for other forms of refractory headache such as migraine, and providing similar functional neurosurgical intervention in the future.

In keeping with the strict selection of surgical candidates, patients receiving DBS for CCH meet the International Headache Society Criteria for CCH and demonstrate failed medical management, including inadequate relief with medical prophylaxis, along with chronic headaches for more than two years [20]. Since its inception, numerous studies have been performed assessing the efficacy of DBS for CCH. The largest single study was published in 2006 by Leone and colleagues, who assessed long-term efficacy in 16 patients who had undergone either ipsilateral or bilateral electrode placement in the posterior inferior hypothalamus [21]. Representative programming settings include: frequency of 180 Hz, voltage of 3 V, and pulse width of 60 microseconds, though optimal settings can differ from patient to patient [24]. Mean follow up of 4 years, 62% of patients remained pain-free with no recurrence of attacks, a dramatic improvement from their baseline functioning [21]. In 3 patients, symptomatology changed from chronic to episodic [21]. Smaller studies ranging from one to six patients report symptomatic improvement in patients as well [25-28]. A recent meta-analysis of 44 patients who had undergone posteromedial hypothalamic DBS found 50% of patients to have a response (defined by at least a 50% reduction in attack frequency and/or severity judged by symptom diary) [29]. Despite the profound improvement of some patients, these studies also highlight side effects and non-responders. In the literature of hypothalamic DBS for CCH, a non-symptomatic ventricular bleed was reported in one patient [14] and one patient died from intracerebral hemorrhage [26]. Side effects related specifically to hypothalamic stimulation include diplopia and weight loss, reported in a small percentage of patients [21]. Another important consideration in these studies is those patients who do not respond or experience symptomatic improvement. With any form of DBS, as mentioned before, the electrode target is a major factor in determining efficacy, and the failure of non-responders may be explained by location of the electrode. Seijo and colleagues recently utilized a modified, more laterally placed hypothalamic target in five patients. At mean follow up of 33 months, two patients were pain-free, two patients had >90% reduction of symptoms, and one had at least 50% reduction in symptoms, indicating the potential for continued anatomical target improvement in any form of DBS [30]. Table 2 is a summary of published studies investigating DBS for CCH.

DBS has also been used for SUNCT, another subtype of TAC that was previously mentioned. SUNCT presents similarly to cluster headaches. It is characterized by episodic attacks of stabbing pain in the orbital, supraorbital, or temporal distributions lasting from seconds to minutes. As the name suggest, SUNCT also causes ipsilateral conjunctival injection and excessive lacrimation [20]. Because SUNCT follows a similar pathophysiologic mechanism to CCH, DBS involving SUNCT has targeted the posterior hypothalamus. However, not as many patients have undergone DBS for SUNCT as it is a less prevalent condition than cluster headache, with one estimate of prevalence of 6.6/100,000 [31]. One patient with refractory SUNCT, as reported by Bartsch and colleagues, was noted to experience significant symptomatic relief after DBS. Prior to DBS, he had failed at least fourteen different medications, occipital nerve block, and microvascular decompression. He experienced multiple episodic attacks every day, often waking him from his sleep.

Since undergoing DBS, the frequency of his attacks has decreased significantly, and he is noted to have improved mood and an absence of side effects. Of note, the patient continued to require oral medication, as the frequency of attacks rises after decreasing medication, highlighting the importance of continued medical management after DBS [32]. Other case reports, totaling three patients, have reported a similar reduction in symptom severity for SUNCT patients undergoing DBS [33, 34].

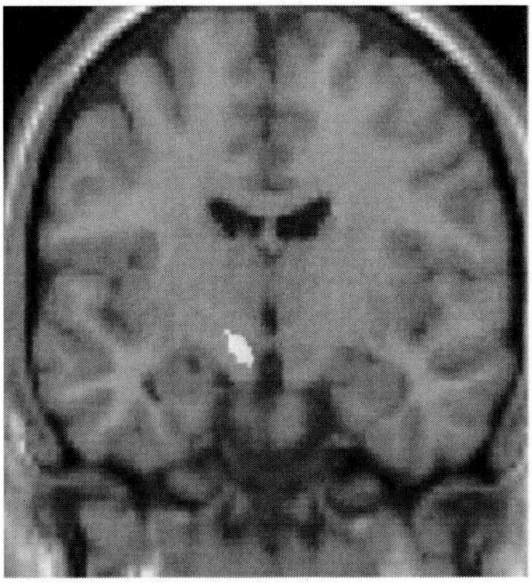

Figure 3. Positron-emission tomography (PET) studies of the brain in patients suffering from all subtypes of TAC demonstrated activation of the ipsilateral posterior hypothalamic grey matter (yellow region) during an acute attack. Replication of these findings defined a clear-cut anatomic target for TAC DBS, which has resulted in an increasing number of patients being treated for refractory TAC. (From May, A., 2005: *Cluster headache: pathogenesis, diagnosis, and management*).

Table 2. Summary of multiple trials of hypothalamic DBS for CCH (from Leone et al. 2008)

Study	# implanted pts	Mean follow up (yrs)	# pain-free or almost pain-free	Percentage improved
Schoenen et al. (2005)	4	4	2	50
D'Andrea et al. (2006)	3	2.5	2	66
Leone et al. (2006)	16	4	10	62
Starr et al. (2007)	4	1	2	50
Bartsch et al. (2008)	6	1.4	3	50
Owen et al. (2007)	1	0.7	1	100
Benabid et al. (2006)	1	1	1	100
Mateos et al. (2007)	2	1	2	100
Totals	50		23	59

Future Directions: DBS for Refractory Migraine?

In speaking of refractory headache disorders, no discussion is complete without considering the most prevalent condition: migraine. Affecting as many as 40 million Americans and 1.3-5.1% of the world population, migraine will typically respond to medical therapeutic options [20, 35]. However, about 3-10% of migraine sufferers will progress to a chronic state, defined by experiencing pain for more than half of the days in each month [36]. Refractory migraine sufferers experience little to no relief from mainstays of medical management, failing trials of multiple treatment options because of inefficacy or inability to tolerate [36]. At this time, the surgical options for migraine are limited. Chronic refractory migraine has not yet been treated with DBS [37], but peripheral neuromodulation has been employed as discussed elsewhere in this book. Methods that have been studied in patients include occipital nerve stimulation (ONS), peripheral trigeminal nerve branch stimulation, and vagal nerve stimulation [36, 38]. There is potential for surgical intervention for chronic, refractory migraine in the future however. Again, for DBS considerations, the identification of a target is the most important first step. Neuroimaging of chronic migraine has demonstrated abnormalities in regions involved in similar trigeminal pathways as those previously mentioned for TAC, along with those regions involved in chronic pain, including anterior cingulate cortex and somatosensory cortex changes [39, 40]. Further delineation of pathways involved in migraine has also suggested involvement of multiple nuclei of the thalamus in modulating pain and photophobia [9]. Moreover, brainstem involvement, particularly of the periaqueductal gray matter (PAG) and dorsolateral pons (DLP), is also shown on neuroimaging analysis [9]. In fact, PAG and sensory thalamus have been successfully explored as targets in DBS for intractable pain [41-43]. The involvement of these regions in both chronic pain and migraine suggest both a common pathway for these pathologies and potential targets for migraine DBS in the future. More research is needed before trials are undertaken.

Conclusion

In conclusion, refractory headache disorders are those that have failed multiple trials of the available medical therapies. Patients with these disorders suffer through daily, debilitating symptomatology. Within this group of patients, properly identified surgical candidates may benefit from the growing field of functional neurosurgical intervention in the form of deep brain stimulation. DBS, which was originally intended as a neurosurgical intervention for chronic, refractory pain, was repurposed in the 1990s for successful application to movement disorders such as Parkinson disease in patients for whom medical therapy has become ineffective. Its application to a variety of other neurological issues is now being explored, including refractory headache disorders. In this field, DBS has been best studied in its application to treatment of the trigeminal autonomic cephalgias, which include chronic cluster headaches. Patients with refractory CCH undergoing DBS have demonstrated a spectrum of symptomatic relief in long-term studies. Combined with the continued improvement of anatomic targets, this represents a promising therapeutic option for the patient who has been suffering for years with no relief from multiple trials of medical management. Though DBS for refractory migraine has not been attempted, its application is currently being studied. Overlap in the pathways involved in pain processing between migraine, TACs, and chronic pain indicates possible therapeutic potential and a possible surgical avenue for relief for a significant number of people suffering from a devastating disorder.

References

[1] Pereira, EA; Green, AL; Aziz, TZ. Deep brain stimulation for pain. *Handb Clin Neurol*, 2013, 116, 277-94.

[2] Wilkinson, HA; Davidson, KM; Davidson, RI. Bilateral anterior cingulotomy for chronic noncancer pain. *Neurosurgery*, 1999, 45(5), 1129-34, discussion 1134-6.

[3] Goadsby, PJ. Pathophysiology of Headache, in Wolff's Headache and other head pain, S.D. Silberstein; et al. Editors. 2008, Oxford University Press: New York. p. xx, 844 p.

[4] Moskowitz, MA. Basic mechanisms in vascular headache. *Neurol Clin*, 1990, 8(4), 801-15.

[5] Akerman, S., & Romero-Reyes, M. Insights into the pharmacological targeting of the trigeminocervical complex in the context of treatments of migraine. *Expert Rev Neurother*, 2013, 13(9), 1041-1059.

[6] Akerman, S, Holland, PR; Goadsby, PJ. Diencephalic and brainstem mechanisms in migraine. *Nat Rev Neurosci*, 2011, 12(10), 570-84.

[7] Moulton, EA; et al. Interictal dysfunction of a brainstem descending modulatory center in migraine patients. *PLoS One*, 2008, 3(11), e3799.

[8] Haines, D. Spinal Trigeminal Pathway: Anterior Trigeminothalamic Tract. 4th ed. Fundamental neuroscience for basic and clinical applications, ed. D.E. Haines and M.D. Ard. 2013, Philadelphia, PA: Elsevier Saunders. xi, 492 p.

[9] Noseda, R; Burstein, R. Migraine pathophysiology: anatomy of the trigeminovascular pathway and associated neurological symptoms, CSD, sensitization and modulation of pain. *Pain*, 2013, 154 Suppl 1.

[10] Reynolds, DV. Surgery in the rat during electrical analgesia induced by focal brain stimulation. *Science*, 1969, 164(3878), 444-5.

[11] Liebeskind, JC; et al. Analgesia from electrical stimulation of the periaqueductal gray matter in the cat: behavioral observations and inhibitory effects on spinal cord interneurons. *Brain Res*, 1973, 50(2), 441-6.

[12] Gasquoine, PG. Localization of function in anterior cingulate cortex: from psychosurgery to functional neuroimaging. *Neurosci Biobehav Rev*, 2013, 37(3), 340-8.

[13] Chiken, S; Nambu, A. Disrupting neuronal transmission: mechanism of DBS? *Front Syst Neurosci*, 2014, 8, p. 33.

[14] Leone, M. Deep brain stimulation in headache. *Lancet Neurol*, 2006, 5(10), 873-7.

[15] Karas, PJ; et al. Deep brain stimulation: a mechanistic and clinical update. *Neurosurg Focus*, 2013, 35(5), p. E1.

[16] NINDS. *NINDS Deep Brain Stimulation for Parkinson's Disease Information Page*. 2014 (cited 2014 11 May).

[17] Umemura, A; et al. Deep brain stimulation for movement disorders: morbidity and mortality in 109 patients. *J Neurosurg*, 2003, 98(4), 779-84.

[18] Chan, DT; et al. Complications of deep brain stimulation: a collective review. *Asian J Surg*, 2009, 32(4), 258-63.
[19] Watson, HC; Bunting-Perry, LK; Heath, SL. *Deep Brain Stimulation Preop Assessment and Teaching*, in *Deep brain stimulation for Parkinson's disease*, G.H. Baltuch and M.B. Stern, Editors. 2007, Informa Healthcare: New York. p. xiii, 349 p.
[20] Hong, J; Roberts, DW. The surgical treatment of headache. *Headache*, 2014, 54(3), 409-29.
[21] Leone, M; et al. Lessons from 8 years' experience of hypothalamic stimulation in cluster headache. *Cephalalgia*, 2008, 28(7), 787-97; discussion 798.
[22] Malick, A, Strassman, RM; Burstein, R. Trigeminohypothalamic and reticulohypothalamic tract neurons in the upper cervical spinal cord and caudal medulla of the rat. *J Neurophysiol*, 2000, 84(4), 2078-112.
[23] Clelland, CD; et al. Common cerebral networks associated with distinct deep brain stimulation targets for cluster headache. *Cephalalgia*, 2014, 34(3), 224-30.
[24] Leone, M; Franzini, A; Bussone, G. Stereotactic stimulation of posterior hypothalamic gray matter in a patient with intractable cluster headache. *N Engl J Med*, 2001, 345(19), 1428-9.
[25] Starr, PA; et al. Chronic stimulation of the posterior hypothalamic region for cluster headache: technique and 1-year results in four patients. *J Neurosurg*, 2007, 106(6), 999-1005.
[26] Schoenen, J; et al. Hypothalamic stimulation in chronic cluster headache: a pilot study of efficacy and mode of action. *Brain*, 2005, 128(Pt 4), 940-7.
[27] Bartsch, T; et al. Hypothalamic deep brain stimulation for cluster headache: experience from a new multicase series. *Cephalalgia*, 2008, 28(3), 285-95.
[28] Sillay, KA; Sani, S; Starr, PA. Deep brain stimulation for medically intractable cluster headache. *Neurobiol Dis*, 2010, 38(3), 361-8.
[29] Franzini, A; et al. Deep brain stimulation of the posteromedial hypothalamus: indications, long-term results, and neurophysiological considerations. *Neurosurg Focus*, 2010, 29(2), p. E13.
[30] Seijo, F; et al. Neuromodulation of the posterolateral hypothalamus for the treatment of chronic refractory cluster headache: Experience in five patients with a modified anatomical target. *Cephalalgia*, 2011, 31(16), 1634-41.
[31] Lambru, G; Matharu, MS. SUNCT and SUNA: medical and surgical treatments. *Neurol Sci*, 2013, 34 Suppl 1, S75-81.
[32] Bartsch, T; et al. Deep brain stimulation of the posterior hypothalamic area in intractable short-lasting unilateral neuralgiform headache with conjunctival injection and tearing (SUNCT). *Cephalalgia*, 2011, 31(13), 1405-8.
[33] Leone, M; et al. Deep brain stimulation to relieve drug-resistant SUNCT. *Ann Neurol*, 2005, 57(6), 924-7.
[34] Lyons, MK; Dodick, DW; Evidente, VG. Responsiveness of short-lasting unilateral neuralgiform headache with conjunctival injection and tearing to hypothalamic deep brain stimulation. *J Neurosurg*, 2009, 110(2), 279-81.
[35] Lionetto, L; et al. Emerging treatment for chronic migraine and refractory chronic migraine. *Expert Opin Emerg Drugs*, 2012, 17(3), 393-406.
[36] Rasskazoff, SY; Slavin, KV. Neuromodulation for cephalgias. *Surg Neurol Int*, 2013, 4(Suppl 3), S136-50.

[37] Magis, D; Jensen, R; Schoenen, J. Neurostimulation therapies for primary headache disorders: present and future. *Curr Opin Neurol*, 2012, 25(3), 269-76.

[38] Perini, F; De Boni, A. Peripheral neuromodulation in chronic migraine. *Neurol Sci*, 2012, 33 Suppl 1, S29-31.

[39] Dasilva, AF; et al. tDCS-induced analgesia and electrical fields in pain-related neural networks in chronic migraine. *Headache*, 2012, 52(8), 1283-95.

[40] Chiapparini, L; et al. Neuroimaging in chronic migraine. *Neurol Sci*, 2010, 31 Suppl 1: S19-22.

[41] Gray, AM; et al. Deep brain stimulation as a treatment for neuropathic pain: a longitudinal study addressing neuropsychological outcomes. *J Pain*, 2014, 15(3), 283-92.

[42] Owen, SL; et al. Deep brain stimulation for the alleviation of post-stroke neuropathic pain. *Pain*, 2006, 120(1-2), 202-6.

[43] Bittar, RG; et al. Deep brain stimulation for pain relief: a meta-analysis. *J Clin Neurosci*, 2005, 12(5), 515-9.

In: Migraine Surgery
Editor: Antonios Mammis
ISBN: 978-1-63321-761-4

Chapter 11

Migraine and Movement Disorders

*Tasneem Peeraully**
Department of Neurology and Neurosciences,
Rutgers New Jersey Medical School, Newark, New Jersey, US

Introduction

There are a number of reports in the scientific literature linking migraine and dopamine. Furthermore, there is evidence that the basal ganglia play a role in pain processing. Pathological alterations in basal ganglia connectivity are primarily implicated in the development of movement disorders. Frequency of migraine has been documented in a number of movement disorders, including essential tremor, Parkinson's disease, and restless legs syndrome. Proposed mechanisms for an association include dopaminergic dysfunction, disruption of brain iron homeostasis, and genetic linkage. [1] In this chapter, the evidence for associations between headache and movement disorders is summarized. Establishing whether or not an association exists may be helpful in identifying potentially shared pathophysiology and application of common treatment strategies.

Basal Ganglia and Migraine

The basal ganglia integrate sensory, emotional and cognitive aspects of pain information via basal ganglia-thalamo-cortical loops. Changes in the basal ganglia activity occur in migraineurs that may account for alterations in cognition and the complex behavioral adaptive responses that characterize migraine. Functional imaging studies demonstrate increased blood

* Corresponding Author: Tasneem Peeraully, MBBS BSc; Assistant Professor; Department of Neurology and Neurosciences; Rutgers New Jersey Medical School; Doctors Office Center, Suite 8100; 90 Bergen Street, Newark, NJ 07103; Phone: 973 972 7407; Fax: 973 972 2559; Email: peerauta@rutgers.edu.

flow in the basal ganglia during migraine attacks, and decreased activation during interictal periods in migraineurs compared to controls. [2]

Migraine aura is likely mediated by cortical spreading depression, a short-lasting depolarization wave that moves across the cortex at a rate of 3–5 millimeters per minute. In a rodent model of migraine with aura, there is reduced neuronal activity in the caudate after induction of cortical spreading depression. [3]

Responses to heat pain stimuli on functional magnetic resonance imaging is significantly lower in the caudate, putamen and pallidum in patients with high frequency of migraine compared to those with low frequency of migraine. However, gray matter volume of the caudate nuclei is significantly larger in the high frequency migraineurs than in the low frequency migraineurs.

Role of Dopamine in Cell Signaling Underlying Migraine

Dopamine is one of several neurotransmitters implicated in migraine. Dopamine may mediate excitatory or inhibitory effects depending upon the receptor activated. D1-like receptors (D1 and D5 receptors) are excitatory whereas D2-like receptors (D2, D3 and D4 receptors) are inhibitory. Dopamine acts in pathogenic mechanisms of migraine, but may also act on certain pathways to protect against migraine.

Dopamine hypersensitivity may explain some migraine features. Premonitory migraine symptoms of yawning, nausea, vomiting and dizziness are attributed to dopaminergic activity. [4] These same symptoms are also seen as side effects of apomorphine, a dopamine agonist, although headaches are not a recognized side effect of dopaminergic therapy. Conversely, D2 receptor antagonists including prochlorperazine and metoclopramide are helpful in management of premonitory migraine symptoms. [5].

In keeping with the theory of migraine as a state of dopamine hypersensitivity, migraineurs demonstrate increased binding affinity of dopamine to platelet D2 receptors in migraineurs. [6, 7]. The Nco1 gene encodes the D2 receptor and has C and T alleles. Increased frequency of the C allele has been demonstrated in migraine with aura, compared to migraine without aura and controls. [8] By contrast, the D4 receptor gene appears to be involved in migraine without aura. Transmission distortion in third exon of the D4 receptor gene and over-represented of allele 4 of D4 receptor gene have been described in migraine without aura. [7]

Single nucleotide polymorphisms in promoter region of dopamine beta hydroxylase (DBH) gene, leading to a C to T substitution, have been associated with migraine. DBH catalyzes conversion of dopamine to norepinephrine. T alleles lower plasma levels of DBH activity and increase availability of dopamine. The TT genotype is associated with a reduced risk of migraine. [9].

The trigeminocervical complex (TCC) conveys somatosensory and visceral information from head and face to the hypothalamus. Aberrant firing of the TCC is involved in migraine. Presence of dopamine receptors in trigeminal ganglion and spinal trigeminal nuclei has been demonstrated in rodents. [10] In rat studies, quinpirole, a centrally acting D2 receptor agonist, inhibits nociceptive transmission at the TCC, whereas centrally acting D2-like receptor antagonists facilitate TCC firing. [11]

Dopaminergic pathways in the brain include nigrostriatal, mesocorticolimbic and tuberoinfundibular pathways. While dopamine modulates control of movement via the nigrostriatal pathway, the tuberoinfundibular pathway is implicated in menstrual migraine. Progesterone stimulates the arcuate nucleus of the hypothalamus, resulting in release of dopamine. Dopamine, in turn, inhibits the anterior pituitary from secreting prolactin. Migrainous women have higher serum prolactin, possibly due to decreased responsiveness to either progesterone or dopamine. [12] Interestingly, cabergoline, a dopamine D2-like receptor agonist, was shown to be useful in improving menstrual-related migraines in a small study.

The A11 nucleus, located in the posterior hypothalamus, sends inhibitory dopaminergic projections to dorsal horn of the spinal cord, modulating trigeminal afferents and inhibiting nociceptive signaling from the TCC. [13] Dysfunction of A11 inhibitory tone has been implicated in migraine but may also play a role in restless legs syndrome (RLS). In mice treated with iron-deficiency diet and 6-OHDA lesions, locomotor activities were increased significantly. This behavior was reversed by administration of ropinirole, a D2/D3 agonist. D2/D3 mRNA and protein levels as well as their binding capacity in the spinal cord were decreased by 6-OHDA lesioning in A11. Combined iron deficiency and 6-OHDA lesions produced a synergistic greater decrease of D2 binding. [14]

Impaired Iron Homeostasis in Migraine and Movement Disorders

Iron forms an essential component in oxygen carrier proteins and many metabolic enzymes. Non-heme iron may be stored as non-toxic ferritin or may be present in a soluble form which can catalyze formation of free radicals which can result in DNA, protein and neuronal cell damage. [15]

Impaired iron homeostasis may be seen in both migraine and certain movement disorders. While Parkinson's disease is complicated by exaggerated iron retention in the substantia nigra pars compacta, restless legs syndrome (RLS) is associated with iron deficiency. [16] Brain iron content is significantly reduced in the substantia nigra, thalamus, putamen and pallidum of RLS patients. [17,18]

In migraine there is evidence for increased brain iron accumulation. [19] Increased iron concentration is found in the periaqueductal grey matter (PAG), putamen, globus pallidus and red nucleus in migraineurs compared to controls, as measured using T2 values on magnetic resonance imaging. Higher iron concentration is correlated with a longer migraine history. It has yet to be elucidated whether the iron accumulation is causative or occurs as a physiologic response to migraine. One theory is that hyperemia during repeated migraine attacks leads to free-radical cell damage and subsequent iron deposition. The PAG is known to be activated during migraine attacks, it has been proposed that iron accumulation further impairs the functions of the brainstem and deep brain nuclei involved in the central anti-nociceptive network in migraineurs. [13]

Parkinson's Disease and Migraine

Parkinson's disease (PD) is a neurodegenerative disorder affecting 1-2% of the population over the age of 60. Intraneuronal alpha-synuclein-positive Lewy bodies are the pathological hallmark of the disease. Involvement of dopaminergic cells in the substantia nigra pars compacta is associated with development of the motor features of PD; bradykinesia, rigidity, tremor, and postural instability. Motor symptoms generally start on one side, with progression to bilateral involvement. Asymmetry is usually preserved, with the side initially involved remaining the most severely affected.

Lifetime prevalence of migraine in PD ranges from 19-23%. [20,21,22] Although PD is more common in older ages when migraine tends to spontaneously remit, it has been proposed that Parkinson's disease might modify the course of migraine. Current migraine is less frequent in PD patients with a lifetime history of migraine compared to age-matched controls with lifetime history of migraine. Prevalence of current migraine ranges from 13-47% in PD vs. 31-68% in controls, Of note, two thirds of PD patients report improvement or remission in migraine after onset of PD motor symptoms. Possible mechanisms for this intriguing observation include a prophylactic effect of chronic dopaminergic therapy and a positive effect of nigral degeneration on migraine pathophysiology. Dopaminergic therapy might be expected to worsen migraine in the latter, unless serotonergic functions of the substantia nigra are primarily implicated. Dopamine agonists are known to have some serotonergic effects and the substantia nigra is known to contain a high concentration of 5HT3 receptors. [23]

Nunes et al. hypothesized that if nigral degeneration does indeed confer protection against migraine, one would expect asymmetry of neurodegeneration in PD would lead to a lower prevalence of headache in the more affected side of the brain, contralateral to the side of symptom onset, in PD migraineurs. [10] True to their expectations, they found a positive correlation between predominant side of headache over the previous year and side of initial PD symptoms in 25 PD patients with migraine. Headache was ipsilateral to the side of motor symptom onset in 84% of PD patients ($p<0.01$).

Cubo et al. proposed that dopaminergic hypersensitivity in migraineurs should predict better response to levodopa in PD patients with migraine compared to those without migraine. They tested their hypothesis in 10 PD patients with migraine and 18 PD controls without migraine. [24] Interestingly, PD patients with migraine showed greater motor improvement with levodopa as measured by the Unified Parkinson's Disease Rating Scale ($p=0.011$). PD patients with migraine were also on lower doses of dopaminergic medication, although the difference was not statistically significant.

Essential Tremor and Migraine

Essential tremor (ET) is defined as a bilateral postural tremor of gradual onset with or without kinetic tremor, involving hands and forearms, gradual in onset, visible, and persistent. Whether or not a link between ET and migraine exists is still debated, with studies yielding conflicting results. Uncontrolled studies implicated an association between migraine and essential tremor (ET), with 26-30% of ET patients reported to have migraine and 17.2% of migraineurs observed to have ET. [25, 26] Approximately 4-5% of the population over age 40 have essential tremor while prevalence of migraine in the general population is estimated to be 7-18%. [27, 28, 29] Given the high prevalence of both disorders, these studies might have detected coexistence rather than comorbidity. In an initial case-control study of 110 ET patients and 110 age and sex matched controls, no significant difference in prevalence or frequency of lifetime migraine was found. Lifetime migraine was reported in 25% of patients with ET and 22% of controls. [30] However, in a Chinese study of 150 ET and 150 matched controls, prevalence of lifetime migraine was 22% and 12.7% respectively, $p=0.035$. [31] In both case-control studies, there was no difference in migraine features between ET migraineurs and control migraineurs. [30, 31] Most tremor characteristics were similar in ET patients with and without migraine although there is a significant female prevalence in patients with ET and migraine.

The *DRD3* gene, on the essential tremor 1 (ETM-1) locus, on chromosome 3q13, encodes the dopamine D3 receptor. *DRD3* is expressed in the basal ganglia, cerebral cortex, cerebellum, and brainstem nuclei. A functional variant of the *DRD3* gene (Ser9Gly, rs6280) is associated with ET, and homozygosity was linked to greater severity and/or earlier onset of symptoms. [31, 32]. Although increased density of lymphocytic D3 receptors have been demonstrated in migraineurs, studies trying to establish a genetic link between ET and migraine have failed to find an association between the *DRD3* gene and migraine. [31,33] While 44/46 ET patients expressed the Ser9Gly variant, there was no significant difference between frequencies of the variant in those with and without migraine. [31]

Tourette's Syndrome and Migraine

Tourette's syndrome (TS) is a common childhood movement disorder characterized by motor and phonic tics. Reported rates of migraine headache in patients with TS range from 17-27%, 4 times higher than the rate of migraine in the general pediatric population. [34,35,36].

The high prevalence of migraine in TS has been explained by serotoninergic system dysregulation, also implicated in TS and obsessive-compulsive disorder (OCD). Barabas et al. speculated that obsessive compulsive features might predict migraine in patients with Tourette's syndrome, although two studies have found no significant association between migraine and comorbid attention deficit hyperactivity disorder or OCD in TS. [25] However, other biochemical abnormalities, including involvement of the dopaminergic system, have been proposed in TS. [35]

In one series of 100 TS patients, there was no significant difference in percentage of patients medicated between those with headache and those with no headache (75% versus 69% respectively). [27] Medication used included antipsychotics, stimulants, anxiolytics, selective serotonin reuptake inhibitors, serotonin-norepinephrine reuptake inhibitors and alpha agonists. Numbers may not have been large enough to detect a difference between types of medication used in the migraine and non-migraine groups.

Restless Legs Syndrome and Migraine

Restless legs syndrome (RLS), is characterized by an urge to move the legs, usually accompanied by an unpleasant sensations in the legs. [37] The discomfort typically occurs in the evening or night, is worse during periods of rest or inactivity, and is relieved by movement. Symptoms respond to dopaminergic drugs. RLS can also be associated with medical conditions such as renal failure, iron deficiency, neuropathy, and pregnancy. [16] Iron supplementation is indicated in the setting of iron deficiency.

RLS is reported to be present in up to a third of migraineurs with studies indicating an increased prevalence of migraine in RLS of 15-23%. [28, 38, 39, 40, 41, 42] Migraineurs with RLS reported premonitory symptoms significantly more often than migraineurs without RLS. [43] Of note, one Italian study found the prevalence of RLS in migraine with aura to be similar to that in headache-free subjects (9.5% and 8.3% respectively).

Looking at mean scores on International Restless Legs Syndrome Severity Grading (IRLSSG) scale, Gozubatik-Celik et al. found severity of RLS was higher in patients with migraine compared to those without headache (23.8 versus 16, $p<0.01$). However, there was no significant difference in RLS severity between migraineurs and those with non-migraine headache. [28] Family history of RLS and headache were also higher in patients with migraine. Interestingly, 36/40 RLS participants with migraine reported improvement in migraine with RLS treatment.

There is also evidence from two populations based studies to support an association between RLS and migraine. As part of the Women's Health Study, 31370 women were followed over a 9-year period, with 22% reporting either prior or current migraine. [41] Those women were found to have an increased risk for RLS compared to those without migraine (14.5% vs. 11.2% respectively, odds ratio 1.22, $p<0.0001$). When migraine subcategorized, the association remained similar for migraine with aura, migraine without aura and those with reports of new migraine, but not for those with prior history of migraine. In a subsequent study of 22,926 male participants recruited from the Physicians' Health Study, 12.3% reported migraine and 7.5% reported RLS. [40] Migraine was associated with an increased risk of RLS, similar to that reported in women (odds ratio 1.20).

In support of a joint underlying pathophysiology, the gene encoding survival motor neuron interacting protein 1 (*SIP1*) on chromosome 14q21 has been found to confer a genetic predisposition to both RLS and migraine without aura in an Italian family. [40] By contrast, no association has been detected between RLS and familial cases of migraine with aura.

Sydenham's Chorea and Migraine

Sydenham's chorea (SC) is an autoimmune disorder characterized by involuntary, non-rhythmic, irregular movements that flow from one body part to another, and is seen as a delayed complication of infection with group A beta-hemolytic streptococcus. Reported to occur in 20-30% of patients with acute rheumatic fever, it is now infrequently seen in developed countries due to early recognition and adequate treatment of the initial pharyngitis. [44] Anti-basal ganglia antibodies are present in patients with SC, but can also be detected in about 13% of patients with RF without an overt movement disorder.

Brazilian investigators made an interesting observation on the frequency of migraine in individuals with SC. Fifty-five participants with SC were compared with 55 participants with rheumatic fever but no movement disorder (RF), and 110 controls. Participants with SC and RF had an increased frequency of migraine (21.8% vs. 18.2% respectively) compared to controls (8.1%). [45] In addition, there was a trend towards migraine with aura occurring with increasing frequency in SC compared to RF (12.7% vs. 1.8%, $p>0.06$).

The investigators proposed that their findings were consistent with the hypothesis that basal ganglia pathology is implicated in migraine, and that the trend towards migraine with aura in SC might reflect greater basal ganglia pathology in SC compared to RF.

Table 1 summarizes the migraine frequency observed in the different movement disorders discussed above.

Table 1. Movement disorders and migraine

Movement disorder	Incidence of migraine compared to controls	References
Essential tremor	Mixed	[25, 26, 30, 31]
Parkinson's disease	reduced	[40, 54, 55]
Tourette's syndrome	increased	[34, 35, 36]
Sydenham's chorea	Increased	[53]
Restless legs syndrome	increased	[28, 38, 39, 40, 41, 42]

Channelopathies

Channelopathies are a group of disorders resulting from mutations in genes that encode proteins involved in ion transportation. They exhibit genotypic and phenotypic heterogeneity, so that mutations in different genes may result in the same clinical symptoms, and different mutations within the same gene may manifest differently. Phenotypes include hemiplegic migraine, movement disorders and epilepsy. Genetic diversity of each ion channel, complex heteromultimeric assembly of channel subunits and post-translational modifications may impact clinical phenotype. [46] The episodic nature of the clinical manifestations of channelopathies might be explained by a low threshold of malfunctioning and increased susceptibility to minor insults.

Familial hemiplegic migraine (FHM) is a rare disorder characterized by migraine with aura including any degree of paresis or hemiparesis, with at least one similarly affected first- or second-degree relative. Inheritance is autosomal dominant with variable penetrance. Causative genes include *CACNA1A* (calcium channel, voltage dependent, P/Q type, alpha-1A subunit), *SCN1A* (sodium channel, neuronal type 1, alpha subunit), and *ATP1A2* (ATPase Na+/K+ transporting, alpha-2 polypeptide), resulting in FHM1, FHM2 and FHM3 respectively (see table 2). [47] In 60% of affected families, the implicated gene is *CACNA1A* located on chromosome 19p13. The FHM1 phenotype is caused by a gain of function mutation in *CACNA1A*. Childhood absence epilepsy and episodic ataxia type 2 are allelic disorders resulting from loss of function mutations in *CACNA1A*, although individuals with FHM1 may have fixed cerebellar signs and progressive ataxia. [18].

Table 2. Ion channel genes implicated in familial hemiplegic migraine and allelic disorders

Gene	Ion channel	Disorders
CACNA1A	Voltage-dependent P/Q type Ca2+ channel, alpha 1A subunit	FHM1, EA2, SCA6, CAE, BPTI, BPVC
ATP1A2	Na+/K+ ATPase, alpha 2 subunit	FHM2,
SCN1A	Voltage-gated fast inactivating Na+ channel	FHM3, GEFS+, SMEI

Key: BPTI – benign paroxysmal torticollis of infancy; BPVC – benign paroxysmal vertigo of childhood; CAE – childhood absence epilepsy; EA2- episodic ataxia type 2; FHM 1 – familial hemiplegic migraine *type 1;* FHM 2 - familial hemiplegic migraine *type 2;* FHM 3 - familial hemiplegic migraine *type 3;* GEFS+ - genetic (generalized) epilepsy and febrile seizures; SCA6 – spinocerebellar ataxia type 6; SMEI - severe myoclonic epilepsy of infancy.

Episodic ataxia type II (EA2) is characterized by episodes of ataxia lasting about 10 minutes triggered by emotional stress or physical exertion. Hemiplegic episodes occur in 10% of individuals. Episodic ataxia II responds to treatment with acetazolamide. Acetazolamide has also been reported as having a beneficial effect in some patients with FHM. [20].

Other paroxysmal movement disorders associated with *CACNA1A* mutations include benign paroxysmal torticollis and benign paroxysmal vertigo of childhood. Benign paroxysmal torticollis is characterized by stereotyped periodic episodes of torticollis lasting hours to days, and typically begins in the first 6 months of life, improving by 2 years, and remitting by 4 years. Associated movements include tortipelvis and ataxia. Associations with familial hemiplegic migraine have been documented. [48].

Benign paroxysmal vertigo of childhood is characterized by recurrent attacks of vertigo, nystagmus and ataxia, with onset between 2 and 5 years. Symptoms may remit in childhood or persist into adolescence. [22].

Antiepileptic drugs acting on ion channels are commonly used in the management of migraine prophylaxis and paroxysmal movement disorders. [18] Lamotrigine, a sodium channel blocker causing decreased release of glutamate, is effective in reducing the frequency and intensity of migraine aura. In a study of 59 patients, including 8 with paresis, 75% had reduction of migraine aura frequency by at least 50%. [49] Other medications used for aura symptoms in hemiplegic migraine include ketamine, an NMDA glutamate receptor antagonist, and intravenous verapamil, a calcium channel blocker. [50] Oral verapamil has been used for prophylaxis in patients with both familial and sporadic hemiplegic migraine with variable results.

PRRT2 Mutations in Hemiplegic Migraine and Paroxysmal Movement Disorders

The *PRRT2* gene on chromosome 16 encodes proline-rich transmembrane protein 2. Mutations in the *PRRT2* gene have been associated with hemiplegic migraine, paroxysmal movement disorder and epilepsy syndromes. Box 1 lists the various paroxysmal disorders associated with mutations of *PRRT2*.

PRRT2 is expressed predominantly in the central nervous system, and is particularly high in the early postnatal period, with low expression before embryonic day 16 and in adulthood. [26] In the postnatal period there is widespread *PRRT2* mRNA expression in the cerebral cortex, cerebellum, hippocampus, and basal ganglia. Thus it is possible that *PRRT2* mutations could manifest different phenotypes in a single individual due to age dependent expression, with remission in adulthood, e.g., epilepsy in infancy and paroxysmal movement disorders in adolescence.

Most *PRRT2* mutations result in premature stop codons and degradation of the mutated messenger RNA, leading to haploinsufficiency. Missense mutations, mostly reported to be closely situated to the transmembrane protein domain, may adversely affect protein function.

PRRT2 protein associates with SNAP-25, a presynaptic protein involved in the docking mechanism of neurotransmitter-containing vesicles, to facilitate exocytosis and release into the synaptic cleft. SNAP-25 may also modulate function of voltage-gated calcium channels. *PRRT2* mutations might alter the properties of voltage gated calcium channels, including $Ca_v2.1$ which is also linked to hemiplegic migraine. [46]

Interestingly, botulinum neurotoxin serotypes A, C and E act by cleaving SNAP-25. One of the proposed mechanisms for botulinum toxin type A in migraine prophylaxis is decreased glutamate-induced mechanical sensitivity of nociceptors and neurogenic vasodilation. Investigators found significantly reduced SNAP-25 in Western blot analysis of injected temporalis muscles and theorized that inhibition of glutamate release reduced provoked CGRP release from muscle nociceptors. [51] Moreover, these effects did not appear to be mediated by muscle weakness as findings were not reproduced with paralysis induced by pancuronium, implicating an alternative mechanism of action in the efficacy of botulinum toxin type A in migraine management.

At least a quarter of families affected and most sporadic cases of hemiplegic migraine do not have a mutation in one of the three FHM genes. [52] One study detected *PRRT2* mutations in 4 out of 101 patients with hemiplegic migraine in whom no mutations in the known FHM genes were identified. [53] Of these four patients, one also developed paroxysmal movement disorder and seizures.

Paroxysmal kinesigenic dyskinesia (PKD) is an autosomal dominant condition with onset in childhood, characterized by brief, frequent attacks of chorea, dystonia, athetosis and ballism, and induced by movement or anticipation of movements. Symptoms respond well to anti-epileptic medications including phenytoin and carbamazepine. [54] Although PKD has similarities with channelopathy PMDs, there has been no association demonstrated with genes encoding channel-related proteins. [55] Studies of Chinese and European populations have identified *PRRT2* mutations in more than 90% of familial cases and 34-45% of sporadic cases of PKD. [22, 56, 57, 58] Three mutations in the *PRRT2* gene have been found in different kindreds with PKD. Two of the mutations cause truncation of the protein, with absence of the transmembrane domain, suggesting resultant loss-of-function.

Benign familial infantile seizures occur in 40% of individuals with PKD. [59,60,61] *PRRT2* mutations identified in 61-96% of families with infantile convulsions and paroxysmal choreoathetosis (ICCA) syndrome in Asian, African-American and Caucasian cohorts and a third of sporadic cases from a Taiwanese study. [25, 62, 63]. Rarely, *PRRT2* mutations may be a cause of episodic ataxia, paroxysmal non-kinesigenic dyskinesia (PNKD), and paroxysmal exertional dyskinesia. [22]

Box 1: Migraine, movement disorders and epilepsy associated with PRRT2 gene mutations

Paroxysmal kinesigenic dyskinesia
Paroxysmal torticollis
Paroxysmal exercise-induced dyskinesia
Paroxysmal non-kinesigenic dyskinesia
Infantile convulsions with choreo-athetosis (ICCA)syndrome
Episodic ataxia
Migraine and hemiplegic migraine
Benign familial infantile seizures
Childhood-absence epilepsy
Febrile seizures

Conclusion

Dopamine plays an important role in the modulation of basal ganglia pathways but the role of dopamine in migraine is still unclear. Both hemiplegic migraine and PMDs may be observed in the channelopathies, indicating that there may be a common underlying genetic mechanism in some cases. Studies of migraine and essential tremor have been conflicting. Discrepancies may be attributed to differences in methodology and few of the studies are population based, with the majority of participants being recruited from tertiary care centers. There is more compelling evidence that the frequency of migraine is increased in Tourette syndrome and restless legs syndrome, and that Parkinson's disease may shorten the course of migraine. Dysregulation of iron metabolism is implicated in migraine, PD and RLS, and may form part of common pathophysiology.

Additional population based studies are needed to further elucidate relationship between migraine and various movement disorders. Greater understanding of potentially shared underlying molecular process will enable better-targeted treatment strategies. Future studies aimed at establishing whether targeted therapies for movement disorders, including deep brain stimulation, alter prevalence of migraine are indicated. Conversely, it remains to be seen whether emerging therapies for migraine alters prevalence of any movement disorders.

References

[1] D'Onofrio F, Barbanti P, Petretta V, Casucci G, Mazzeo A, Lecce B, Mundi C, Cologno D. Migraine and movement disorders. *Neurol Sci.* 2012 May;33 Suppl 1:S55-9. doi: 10.1007/s10072-012-1042-9. Review. PubMed PMID: 22644172.

[2] Kobari M, Meyer JS, Ichijo M, Imai A, Oravez WT. Hyperperfusion of cerebral cortex, thalamus and basal ganglia during spontaneously occurring migraine headaches. *Headache.* 1989 May;29(5):282-9.

[3] Seghatoleslam M, Ghadiri MK, Ghaffarian N, Speckmann EJ, Gorji A. Cortical spreading depression modulates the caudate nucleus activity. *Neuroscience.* 2014 May 16;267:83-90. doi: 10.1016/j.neuroscience.2014.02.029. Epub 2014 Mar 6.

[4] Headache Classification Committee of the International Headache Society (IHS). The International Classification of Headache Disorders, 3rd edition (beta version). *Cephalalgia.* 2013 Jul;33(9):629-808.

[5] Charbit AR, Akerman S, Goadsby PJ. Dopamine: what's new in migraine? *Curr Opin Neurol.* 2010 Jun;23(3):275-81.

[6] D'Andrea G, Granella F, Perini F, Farruggio A, Leone M, Bussone G. Platelet levels of dopamine are increased in migraine and cluster headache. *Headache.* 2006 Apr;46(4):585-91.

[7] Shukla R, Khanna VK, Vinod P, Sankhwar ML, Yadav RS. Platelet dopamine: D2 receptor binding in patients with migraine. *Cephalalgia.* 2009 May;29(5):532-8.

[8] Peroutka SJ. Dopamine and migraine. *Neurology.* 1997 Sep;49(3):650-6.

[9] Fernandez F, Colson N, Quinlan S, MacMillan J, Lea RA, Griffiths LR. Association between migraine and a functional polymorphism at the dopamine beta-hydroxylase locus. *Neurogenetics.* 2009 Jul;10(3):199-208.

[10] Nunes JC, Costa Bergamaschi EN, Freitas FC, Diaz AP, Queiroz LP, Debona R, Prediger RD, Linhares MN, Lin K, Walz R. Prevalence of headache in patients with Parkinson's disease and its association with the side of motor symptom onset. *Neurol Sci.* 2014 Apr;35(4):595-600.

[11] Charbit AR, Akerman S, Goadsby PJ. Comparison of the effects of central and peripheral dopamine receptor activation on evoked firing in the trigeminocervical complex. *J Pharmacol Exp Ther.* 2009 Nov;331(2):752-63.

[12] Cavestro C, Rosatello A, Marino MP, Micca G, Asteggiano G. High prolactin levels as a worsening factor for migraine. *J Headache Pain.* 2006 Apr;7(2):83-9.

[13] Charbit AR, Akerman S, Holland PR, Goadsby PJ. Neurons of the dopaminergic/calcitonin gene-related peptide A11 cell group modulate neuronal firing in the trigeminocervical complex: an electrophysiological and immunohistochemical study. *J Neurosci.* 2009 Oct 7;29(40):12532-41.

[14] Zhao H, Zhu W, Pan T, Xie W, Zhang A, Ondo WG, Le W. Spinal cord dopamine receptor expression and function in mice with 6-OHDA lesion of the A11 nucleus and dietary iron deprivation. *J Neurosci Res.* 2007 Apr;85(5):1065-76.

[15] Kruit MC, Launer LJ, Overbosch J, van Buchem MA, Ferrari MD. Iron accumulation in deep brain nuclei in migraine: a population-based magnetic resonance imaging study. *Cephalalgia.* 2009 Mar;29(3):351-9.

[16] Peeraully T, Tan EK. Linking restless legs syndrome with Parkinson's disease: clinical, imaging and genetic evidence. *Transl Neurodegener.* 2012 Feb 27;1(1):6.

[17] Ayton S, Lei P. Nigral iron elevation is an invariable feature of Parkinson's disease and is a sufficient cause of neurodegeneration. *Biomed Res Int.* 2014;2014:581256. doi: 10.1155/2014/581256. Epub 2014 Jan 16. PubMed PMID: 24527451; PubMed Central PMCID: PMC3914334.

[18] Rizzo G, Manners D, Testa C, Tonon C, Vetrugno R, Marconi S, Plazzi G, Pizza F, Provini F, Malucelli E, Gramegna LL, Lodi R. Low brain iron content in idiopathic restless legs syndrome patients detected by phase imaging. *Mov Disord.* 2013 Nov;28(13):1886-90.

[19] Kruit MC, van Buchem MA, Launer LJ, Terwindt GM, Ferrari MD. Migraine is associated with an increased risk of deep white matter lesions, subclinical posterior circulation infarcts and brain iron accumulation: the population-based MRI CAMERA study. *Cephalalgia*. 2010 Feb;30(2):129-36.

[20] Lorentz IT. A survey of headache in Parkinson's disease. *Cephalalgia.* 1989 Jun;9(2):83-6.

[21] Nunes JC, Costa Bergamaschi EN, Freitas FC, Diaz AP, Queiroz LP, Debona R, Prediger RD, Linhares MN, Lin K, Walz R. Prevalence of headache in patients with Parkinson's disease and its association with the side of motor symptom onset. *Neurol Sci.* 2014 Apr;35(4):595-600.

[22] Rasmussen BK, Jensen R, Schroll M, Olesen J. Epidemiology of headache in a general population--a prevalence study. *J Clin Epidemiol.* 1991;44(11):1147-57.

[23] Castro ME, Pascual J, Romón T, del Arco C, del Olmo E, Pazos A. Differential distribution of [3H]sumatriptan binding sites (5-HT1B, 5-HT1D and 5-HT1F receptors) in human brain: focus on brainstem and spinal cord. *Neuropharmacology*. 1997 Apr-May;36(4-5):535-42.

[24] Cubo E, Kompoliti K, Leurgans SE, Raman R. Dopaminergic hypersensitivity in patients with Parkinson disease and migraine. *Clin Neuropharmacol.* 2004 Jan-Feb;27(1):30-2.

[25] Biary N, Koller W, Langenberg P. Correlation between essential tremor and migraine headache. *J Neurol Neurosurg Psychiatry.* 1990 Dec;53(12):1060-2.

[26] Bain PG, Findley LJ, Thompson PD, Gresty MA, Rothwell JC, Harding AE, Marsden CD. A study of hereditary essential tremor. *Brain*. 1994 Aug;117 (Pt 4):805-24.

[27] Barbanti P, Fabbrini G, Vanacore N, Rum A, Lenzi GL, Meco G, Cerbo R. Dopamine and migraine: does Parkinson's disease modify migraine course? *Cephalalgia.* 2000 Oct;20(8):720-3.

[28] Gozubatik-Celik G, Benbir G, Tan F, Karadeniz D, Goksan B. The prevalence of migraine in restless legs syndrome. *Headache.* 2014 May;54(5):872-7.

[29] Barbanti P, Fabbrini G, Vanacore N, Rum A, Lenzi GL, Meco G, Cerbo R. Dopamine and migraine: does Parkinson's disease modify migraine course? *Cephalalgia.* 2000 Oct;20(8):720-3.

[30] Barbanti P, Fabbrini G, Aurilia C, Defazio G, Colosimo C, Berardelli A. No association between essential tremor and migraine: a case-control study. *Cephalalgia.* 2010 Jun;30(6):686-9.

[31] Hu Y, Tang W, Liu R, Dong Z, Chen X, Pan M, Yu S. Higher prevalence of migraine in essential tremor: A case-control study. *Cephalalgia.* 2014 Apr 11.

[32] Jeanneteau F, Funalot B, Jankovic J, Deng H, Lagarde JP, Lucotte G, Sokoloff P. A functional variant of the dopamine D3 receptor is associated with risk and age-at-onset of essential tremor. *Proc Natl Acad Sci U S A.* 2006 Jul 11;103(28):10753-8. Epub 2006 Jun 29.

[33] Garcia-Martin E, Martinez C, Serrador M, Alonso-Navarro H, Navacerrada F, Agundez J, Jimenez-Jimenez F. Dopamine receptor 3 (DRD3) polymorphism and risk for migraine. *European Journal of Neurology.* 2010,17:1220-1223.

[34] Barabas G, Matthews WS, Ferrari M. Tourette's syndrome and migraine. *Arch Neurol.* 1984 Aug;41(8):871-2.

[35] Kwak C, Vuong KD, Jankovic J. Migraine headache in patients with Tourette syndrome. *Arch Neurol.* 2003 Nov;60(11):1595-8.

[36] Ghosh D, Rajan PV, Das D, Datta P, Rothner AD, Erenberg G. Headache in children with Tourette syndrome. *J Pediatr.* 2012 Aug;161(2):303-7.e6.

[37] Allen RP, Picchietti D, Hening WA, Trenkwalder C, Walters AS, Montplaisi J. Restless legs syndrome diagnosis and epidemiology workshop at the National Institutes of Health; International Restless Legs Syndrome Study Group. Restless legs syndrome: diagnostic criteria, special considerations, and epidemiology. A report from the restless legs syndrome diagnosis and epidemiology workshop at the National Institutes of Health. *Sleep Med.* 2003;4:101–19.

[38] Gupta R, Lahan V, Goel D. Primary headaches in restless legs syndrome patients. *Ann Indian Acad Neurol.* 2012 Aug;15(Suppl 1):S104-8.

[39] d'Onofrio F, Bussone G, Cologno D, Petretta V, Buzzi MG, Tedeschi G, Bonavita V, Cicarelli G. Restless legs syndrome and primary headaches: a clinical study. *Neurol Sci.* 2008 May;29 Suppl 1:S169-72.

[40] Rhode AM, Hösing VG, Happe S, Biehl K, Young P, Evers S. Comorbidity of migraine and restless legs syndrome--a case-control study. *Cephalalgia.* 2007 Nov;27(11):1255-60.

[41] Winter AC, Schürks M, Berger K, Buring JE, Gaziano JM, Kurth T. Migraine and restless legs syndrome in men. *Cephalalgia.* 2013 Jan;33(2):130-5.

[42] Schürks M, Winter AC, Berger K, Buring JE, Kurth T. Migraine and restless legs syndrome in women. *Cephalalgia.* 2012 Apr;32(5):382-9.

[43] Cologno D, Cicarelli G, Petretta V, d'Onofrio F, Bussone G. High prevalence of Dopaminergic Premonitory Symptoms in migraine patients with Restless Legs Syndrome: a pathogenetic link? *Neurol Sci.* 2008 May;29 Suppl 1:S166-8. doi

[44] Eshel G, Lahat E, Azizi E, Gross B, Aladjem M. Chorea as a manifestation of rheumatic fever--a 30-year survey (1960-1990). Eur J Pediatr. 1993;152(8):645-6.

[45] Teixeira AL Jr, Meira FC, Maia DP, Cunningham MC, Cardoso F. Migraine headache in patients with Sydenham's chorea. *Cephalalgia.* 2005 Jul;25(7):542-4.

[46] Peeraully T, Tan EK, Kaji R. The Borderland between Epilepsy and Movement Disorders. Poewe & Jankovic: Movement Disorders in Neurologic & Systemic Disease, *Cambridge University Press,* April 2014

[47] Dichgans M, Freilinger T, Eckstein G, Babini E, Lorenz-Depiereux B, Biskup S, Ferrari MD, Herzog J, van den Maagdenberg AM, Pusch M, Strom TM. Mutation in the neuronal voltage-gated sodium channel SCN1A in familial hemiplegic migraine. *Lancet.* 2005;366(9483):371-7.

[48] Gelfand AA. Migraine and childhood periodic syndromes in children and adolescents. *Curr Opin Neurol.* 2013 Jun;26(3):262-8.

[49] Lampl C, Katsarava Z, Diener HC, Limmroth V. Lamotrigine reduces migraine aura and migraine attacks in patients with migraine with aura. *J Neurol Neurosurg Psychiatry.* 2005 Dec;76(12):1730-2.

[50] Russell MB, Ducros A. Sporadic and familial hemiplegic migraine: pathophysiological mechanisms, clinical characteristics, diagnosis, and management. *Lancet Neurol.* 2011 May;10(5):457-70

[51] Gazerani P, Au S, Dong X, Kumar U, Arendt-Nielsen L, Cairns BE. Botulinum neurotoxin type A (BoNTA) decreases the mechanical sensitivity of nociceptors and inhibits neurogenic vasodilation in a craniofacial muscle targeted for migraine prophylaxis. *Pain.* 2010 Dec;151(3):606-16.

[52] Méneret A, Gaudebout C, Riant F, Vidailhet M, Depienne C, Roze E. PRRT2 mutations and paroxysmal disorders. *Eur J Neurol.* 2013 Jun;20(6):872-8.

[53] Riant F, Roze E, Barbance C, Méneret A, Guyant-Maréchal L, Lucas C, Sabouraud P, Trébuchon A, Depienne C, Tournier-Lasserve E. PRRT2 mutations cause hemiplegic migraine. *Neurology.* 2012 Nov 20;79(21):2122-4.

[54] Bernard G, Shevell MI. Channelopathies: a review. *Pediatr Neurol.* 2008 Feb;38(2):73-85.

[55] Lee HY, Huang Y, Bruneau N, Roll P, Roberson ED, Hermann M, Quinn E, Maas J, Edwards R, Ashizawa T, Baykan B, Bhatia K, Bressman S, Bruno MK, Brunt ER, Caraballo R, Echenne B, Fejerman N, Frucht S, Gurnett CA, Hirsch E, Houlden H, Jankovic J, Lee WL, Lynch DR, Mohamed S, Müller U, Nespeca MP, Renner D, Rochette J, Rudolf G, Saiki S, Soong BW, Swoboda KJ, Tucker S, Wood N, Hanna M, Bowcock A, Szepetowski P, Fu YH, Ptáček LJ. Mutations in the novel protein PRRT2 cause paroxysmal kinesigenic dyskinesia with infantile convulsions. *Cell Rep.* 2012;1(1):2-12.

[56] Chen WJ, Lin Y, Xiong ZQ, Wei W, Ni W, Tan GH, Guo SL, He J, Chen YF, Zhang QJ, Li HF, Lin Y, Murong SX, Xu J, Wang N, Wu ZY. Exome sequencing identifies truncating mutations in PRRT2 that cause paroxysmal kinesigenic dyskinesia. *Nat Genet.* 2011 Nov 20;43(12):1252-5.

[57] Wang JL, Cao L, Li XH, Hu ZM, Li JD, Zhang JG, Liang Y, San-A, Li N, Chen SQ, Guo JF, Jiang H, Shen L, Zheng L, Mao X, Yan WQ, Zhou Y, Shi YT, Ai SX, Dai MZ, Zhang P, Xia K, Chen SD, Tang BS. Identification of PRRT2 as the causative gene of paroxysmal kinesigenic dyskinesias. *Brain.* 2011 Dec;134(Pt 12):3493-3501.

[58] Li J, Zhu X, Wang X, Sun W, Feng B, Du T, Sun B, Niu F, Wei H, Wu X, Dong L, Li L, Cai X, Wang Y, Liu Y. Targeted genomic sequencing identifies PRRT2 mutations as a cause of paroxysmal kinesigenic choreoathetosis. *J Med Genet.* 2012 Feb;49(2):76-8.

[59] Rochette J, Roll P, Fu YH, Lemoing AG, Royer B, Roubertie A, Berquin P, Motte J, Wong SW, Hunter A, Robaglia-Schlupp A, Ptacek LJ, Szepetowski P. Novel familial cases of ICCA (infantile convulsions with paroxysmal choreoathetosis) syndrome. *Epileptic Disord.* 2010 Sep;12(3):199-204.

[60] Espeche A, Cersosimo R, Caraballo RH. Benign infantile seizures and paroxysmal dyskinesia: A well-defined familial syndrome. *Seizure.* 2011 Nov;20(9):686-91.

[61] Szepetowski P, Rochette J, Berquin P, Piussan C, Lathrop GM, Monaco AP. Familial infantile convulsions and paroxysmal choreoathetosis: a new neurological syndrome linked to the pericentromeric region of human chromosome 16. *Am J Hum Genet.* 1997 Oct;61(4):889-98.

[62] Heron SE, Grinton BE, Kivity S, Afawi Z, Zuberi SM, Hughes JN, Pridmore C, Hodgson BL, Iona X, Sadleir LG, Pelekanos J, Herlenius E, Goldberg-Stern H, Bassan H, Haan E, Korczyn AD, Gardner AE, Corbett MA, Gécz J, Thomas PQ, Mulley JC, Berkovic SF, Scheffer IE, Dibbens LM. PRRT2 mutations cause benign familial infantile epilepsy and infantile convulsions with choreoathetosis syndrome. *Am J Hum Genet*. 2012 Jan 13;90(1):152-60.

[63] Lee YC, Lee MJ, Yu HY, Chen C, Hsu CH, Lin KP, Liao KK, Chang MH, Liao YC, Soong BW. PRRT2 mutations in paroxysmal kinesigenic dyskinesia with infantile convulsions in a Taiwanese cohort. *PLoS One*. 2012;7(8):e38543.

In: Migraine Surgery
Editor: Antonios Mammis

ISBN: 978-1-63321-761-4

Chapter 12

Migraine and Exercise

*Katherine J. Zehr**
Synergy Fitness Clubs, Astoria, New York, US

Migraines affect tens of thousands of people and can be downright debilitating for many. With no outright cure, this paints a dismal picture for migraine sufferers. In fact, they are documented as some of the most dissatisfied of all medical patients, with approximately half of them discontinuing treatment due to this fact [1]. Since exercise or similar physical exertion can often be a trigger for migraine sufferers, many who experience them regularly avoid engaging in such activity, despite the fact that it is a pivotal component to a healthy lifestyle [2]. There is no doubt that migraine sufferers cannot and should not put their physical fitness aside for fear of inducing an attack. Fortunately, there is evidence suggesting that not only can those living with migraines exercise routinely, but also that doing so can be part of a preventative treatment plan [2]. While this conclusion remains quite controversial among medical professionals and neuroscientists, a structured exercise regimen may be a viable option for migraine patients looking for a prophylactic other than prescription drugs, or as part of a combined treatment plan.

During a randomized controlled study, a Swedish headache clinic found that migraine patients who were put on a routine exercise program experienced a reduction in migraine frequency each month that was almost identical to patients who had been put on the prophylactic topiramate or relaxation therapy [2]. The exercise group of patients who participated in the study performed forty minutes of cardiovascular activity on an indoor stationary bicycle, three times per week, guided by a physiotherapist. Another portion of participants engaged in individualized relaxation therapies with a physiotherapist once a week, with the addition of self-performed relaxation techniques involving breathing and stress-management exercises at home with a CD. The last group of patients was given the highest tolerable dose (up to 200mg per day) of the drug topiramate. While the topiramate users in the study experienced the highest mean reduction in intensity of pain, the absolute

* Corresponding Author: Katherine J. Zehr, B.A.; Synergy Fitness Clubs; 23-35 Broadway; Astoria, NY 11106; 718 267-7700; kjzehr89@gmail.com.

difference was so slight that the conclusion of those running the trial was that it is hardly clinically relevant [2].

Another study performed in Turkey measured the changes and effects of aerobic exercise with plasma beta-endorphin levels in migraine patients without aura, with findings that also point to exercise as being highly beneficial for migraine patients [3]. In this study, the initial session was performed on a treadmill, followed by an in-home aerobic exercise program performed for six weeks without supervision. The neurologists who ran the study believe that the improvement seen in the reduction of migraine frequency and intensity in patients was due to the increase in beta-endorphin levels, especially because the participants who experienced the most benefit were those who had the lowest basal (pre-exercise) beta-endorphin levels. In their discussion of the results, however, they do concede that neither the changes in beta-endorphin levels, nor any other single influence, are likely solely responsible for the benefits that exercise causes for migraine sufferers. They instead hypothesize that the positive effects of exercise experienced by migraine patients are due to a combinations of many factors, such as improved cardiovascular and cerebrovascular fitness and relief of psychological conditions like depression and anxiety [3].

According to some experts, the key seems to be the use of a structured routine, according to which the individual adheres to a regular schedule, exercising on the same days and times each week. Robert Cowan, M.D. of the Keeler Center for the Study of Migraine, states that for most patients it is "how and when" that can make the difference between whether exercise will precipitate a migraine or not [4]. He has found that patients who exercise daily or several times a week, at the same time on the same days each week, and who incorporate low-impact aerobic activity into their routines, are not only able to exercise without triggering migraines, but generally find a reduction in the intensity, duration, and frequency of their migraines. This is consistent with the research findings of the groups in Sweden and Turkey, no matter how limited the scientific data may be at this time. Cowan surmises that this is due to the rise of endorphin levels during exercise, which raises pain thresholds, and once again his assumptions are in accordance with the study of migraine and changes in plasma beta-endorphin levels discussed previously [4]. The positive effects of increased endorphin production and release is the same reason exercise is recommended as part of a comprehensive treatment plan for those who suffer from anxiety and/or depression, as the same peptides that raise pain tolerance also contribute to feelings of satisfaction, peace of mind, and emotional stability [5].

In addition to working out according to a habitual schedule, Cowan stresses the import of a proper physical warm up as a precursor to more intense exercise to avoid the onset of a migraine [4]. This is also reflected in early research findings from the doctors who conducted the study in Sweden, and is recommended by most headache and migraine resources [6, 7]. In reality, a proper warm up and cool-down are key for every exerciser, as it prepares the body and the brain for physical exertion and prevents injury to muscles, tissues, and joints. But it seems to be especially useful to those who tend to experience migraines and other types of headaches when they work out. The American Council on Exercise defines a warm-up as "a period of lighter exercise preceding the conditioning phase of the exercise bout, and should last for 5-10 minutes for most healthy adults" [8]. Low intensity cardiovascular activity should be the starting point for every workout, and perhaps followed by dynamic, active stretching. Cowan stresses that performing stretches for the neck and shoulders prior to exercising may be extremely helpful to migraine sufferers [4]. The highest intensity portion of any exercise session should only begin after such a warm-up has been executed. Static stretching, meaning stretching that involves holding a fixed position for a minute or more, should be conducted at the conclusion of the workout, when the body is warm and supple, so as to prevent tears and other types of injury or discomfort. If one takes the time to go through a proper warm up and systematically build toward higher intensity activity, and then slowly cool the body down after its completion, they may experience less of a connection between exercise and the onset of a migraine, and will certainly prevent other damage to the body [4].

To determine what to avoid when exercising so as to prevent triggering a migraine, it can be very helpful to keep a headache diary [4,7]. Any time a migraine is triggered during or shortly after exercising, it should be noted, along with what specific exercises were performed, for how long, at what intensity, as well as what was eaten before exercising and any other potentially relevant information. Hydration also plays a large role in whether or not a migraine may be induced because of exercise, and Dr. Cowan cautions that dehydration coupled with exercise can not only trigger a migraine, but make it much worse [4]. What specifically during exercise may or may not cause a migraine will likely vary based on the individual.

Though the numbers from the discussed research and other similar studies of exercise and migraines do not lie, the scientific reasons for how and why a regular exercise program has been shown to help prevent migraines has not yet been determined, causing many professionals to conclude that this theory lacks efficacy. In fact, doctors Volker Busch and Charly Gaul write, “Strictly speaking, none of the present studies met valid criteria of good clinical practice” and ultimately determine that the current evidence available “refers to anecdotal reports and observational studies” and is not sufficient to classify an exercise program as a migraine prophylactic without further research [9]. While this may be true, it cannot be overlooked that each study, regardless of program design and methodology, reported some type of relief among the patients following aerobic exercise programs. Even if the *why* has not been discovered, the fact remains that the patients experienced fewer migraines and lower pain intensity, and in addition they were enjoying the host of other benefits that regular exercise induces, such as higher oxygen uptake, increased energy, lower body mass, and an overall improvement in quality of life [2, 3, 6]. Though the lack of physiological and neurological proof may not satisfy all medical professionals, the reported relief and reduction of pain should be enough to convince patients that engaging in regular, moderate intensity exercise will be of benefit to them. Even if a reduction in migraine frequency is not experienced through routine exercise, an elevated pain threshold will almost certainly occur due to the increased production of beta-endorphins, resulting in better tolerance for the pain patients encounter during migraines.

One could speculate that this will also lead to an improved state of mind among migraine sufferers regarding their pain, as those same beta-endorphins aid and abet in the relief of depression and similar psychological issues that are often experienced by those with chronic pain [5]. More research and scientific evidence may well be required to explain the phenomena associated with exercise as a prophylactic measure for migraine patients, but patients need not wait in order to start reaping the benefits of it.

References

[1] Lemstra, Mark; Stewart, Brad; Olszynski, W.P. "Effectiveness of Multidisciplinary Intervention in the Treatment of Migraine: A Randomized Clinical Trial." *Headache: The Journal of Head & Face Pain.* 2002 October; 845-854. Academic Search Premier. Web. 28 May 2014.

[2] Varkey, Emma; Cider, Asa; Carlsson, Jane; Linde, Mattias. "Exercise as migraine prophylaxis: A randomized study using relaxation and topiramate as controls." *Cephalalgia.* 2011 October; 31(14): 1428–1438. SAGE Choice. Web. 28 May 2014.

[3] Koseoglu, E.; Akboyraz, A.; Soyuer, A.; Ersoy, AO. "Aerobic exercise and plasma beta endorphin levels in patients with migrainous headache without aura." *Cephalalgia.* 2003; 23: 972-976. Academic Search Premier. Web. 28 May 2014.

[4] Cowan, Robert, M.D. The Keeler Migraine Method: A Groundbreaking, Individualized Program from the Renowned Headache Treatment Clinic. New York: Penguin Group, 2008. Google Books. Web. 27 May 2014.

[5] Sarris, Jerome; O'Neil, Adrienne; Coulson, Carolyn E.; Schweitzer, Isaac; Berk, Michael. "Lifestyle Medicine for Depression." *BMC Psychiatry* 2014, 14:107. Academic Search Premier. Web. 1 June 2014.

[6] Varkey, Emma; Cider, Asa; Carlsson, Jane; Linde, Mattias. "A Study to Evaluate the Feasibility of an Aerobic Exercise Program in Patients With Migraine." *Headache.* 2009 April; 563-570. Academic Search Premier. Web. 28 May 2014.

[7] "Migraine Fact Sheets: Exercise and Migraines." www.migrainetrust.org. The Migraine Trust. 2012. Web. 1 June 2014.

[8] ACE Personal Trainer Manual: The Ultimate Resource for Fitness Professionals. 4th ed. San Diego: American Council on Exercise, 2010. Print.

[9] Busch, Volker; Gaul, Charly. "Exercise in Migraine Therapy – Is there Any Evidence for Efficacy? A Critical Review." *Headache.* 2008 June;48:890-899. Academic Search Premier. Web. 28 May 2014.

[10] "Exercise May Help Prevent Migraines." *PT in Motion.* 2012 March; 4 (2): 12-12. Academic Search Premier. Web. 28 May 2014.

In: Migraine Surgery
Editor: Antonios Mammis

ISBN: 978-1-63321-761-4

Chapter 13

Alternative and Complementary Treatments

Jennifer Gyi*[*1], BranDee N. Gentile[1] and Dennis Grech[2]

[1]Department of Neurological Surgery, Rutgers New Jersey Medical School, Newark, New Jersey, US

[2]Department of Anesthesiology, Rutgers New Jersey Medical School, Newark, New Jersey, US

Introduction to Acupuncture

Acupuncture is one of the oldest forms of healing practices in the world. It has been used within the Chinese health care system for the past 2,500 years and is widely used to treat and prevent migraine attacks. Due to its low side effect profile, it is a good option for many patients who fail more conventional treatments. International health organizations such as the World Health Organization (WHO) have recognized the use of acupuncture to produce strong analgesic effects and have validated its use for acute and chronic ailments; including migraine headaches.

Keywords: Acupuncture, Acupoint, Auriculotherapy, Nogier, Traditional Chinese Medicine, Complementary Medicine, Meridian

* Corresponding Author: Jennifer Gyi, D.O. Assistant Professor, Department of Neurological Surgery, Rutgers New Jersey Medical School, 90 Bergen Street, Suite 8100, Newark, New Jersey 07103, 973 972-2323, jg1096@njms.rutgers.edu

Definitions

Cun – one cun is equal to the space between the distal interphalangeal joint and the proximal interphalangeal joint on the middle finger
GB – gall bladder meridian
LI – Large intestine meridian
LU – Lung meridian
LV – Liver meridian
ST – Stomach meridian
P – Pericardium

Mechanism of Action

Acupuncture is an essential part of Traditional Chinese Medicine (TCM). The Chinese developed the concept of qi as early as second century BC. Qi (pronounced 'chee') is the life energy that flows through the twelve organs and twelve meridians. (Figure 1) Qi is related to a patient's balance of Ying and Yang (Figure 2).

It is believed that blockages or disruptions along the meridian can occur which can lead to a pathological stagnation of blood and qi. This prevents proper flow to the organs and to the different areas of the body. There are 359 acupoints that can be stimulated along the meridians to unblock the disturbances, thus allowing proper qi to flow to the organs and the different areas of the body, ultimately bringing a balance between Ying and Yang. The effectiveness of acupuncture can be broken into four separate categories: inhibitory systems of the CNS, serotonin and noradrenaline, the anti-inflammatory effect, and non-specific effects.

Inhibitory Systems

The prefrontal cortex, rostral anterior cingulate cortex (rACC) and the brainstem have been identified as structures within the CNS that form a network for pain perception through the use of functional MRI (fMRI) and PET studies. It is believed that acupuncture activates the same network and is supported by studies in which electroacupuncture-induced analgesia was inhibited (1).

Serotonin & Noradrenalin

According to Endres et al. acupuncture analgesic effects could be caused by serotonergic projections from the raphe nucleus to the higher centers of the CNS and descending projections to the spinal cord, in conjunction with noradrenaline. However, chemical or mechanical destruction of the nucleus raphe magnus, which contains most of the brain's serotonin cells, reduces acupuncture analgesia. Endres et al. also suggested that a pharmacological blockade of serotonin synthesis and blockade of serotonin receptors inhibit acupuncture analgesia and that if serotonin is applied systemically or directly in the CNS, acupuncture analgesia is magnified.

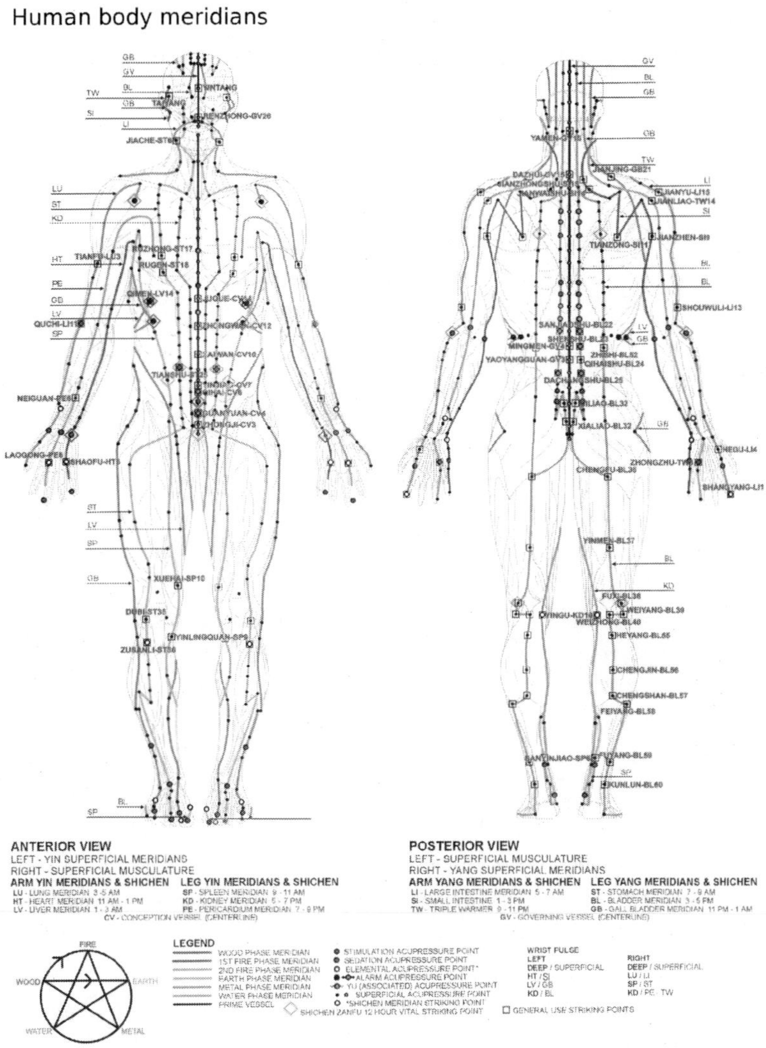

Figure 1.

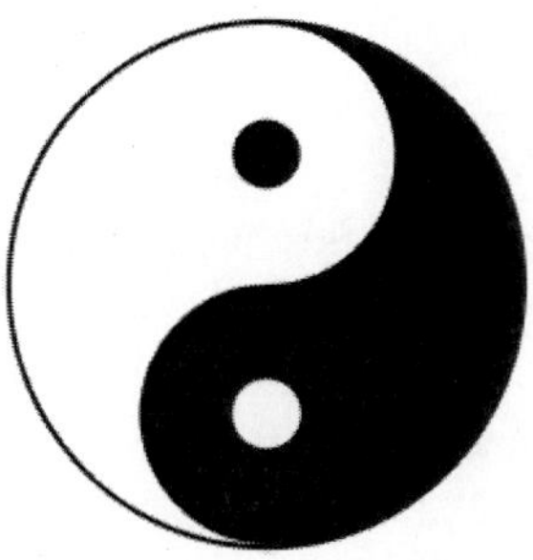

Figure 2.

Anti-inflammatory Effect

Lao et al. demonstrated an anti-inflammatory effect at acupoint GB-30 when compared to sham acupoints. GB-30 is located in the gluteal region between the greater trochanter and the sacral hiatus [2]. A low frequency of 10 Hz electroacupuncture resulted in an effect that lasted for days, whereas a frequency of 100 Hz lasted a few hours. Mediated by ACTH and endorphins, it was observed that the anti-inflammatory effect was effective centrally and also at the site locally. Recent studies have shown that endorphins are secreted centrally as well as peripherally, which demonstrates a decrease in pain.

Nonspecific Effects in Acupuncture

The use of a control group receiving sham acupuncture is important in order to determine the differences between the effects of specific known acupuncture points along the meridians and the effect of nonspecific points with superficial skin penetration. There are many psychological effects of acupuncture, which can include, but are not limited to: positive patient expectations [3], negative expectations about traditional medicine [1], response to an increase level of care, the idea of partaking in a 'healing ritual' [4], the experience of having an invasive technique used as treatment [3], and emotional variables; including anxiety.

The differences between true acupuncture and sham acupuncture results are important in determining if the location of the acupoint is important, whether or not the depth of the needle matters (sham acupuncture uses needles at the superficial level only), or if the elicitation of the de qi sensation (slight tingling or heat) is required for a decrease in pain. The de qui sensation is not important in sham acupuncture and is used to represent insufficient stimulation.

Important Acupoints for Treating Headaches/Migraines

Acupuncture treatment is tailored to each patient based on the diagnostic tools and principles of Traditional Chinese Medicine (TCM). These include a detailed patient history and examination of the patient's pulses and tongue.

An acupuncture treatment regimen consists of needling at various locations along key meridians on the body. Utilizing 26-34 gauge acupuncture needles, the practioner inserts the needles at various depths, ranging from 2mm to 2.5cm. The depth of the needle is dependent upon the site and angle of insertion. Electrical current can be applied to the needles as well as an herbal preparation known as Moxa. The treatments are prepared according to the principles of the ancient text of the Nei Jing, which dates back to 305 B.C.

A brief description of the common acupuncture points is listed below. Many of the same acupoints are utilized in different combinations that will have a different effect upon the patient. Common acupoint combinations are summarized in Table 1.

Zhong Wan CV-12 is easily located 4 cun above the umbilicus. CV-12 is indicated for all digestive issues including those related to stress, such as nervous stomach [5]. This acupoint can also be used to treat insomnia and anxiety, particularly those from worrying and overthinking. Those patients in advance stages of pregnancy should not have this acupoint utilized [5].

Hanyan GB-4 is commonly used in the treatment of one-sided headaches. It is located within the hairline and directly under ST-8 [5]. It is suggested that this site always be palpated with one-sided headache and needled if tender [5].

Table 1. Common acupoint combinations used for treating migraines and their related symptoms

Common Migraine Acupoints	Acupoints for specific treatment of headache and vomiting	Acupoints for specific treatment of headache, nausea, and loss of appetite
CV-12	x	x
GB-4		
GB-8		x
GB-14		
GB-20		x
GB-34		
GB-37		
GV-20	x	x
LI-4	x	x
LI-11		
LV-3		
P-6	x	
ST-8	x	x
ST-36	x	x

Shuaigu GB-8 located one cun above Jiaosun SJ-20; which is located directly above the middle of the ear. This acupoint is an important point for treating one-sided headaches, specifically parietal or temporal headaches. It is also the main point on the head to treat those with headache-induced vomiting [5].

Pain in the forehead or pain in the supraorbital ridge can be treated with the acupoint Yangbai GB-14. This acupoint can be located on the forehead, directly above the pupil, and 1 cun above the midpoint of the eyebrow [5]. The large intestine and stomach channels, which are associated with the forehead area, meet at this point. GB-14 is indicated for pain in the forehead; specifically for frontal headaches and frontal sinusitis [2] and eye twitching.

Fengchi GB-20 is the single most important acupuncture point in the treatment of headache (5), regardless of the etiology or channels involved. It is located below the occiput and the nuchal line [2] between the origins of the sternocleidomastoid and trapezius muscles. Due to its location between the head and body Fengchi GB-20 is positioned to treat all diseases of the head, brain, and sensory organs [5]. This is a particularly beneficial point to treat for those suffering from generalized headaches, hypertension, and dizziness. Dependent on the symptoms that the patient is having, the needle placement can be directed towards other acupoints for best relief [5].

Yang Ling Quan GB-34 is located anteriorly and inferiorly to the head of the fibula. This site has a variety of indications, but for the purposes in this chapter it is utilized for the treatment of pain, nausea, and vomiting. GB-34 is the strongest of all the gall bladder acupoints [2]. Guang Ming GB-37 is located on the anterior border of the fibula and 5 cun above the tip of the external malleolus [2]. Clinically it is indicated for treatment of blurry vision and headaches; which affect the region around the eyes and specifically headaches that are located in the temporal, infraorbital, and supraorbital regions of the head [5].

The most important yang point of the body is located at Bai Hui GV-20 [5]. It is the highest of all points being at the apex of the head. This is the main point indicated for one-sided headache, headache, heavy feeling of the head, dizziness, eye pain, tinnitus, and pain at the vertex [5]. He Gu LI-4 is located centrally on the radial side of the second metacarpal bone, on the belly of the first interosseous dorsalis muscle [2]. This acupoint is indicated for the treatment of frontal or sinus headaches and chronic pain. LI-4 should not be used in pregnant women because it could induce labor [5].

Qu Chi LI-11 is easily located when the elbow is slightly flexed. The point is found by starting at the center of the transverse cubital crease then moving laterally to the lateral epicondyle of the humerus (5). LI-11 is found halfway between those two points. This point is used to treat headache, dizziness, redness, swelling and pain of the eye, and blurring vision [5].

Tai Chong LV-3 is located on the dorsum of the foot and is easily palpated within the depression that is just distal to the first and second metatarsal bone junction [2]. This acupoint is important in the treatment of headaches, dizziness, blurred vision, painful eyes, nausea, and vomiting. It can also be used as a treatment point to assist with calming of anger, irritability, insomnia, and anxiety. LV-3 is the strongest acupoint within the Liver meridian [2].

Neiguan P-6 is located 2 cun above the transverse crease of the wrist on the palmer side [5]. It is found between the palmaris longus and flexor carpi radialis tendons. This acupoint is extremely useful in the treatment of nausea, vomiting, depression, and dizziness [5].

Touwei ST-8 is the meeting point of the stomach channel, gall bladder channel, and the Yang Linking vessel; it is located directly above ST-7 and a .5 cun from the anterior hairline at the anterior of the forehead [5]. This site is indicated to treat headache, splitting headache with fever and chills, dizziness, eye pain, and blurry vision [2].

Zu san li ST-36 is located 3 cun below the inferior pole of the patella [2], and one finger width laterally from the tibia [5]. This acupoint is commonly used to treat gastrointestinal discomfort, nausea, vomiting, stress, and fatigue. It is also an important point in traditional Chinese practice to promote health and longevity, due to being one of the strongest acupoints on the body [2].

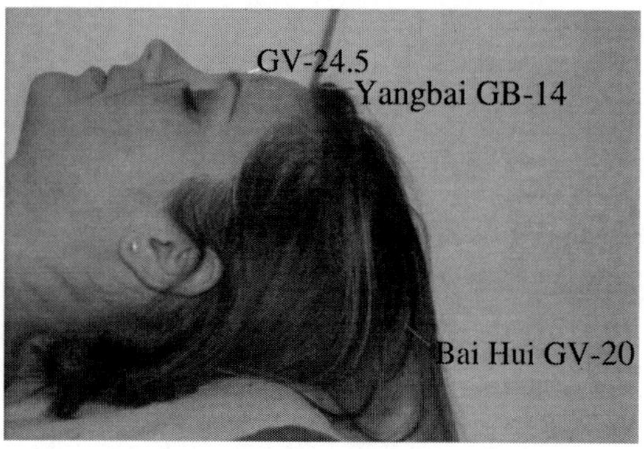

Figure 3.

Auriculotherapy

Auriculotherapy, or ear acupuncture, is also a powerful treatment modality. It is based on the concept that the ear is a microsystem; which can control the entire body. The auricle, or outer portion of the ear, is the locus for a multitude of acupoints which, when stimulated, can have profound effects on a variety of patient ailments; including migraine headaches [6].

Auriculotherapy was first described by the French neurologist, Paul Nogier. In 1957 he published the Treatise of Auriculotherapy. These developments were made using clinical trials based in a phrenological method of projection of a fetal Homunculus on the ear for reference of complaints and points for treatment [6]. (Figure 3)

Placing needles on the corresponding ear points while simultaneously placing needles on the patient's body acupuncture points can improve the efficacy of treatment. Patients often report a decreased frequency and intensity of migraine headaches after a few sessions of acupuncture. Most patients treated with acupuncture report a decrease in medication usage and cessation of nausea, vomiting, or photophobia [6].

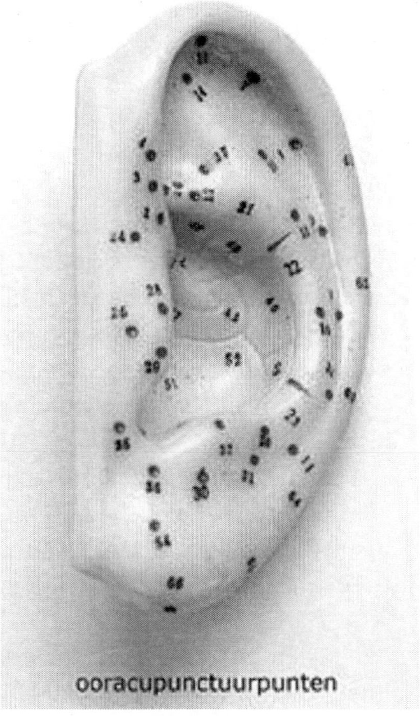

Figure 4.

Supporting Literature

There are a multitude of scientific publications that support the use of acupuncture for the treatment of migraine headaches. Below is a sampling of the most significant findings in the literature.

The objective of the study by Linde et al., was to investigate the effect of acupuncture on migraine pain when compared to sham acupuncture and no acupuncture. The study sample had 3 randomized groups, N= 302 patients (88% women), with an average age of 43 years [9], with migraine headaches, which was based on the International Headache Society criteria. The patients were at eighteen outpatient centers in Germany. The two acupuncture groups, true acupuncture and sham acupuncture, received twelve total sessions over an eight-week time frame. Participants completed headache diaries four weeks prior to the study to twelve weeks after randomization, then again from week twenty-one to twenty-four after randomization. The study concluded that there was no difference between the true acupuncture and the sham acupuncture groups (0.0 days, 95% confidence interval, -0.7 to 0.7 days; $P = .96$) however, both true and sham acupunctures were more effective in decreasing migraine pain than the control group [7].

A 2009 Cochrane review of acupuncture and prophylaxis for migraine headaches analyzed 22 randomized controlled trials (RCTs) with 4,419 participants. Six of the trials compared true acupuncture without prophylactic treatment. Fourteen trials compared true acupuncture to sham acupuncture and four trials looked at acupuncture with proven drug regiments. It was found that after four months of true acupuncture participants reported a decrease in migraines when compared with drug treatment (standard mean difference [SMD] = –0.26; 95% confidence interval [CI], –0.41 to –0.11), and compared with no treatment (SMD = –0.43; 95% CI, –0.60 to –0.27). True acupuncture was determined to be as effective as proven drug regiments, but not statistically more effective than sham acupuncture (SMD = –0.18; 95% CI, –0.44 to 0.07) [8].

Pickett put forth a review in 2010, “Acupuncture for Migraine and Recurrent Headaches”. One study stated that patients who were in the behavioral study group reported less medication use and fewer headaches than the acupuncture group. Another study said that patients on metoprolol suffered more side effects but less frequency, duration, and intensity of headaches when compared to the acupuncture group. A third paper showed the number of patients receiving true acupuncture having >50% symptom reduction was 16 out of 20, whereas the number of patients receiving sham acupuncture having >50% symptom reduction was only 3/20. Their conclusion was that while the small sample sizes and overall quality of the studies prohibited them from making a straightforward recommendation of acupuncture, the treatment seems to be relatively safe in the hands of qualified providers.

Lastly, a study published in the British Medical Journal “Acupuncture for Chronic Headache in Primary Care - A Large Pragmatic, Randomized Trial.” For this study, a Cochrane review of twenty-six randomized trials of acupuncture for headache was performed. The authors concluded that although existing evidence supports the value of acupuncture, the quality and amount of evidence are not fully convincing. The parameters evaluated for each patient included headache, health status, sick days, and the use of resources for treatment of with chronic headache. A sample of 401 patients with chronic headache, predominantly migraine was selected. Patients were allocated to two separate groups, acupuncture or non-acupuncture, by using a biased coin. This was used to minimize age, sex, diagnosis, headache score at baseline, and duration of headache disorder variables. Patients in the acupuncture group received 12 treatments in addition to standard care from their general practitioner. Patients in the non-acupuncture group received general care from their general practioner only. The acupuncture point prescriptions used were individualized to each patient. The study was modeled on a double blind, placebo controlled trial. However, one limitation was that patients were not blinded and may have given biased assessments of their headache scores. Measures to minimize bias included minimal contact between trial participants and study team members and educating patients about bias. Patients completed a daily diary of headache and medication for four weeks at baseline then at three months and one year after randomization. Severity ranked on 6 point Likert scale: 0- "no headache", 3- "headache is painful, but I can do my job or usual tasks", 5- "intense incapacitating headache." Their conclusion was that acupuncture leads to persistent, clinically relevant benefits for primary care patients with chronic headache, particularly migraine. In addition, they stated that expansion of NHS (National Coordinating Centre for Health Technology Assessment) acupuncture services should be considered. Improvements in quality of life, decreases in use of medication visits to general practitioners, and reductions in days off sick were all observed.

The above articles only represent a few of the research studies completed for the treatment of migraines with acupuncture. Further research needs to be completed to further dissect the analgesic and physiological effects of acupuncture.

Osteopathic Manipulation for Migraines

The efficacy of Osteopathic Manipulation for the treatment of migraine headaches is another option for patients seeking alternative treatments for migraines. In the *Journal of Alternative and Complementary Medicine,* a randomized controlled placebo trial was performed. The study concluded that osteopathic medicine decreased pain intensity, reduced the number of days missed from work, disability, and improved quality of life in women with migraines. The article was not specific except to say that the osteopathic physician used manual, visceral and cranial techniques [9]. Recently in a March 2013 issue of the *International Journal of Osteopathic Medicine* a study showed a significant difference between the Osteopathic Manipulation Treatment (OMT) group compared to drug and sham therapy. OMT is considered a valid treatment for the management of patients suffering from migraine headaches.

Osteopathic physicians must make an osteopathic diagnosis before treating a patient. In order to form an osteopathic diagnosis the physician will palpate the various sutures of the skull and assess for any cranial motion. After developing a diagnosis, the osteopathic physician can treat the patient for a variety of indications using facial effleurage, venous sinus drainage, frontal lift, parietal lift, sphenobasilar synchondrosis compression decompression, trigeminal self-stimulation, sphenopalatine ganglion stimulation, temporal decompression, TMJ compression/decompression, occipital decompression, and balanced membranous tension. There has been published literature that suggests osteopathic manipulation has some benefit for tension and migraine headaches similar to amitriptyline.

Facial effleurage can be used to treat patients with tension headaches and upper respiratory congestion [10]. Four different types of effleurage are described below. These include Lateral Effleurage, Frontal Effleurage, Maxilla Effleurage, and Mandible Effleurage. Contraindications include, but are not limited to intracranial bleed, craniofacial fracture, central nervous system (CNS) malignancy, CNS infection, and cystic acne. These techniques can be performed in either a seated or supine position and the practioner can either stand to the side of the patient or at the head of the table [10].

To begin lateral effleurage, the practioner should place their fingertips inferior to the patient's ears and firmly slide them inferiorly toward the medial clavicles. When performing this technique the practioner should avoid applying pressure on the carotid arteries. This technique can be repeated as often as needed to facilitate lymphatic drainage. When performing frontal effleurage, the practioner should place their thumbs (or fingertips) at the midline of the forehead and firmly slide them laterally toward the ears. In order to perform maxilla effleurage the practioner places their thumbs (or fingertips) at the bridge of the patient's nose and firmly slides them laterally toward the angle of the mandible. For mandible effleurage the practioner should place their thumbs (or fingertips) at the midline of the mandible and firmly slide laterally towards the angles of the mandible. Any combination of the effleurage techniques described above can be used to promote lymphatic drainage [10].

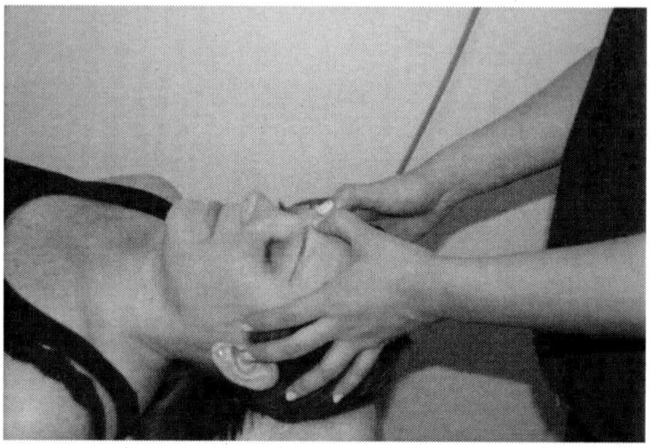

Figure 5. Frontal Effleurage.

The Venous Sinus Drainage technique consists of four different parts (10). These parts can be combined to aid in the treatment of headaches and upper respiratory congestion. Contraindications include intracranial bleeding, craniofacial fracture, CNS malignancy, and/or CNS infections. In order to perform this technique the patient should be lying down in the supine position. The practioner should be seated in a chair at the head of the table. The first step starts with the transverse sinus. The practioner should align their fingertips along the superior nuchal ridge with the fifth fingers on the inion. Pressure should be exerted slightly superiorly and laterally until the tissue gives. Step two consists of the practioner aligning their fingertips on both sides of the midline of the occipital bone with the fifth fingers on the inion. Pressure should again be applied slightly anteriorly and laterally until the tissue gives. During the third step, the practioner should cross their thumbs and palpate the opposite parietal bone on either side of the sagittal suture at lambda. Slight inferior and lateral pressure should be applied until the tissue gives. This should be repeated moving anteriorly along the sagittal suture until reaching bregma. The practioner should then move their fingertips alongside the metopic suture or along the midline of the frontal bone. Slight posterior and lateral pressure should then be applied until the tissue gives.

The Frontal Lift technique is utilized for patients that suffer predominately from restricted mobility associated with headache, depression, sinus congestion, and pediatric development abnormalities [10]. Contraindications could include intracranial bleed, craniofacial fracture, CNS malignancy, and CNS infection. In order for this technique to be performed the patient should be lying in the supine position and the practioner should be seated at the head of the table. The practioner palpates along the frontal bone just posterior to the orbital ridge bilaterally and feels for the cranial rhythmic impulse. Gentle pressure should be applied anteriorly to identify the restricted frontal mobility. The frontal bone ought to be lifted until slight give is equal on bilateral sides. Re-examination of the patient must be completed post manipulation in order to assess for any change in mobility [10].

The Parietal Lift is a technique that can be used for patients that suffer from parietal mobility issues often associated with headache, upper respiratory congestion, and pediatric development abnormalities [10]. Contraindications include intracranial bleed, craniofacial fracture, CNS malignancy, and CNS infection. The patient needs to be lying in a supine position and the practioner should be seated at the head of the table. The practioner's thumbs are then placed at the top of the patient's head and their fingertips should gently palpate the lateral aspect of the parietal bones, just superior to the squamous sutures. The cranial rhythmic impulse must be located and used to identify restricted parietal mobility. The parietal bones should have gentle pressure applied until slight give is equal bilaterally. Then the parietal bones need to be lifted gently in a superior fashion. Slight give should be equal on either side. The practioner should then re-examine the patient.

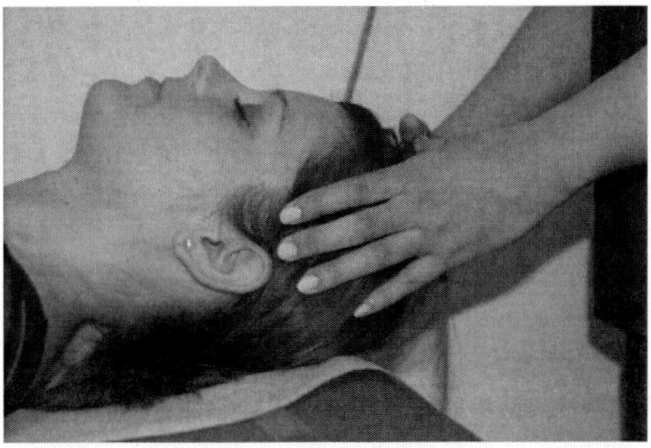

Figure 6. Parietal Lift.

The Spenobasilar Synchrondrosis (SBS) Compression-Decompression technique is indicated for diminished cranial rhythmic impulse amplitude related to headache, mood disorders, cranial nerve entrapment, upper respiratory congestion, and pediatric development abnormalities [10]. Relative contraindications include intracranial bleed, craniofacial fracture, CNS malignancy, and CNS infection. The patient needs to be lying in a supine position and the practioner should be seated at the head of the table. The practioner should grasp the patient's head using either the posterior temporal or the frontooccipital hold and gently compress the sphenobasilar synchondrosis (SBS). This is completed by moving the sphenoid greater wings posteroinferiorly and the occiput anterosuperiorly until slight give is felt bilaterally. After slight give is felt, the practioner should decompress the SBS by lifting the sphenoid greater wings anterosuperiorly and the occiput posteroinferiorly until slight give is felt again bilaterally. The practioner should then slowly release the decompression and re-examine the patient's cranial rhythmic impulse. Mobility of the sphenoid and occiput should also be re-examined.

Trigeminal Self Stimulation can be taught to patients that suffer from nasal congestion. After being taught the proper technique, the patient can perform this rather easily and as often as needed [10]. The patient should be instructed to palpate their eyebrow and slide their finger laterally until feeling a tender depression. Once the area is located, rotatory pressure should be applied for 10 seconds. Then the patient should move their fingertip to the top of their nose. Instruct the patient to slide their finger down the side of their nose until the feel another tender depression. Exert rotatory pressure for 10 seconds. The patient can repeat on either side as often as needed to relieve nasal congestion.

Sphenopalatine Ganglion Stimulation is indicated for use with upper respiratory congestion symptoms [10]. Relative contraindications include craniofacial fractures, intracranial bleed, CNS malignancy, and CNS injection. In order to perform this technique, the patient should be lying comfortably in the supine position and the practioner should be standing on one side of the patient and should also be wearing gloves. Using the fifth finger, palpate along the outside of the upper molars, moving posteriorly and then superiorly. The practioner should feel a small depression in the back of the mouth. Once the depression is located, exert slight pressure until tender or have the patient flex their head into the practioner's finger to tolerance for 3 seconds. This should be repeated 3-5 times or until the patient starts tearing on the side the practioner is working on. Repeat on the opposite side if needed.

Patients complaining of otitis media, TMJ syndrome, restricted temporal mobility associated with headache, and/or tinnitus can be treated with a Temporal Decompression technique [10]. Relative contraindications include intracranial bleed, craniofacial fracture, CNS malignancy, and/or CNS infection. The patient should be lying comfortably in a supine position and the practioner should be seated at the head of the table. Once positioned the practioner should gently grasp ahold of the patients earlobes between their thumbs and fingertips; then gently pull the ears in a posterolateral direction until a slight give is felt and is equal on both sides. Once the give is felt by the practioner; temporal mobility should be re-examined.

Patients suffering from temporomandibular joint (TMJ) restriction related to TMJ pain, mandible restriction, and/or neck pain could benefit from a TMJ Compression/ Decompression technique. Contraindications for this technique would be craniofacial fracture. For this technique the patient should be lying comfortably in the supine position and the practioner should be seated at the head of the table. Once positioned, the practioner should place their fingertips under the body of the mandible, and then gently pull superiorly toward the TMJ until slight give is felt equally on either side. The practioner should then move their fingertips to the lateral mandible and gently push it inferiorly away from the TMJ until a slight give is again felt equally on either side. The practioner should then re-examine the patient for TMJ mobility. If there is improvement, the practioner should consider prescribing TMJ self-mobilization techniques for further relief.

Occipital Decompression can be used to treat infant patient's with restricted occipital mobility associated with infant feeding disorders, colic, and congenital muscular torticollis [10]. Relative contraindications include intracranial bleed, craniofacial fracture, CNS malignancy, and/or CNS infections. The infant patient should be lying supine on a table and the practioner should be seated at the head of the table. The practioner should then place their index fingers on the infant's mastoid processes, their middle fingers on the infant's occipital condyles, and their ring fingers on the infant's supraocciput. The practioner should then gently pull the occiput in a posterior then lateral direction and should be resisting any mastoid process movement until the practioner feels an equal give within the occiput. The practioner should then re-examine the infant patient for any changes in occipital mobility.

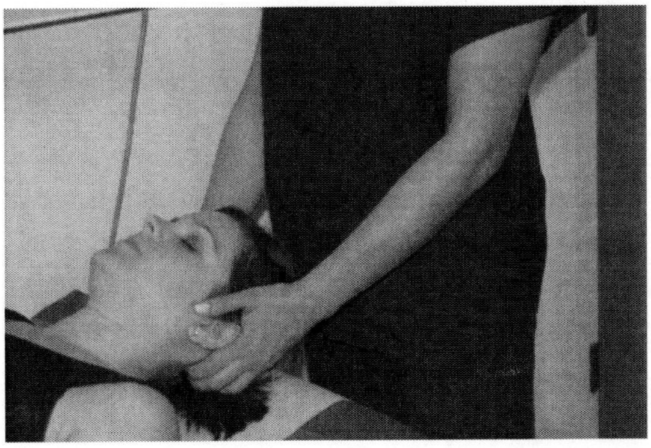

Figure 7. Occipital Decompression.

Patients with asymmetrical or diminished cranial rhythmic impulse (CRI) related to headache and/or cranial nerve entrapment could possibly benefit from the Balanced Membranous Tension technique [10]. Relative contraindications of this technique are intracranial bleed, craniofacial fracture, CNS malignancy, and CNS infection. With this technique the patient lies supine on an examining table and the practioner is seated at the head of the table and using the vault hold to palpate the cranial rhythmic impulse (CRI). The practioner is seated in this position in order to best identify any asymmetry of motion secondary to intracranial membranous strain. The practioner should use their hands to exaggerate membranous asymmetry and resist return to neutral until the CRI stops at a still point. This position should be maintained until the CRI returns. The practioner should then gently follow it back to neutral before releasing any pressure. The patient should then be re-examined to determine CRI and return of symmetry.

The Balanced Membranous Tension technique requires the practioner to know how to position their hands in the Vault Hold. The Vault Hold requires the practioner to be seated at the head of the table. Their index fingers should be located over the sphenoid greater wings, third and fourth fingertips anterior and posterior to the ears and their fifth fingertips should be placed on the occipital bone. The practioner's thumbs should be resting gently on the vertex of the head. Cranial rhythmic impulse should then be evaluated for rate, amplitude, and symmetry [10].

Herbal Preparations, Vitamins, Minerals and Other Interventions

According to American Academy of Neurology (AAN), petasites (butterbur) is a very effective for migraine prevention. Petasites was originally used by the Native American people for the treatment of headaches and inflammation. The chemical petsin and isopetsin inside the butterbur is believed to have benefits in treating headaches. Petasites have a level A recommendation from AAN and the American Headache Society (AHS) for the treatment of headaches. However, it is noted that Butterbur contains components of a toxic hepatic chemical called pyrrolizidine alkaloids.

Riboflavin (vitamin B2), magnesium, and MIG-99 (feverfew) are effective in the prophylaxis of migraine. Riboflavin plays a key role in maintaining health of humans; it is required in different cellular processes. An important role that riboflavin plays is for the metabolism of fats, ketone bodies, carbohydrates, and proteins. Riboflavin can be found in a variety of products including, dairy, liver, kidneys, legumes, yeast, mushrooms, and almonds.

Magnesium plays an important role in migraine pathogenesis. A study published in the Journal of Neural Transmission in May 2012, found that up to fifty percent of migraine patients may suffer from a magnesium deficiency. Routine blood test is not a good representation of the body's magnesium storage. Less than two percent of the body's magnesium is in the extracellular space. Sixty-seven percent of magnesium is in bone and the other thirty-one percent is located intracellularly. Having low magnesium causes depression by affecting serotonin receptor function and affects the synthesis/release of neurotransmitters. Treating patients with oral and intravenous magnesium is safe, inexpensive, and highly effective.

MIG-99 or feverfew is a daisy-like plant that grows in Eastern Europe. Traditional uses of feverfew have included fevers, headaches, stomachaches, toothaches, insect bites, infertility, and other gynecological problems. Side effects of feverfew include canker sores, irritation of the oral cavity, loss of taste, nausea, digestive issues, and bloating. Pregnant women should not take feverfew because it can cause premature delivery.

According to American Academy of Neurology (AAN), petasites (butterbur) is a very effective for migraine prevention. Petasites was originally used by the Native American people for the treatment of headaches and inflammation. The chemical petsin and isopetsin inside the butterbur is believed to have benefits in treating headaches. Petasites have a level A recommendation from AAN and the American Headache Society (AHS) for the treatment of headaches. However, it is noted that Butterbur contains components of a toxic hepatic chemical called pyrrolizidine alkaloids.

Tai Chi and Treatment of Headache

Tai Chi is a traditional Chinese exercise, which improves health by changes in mental focus, breathing, coordination, and relaxation. The goal of Tai Chi is to the "rebalance" the body and allows self-healing. Several review articles have demonstrated that tai chi improves balance, prevent falls, improves musculoskeletal function, cardiovascular and respiratory function, and immune function. The study completed by Abbot *et al.* focused on tension type headaches and muscle tightness caused by stressed. Therefore, if tai chi can cause relaxation, breathing, focus and coordination, it will not only treat the symptoms but also treat the main source of the problem.

Conclusion

Complementary Alternative Medicine is a holistic approach to patient care and differs from the approach of traditional conventional medicine. It offers a large range of benefits, often with fewer side effects. Integration of both CAM and conventional medical treatment will allow patients to have safer, affordable, and more effective treatment plan for patients with migraines in the future.

References

[1] Endres, H. G., Diener, H., & Molsberger, A. Role of acupuncture in the treatment of migraine. *Expert Review of Neurotherapeutics*, *7*, 1121-1135. Retrieved May 30, 2014.

[2] Helms, J. M., Elorriaga-Claraco, A., & Ng, A. (2010). *Point Locations and Functions* (4 ed.). Berkeley: Medical Acupuncture Publishers.

[3] Moerman DE, Jonas WB. Deconstructing the placebo effect and finding the meaning response. *Ann. Int. Med.* 136(6), 471-476 (2002).

[4] Kaptchuk TJ. The placebo effect in alternative medicine: can the performance of a healing ritual have clinical significance? *Ann. Int. Med.* 136(11), 817-825 (2002).

[5] Deadman, P., Al-Khafaji, M., & Baker, K. Some acupuncture points which treat headache. *Journal of Chinese Medicine*, *56*, 1-18. Retrieved May 30, 2014.

[6] Helms, J. M. (1995). *Acupuncture energetics: a clinical approach for physicians.* Berkeley, Calif., U.S.A.: Medical Acupuncture Publishers.

[7] Linde K, Streng A, Jürgens S, Hoppe A, Brinkhaus B, et al. "Acupuncture for Patients With Migraine: A Randomized Controlled Trial. *JAMA: The Journal of the American Medical Association.* 2005; 293:2118-2125.

[8] Pickett, H., & Blackwell, J. Acupuncture for Migraine Headaches. *American Family Physician*, *81*, 1036-1037. Retrieved May 30, 2014, from http://www.aafp.org/afp/2010/0415/p1036.html.

[9] Voigt, K., Liebnitzky, J., Burmeister, U., Sihvonen-Riemenschneider, H., Beck, M., Voigt, R., et al. Efficacy of Osteopathic Manipulation Treatment of Female Patients with Migraine: Results of a Randomized Controlled Trial. *The Journal of Alternative and Complementary Medicine*, *17*, 225-230.

[10] Beatty, D., Li, T. S., Steele, K., Comeaux, Z., Garlitz, J., Kribs, J., & Lemley, W. (2011). *The Pocket Manual of OMT - Osteopathic Manipulative Treatment for Physicians*. (2nd ed., pp. 230, 235-238, 240-242, 244-247, 250-251). Philadelphia, PA: Wolters Kluwer Health.

[11] Abbott RB, Hui KK, Hays RD, Li MD, Pan T. A randomized controlled trial of Tai Chi for tension headaches. *Evidence-Based Complementary and Alternative Medicine*. 2007;4(1):107–113.

[12] Acupuncture Points. (2014, January 1). Retrieved May 30, 2014, from http://www.yinyanghouse.com/acupuncturepoints/st1.

[13] Acupuncture for Migraine and Recurrent Headaches. Med Article. 2014.

[14] Grech D, Gorgy G. Acupuncture as a Complementary Treatment for Migraine Headaches. *Austin J. Anesthesia and Analgesia*. 2014;2(3): 3.

[15] Herbs at a Glace: Feverfew. (2006, December 1). . Retrieved April 1, 2014, from http://nccam.nih.gov/health/feverfew.

[16] International Headache Society. International Classification of Headache Disorders. Cephalalgia. 2013; 33: 629-808.

[17] Lao L, Zhang RX, Zhang G, Wang X, Berman BM, Ren K. A parametric study of electroacupuncture on persistent hyperalgesia and Fos protein expression in rats. *Brain Res.* 1020(1,2), 18-29 (2004).
[18] Linde K, Allais G, Brinkhaus B, Manheimer E, Vickers A, White AR. Acupuncture for migraine prophylaxis. *Cochrane Database Syst. Rev*. 2009;(1):CD001218.
[19] National Center for Complementary and Alternative Medicine. *Acupuncture.* National Institutes of Health Web Site. Accessed at http://nccam.nih.gov/health/acupuncture/introduction.htm on May 30, 2014.
[20] Pan, T. A Randomized Controlled Trial of Tai Chi for Tension Headaches. *Evidence-based Complementary and Alternative Medicine*, *4*, 107-113.
[21] Sharma, Krisha (2013) Acupuncture for Migraine Simplified.
[22] The Journal of Traditional Eastern Health and Fitness. http://www.qi-journal.com/acupuncture.asp?-token.D=Article&-MaxRecords=1&-SkipRecords=3&-Op=bw&Name=Acupuncture%20FAQ
[23] Vickers AJ. Acupuncture for Chronic Headache in Primary Care: Large, Pragmatic, Randomised Trial. BMJ. 2004; 328:744.

In: Migraine Surgery
Editor: Antonios Mammis
ISBN: 978-1-63321-761-4

Chapter 14

The Business and Economics of Migraine Surgery

***Aaron F. Hajart**[*1,2,3,4] and Michelle Armonda[1,4]*
[1]Rutgers New Jersey Medical School,
Rutgers Neurological Institute of New Jersey, Newark, New Jersey, US
[2]Departments of Neurological Surgery,
Otolaryngology-Head and Neck Surgery[3], and Neurology,[4]
Rutgers New Jersey Medical School, Newark, New Jersey, US

Introduction

The use of a variety of surgical and interventional treatments for intractable migraine headaches has evolved over the last few decades and has contributed to the growth of the field. While literature for the support of these treatments continues to expand, the business aspect of the care is still an evolving area. The total financial burden of treatment for migraines in the United States is over $13 billion per year. [1] The economic contribution to the health care system is about $1 billion dollar each year. [2] This presents a considerable economic impact to the United States health care system and is a major reason this field has evolved at a considerable rate.

The major challenge in the treatment of migraines is the considerable cost of care over the life of the patient. Annually, the cost of care for migraine sufferers can be as high as $7,089 [3] to $7,750 [4]. Faber et al. found that after Botulinum Toxin injections the annual cost of medical care was reduced by $3,949.70 on average to $1,997.26 per year. [5] Chronic Migraine suffers reported that in-direct costs from the loss of work productivity represented about 70% of the total economic burden of their pathology. [6]

* Corresponding Author: Aaron F. Hajart, MS, ATC, Rutgers Neurological Institute of New Jersey, 90 Bergen St. Suite 8100, Newark, NJ 07103, (o) 973-972-2341, hajartaf@njms.rutgers.edu

Keywords: Migraine, Insurance, Acupuncture, Surgery, Pharmological, Neurostimulation, Coding, Billing, Healthcare, Patient Care, Electrodes, Cost effectiveness

Insurance Coverage

One of the main challenges for the business aspect of migraine surgery is lack of consistent insurance coverage regulations. As of May 2014, 42 of the nationwide Medicare contractors had a Local Coverage Determination that approved Botulinum Toxin for the treatment of Migraines. The use of Botulinum Toxin for the treatment of intractable migraines became a very common modality when approved by the U.S. Food and Drug Administration on October 15, 2010. The administration of Botulinum Toxin for migraine sufferers is also well covered by private insurers.

The long-term use of Botulinum Toxin, however, has financial challenges. An analysis of the pre and post-treatment costs associated with Botulinum Toxin show that it did not demonstrate a reduction in total healthcare costs and more importantly had no impact on the use of migraine-related medications. [7] This will be an important consideration as more insurance plans are now collecting outcomes data and applying this when determining coverage of current and new therapies.

While the use and coverage for Botulinum Toxin is widespread, only three states (California, Hawaii, and Nevada) and three territories (America Samoa, Guam, and Northern Mariana) have a Local Coverage Determination that approves the use of Peripheral Nerve Stimulation (PNS) for treatment of intractable migraines (Table 1). Many local commercial payers still exclude the use of Neurostimulation for the treatment of intractable migraines but this seems to be changing. Major payers are starting to add the use of Peripheral Nerve Stimulation to their medical management guidelines for patients with persistent Headache-Facial Pain (ICD-9 784.0). [8] Coverage determinations have and will continue to present challenges for the use of Neurostimulation in migraine suffers but the tide has turned in recent years which may allow for more wide spread coverage of PNS in the near future.

Although there is some opportunity of insurance coverage for the use of peripheral nerve stimulation and potentially occipital nerve stimulation as a form of treatment for intractable migraines, the insurance coverage for surgical deactivation of migraine trigger sites is currently far behind other surgical interventions. Surgical Deactivation is a recent alternative to the treatment of migraines that has had some positive clinical trial research supporting its use. [9] Currently however, it is not typically covered by commercial insurance at this time. [10] There are still considerable amounts of questions as to the efficacy of this treatment that need to be addressed which will impact the opportunity for this treatment to be considered medically necessary. [11] Until research is able to demonstrate consistent effectiveness, the opportunity for insurance approval of this procedure is not likely to change in the long term.

The use of Acupuncture for the treatment of migraines has been well researched and supported in literature. As a result, acupuncture is commonly covered by commercial insurances. Aetna [12], some local Blue Cross and Blue Shield plans [13], Cigna [14], and many other local and national payers typically pay for acupuncture as a treatment of chronic migraines. A recent analysis of the cost of acupuncture versus the impact to Quality Adjusted Life Year was found to be below the threshold of patients' willingness to pay for care [15].

Table 1. Medicare Coverage for Migraine Surgery

Medicare Contractor	LCD ID Number	Coverage Region	Covered Service	Coverage
Noridian Healthcare Solutions, LLC	L33714	California-Northern	PNS	"PNS of occipital nerves for occipital neuralgia, post-surgical neuropathic pain, cervicogenic headaches and treatment resistant migraines."
Noridian Healthcare Solutions, LLC	L33714	California-Southern	PNS	"PNS of occipital nerves for occipital neuralgia, post-surgical neuropathic pain, cervicogenic headaches and treatment resistant migraines."
Noridian Healthcare Solutions, LLC	L33714	American Samoa, Guam, Hawaii, Northern Mariana Islands	PNS	"PNS of occipital nerves for occipital neuralgia, post-surgical neuropathic pain, cervicogenic headaches and treatment resistant migraines."
Noridian Healthcare Solutions, LLC	L33714	Nevada	PNS	"PNS of occipital nerves for occipital neuralgia, post-surgical neuropathic pain, cervicogenic headaches and treatment resistant migraines."
Wisconsin Physicians Service Insurance Corporation	L28555	Missouri	Botulinum toxin	"Botulinum toxin for the treatment of MIGRAINE headaches"
Wisconsin Physicians Service Insurance Corporation	L28555	Iowa	Botulinum toxin	"Botulinum toxin for the treatment of MIGRAINE headaches"
Wisconsin Physicians Service Insurance Corporation	L28555	Kansas	Botulinum toxin	"Botulinum toxin for the treatment of MIGRAINE headaches"
Wisconsin Physicians Service Insurance Corporation	L28555	Nebraska	Botulinum toxin	"Botulinum toxin for the treatment of MIGRAINE headaches"
Wisconsin Physicians Service Insurance Corporation	L28555	Indiana	Botulinum toxin	"Botulinum toxin for the treatment of MIGRAINE headaches"
Wisconsin Physicians Service Insurance Corporation	L28555	Michigan	Botulinum toxin	"Botulinum toxin for the treatment of MIGRAINE headaches"
Noridian Healthcare Solutions, LLC	L33513	California-Northern	Botulinum toxin	"Botulinum Toxin Type A (Botox-onabotulinumtoxinA) is covered for prophylaxis of headaches in adult patients with chronic MIGRAINE (≥15 days per month"with headache lasting 4 hours a day or longer)."
Noridian Healthcare Solutions, LLC	L33513	California-Southern	Botulinum toxin	"Botulinum Toxin Type A (Botox-onabotulinumtoxinA) is covered for prophylaxis of headaches in adult patients with chronic MIGRAINE (≥15 days per month"with headache lasting 4 hours a day or longer)."

Table 1. (Continued)

Medicare Contractor	LCD ID Number	Coverage Region	Covered Service	Coverage
Noridian Healthcare Solutions, LLC	L33513	American Samoa, Guam, Hawaii, Northern Mariana Islands	Botulinum toxin	"Botulinum Toxin Type A (Botox-onabotulinumtoxinA) is covered for prophylaxis of headaches in adult patients with chronic MIGRAINE (≥15 days per month"with headache lasting 4 hours a day or longer)."
Noridian Healthcare Solutions, LLC	L33513	Nevada	Botulinum toxin	"Botulinum Toxin Type A (Botox-onabotulinumtoxinA) is covered for prophylaxis of headaches in adult patients with chronic MIGRAINE (≥15 days per month"with headache lasting 4 hours a day or longer)."
Noridian Healthcare Solutions, LLC	L24280	Washington	Botulinum toxin	"the prophylaxis of headaches in adult patients with Chronic MIGRAINE (≥ 15 days per month with headache lasting 4 hours a day or longer."
Noridian Healthcare Solutions, LLC	L24280	Arizona	Botulinum toxin	"the prophylaxis of headaches in adult patients with Chronic MIGRAINE (≥ 15 days per month with headache lasting 4 hours a day or longer."
Noridian Healthcare Solutions, LLC	L24280	Montana	Botulinum toxin	"the prophylaxis of headaches in adult patients with Chronic MIGRAINE (≥ 15 days per month with headache lasting 4 hours a day or longer."
Noridian Healthcare Solutions, LLC	L24280	North Dakota	Botulinum toxin	"the prophylaxis of headaches in adult patients with Chronic MIGRAINE (≥ 15 days per month with headache lasting 4 hours a day or longer."
Noridian Healthcare Solutions, LLC	L24280	Utah	Botulinum toxin	"the prophylaxis of headaches in adult patients with Chronic MIGRAINE (≥ 15 days per month with headache lasting 4 hours a day or longer."
Noridian Healthcare Solutions, LLC	L24280	Wyoming	Botulinum toxin	"the prophylaxis of headaches in adult patients with Chronic MIGRAINE (≥ 15 days per month with headache lasting 4 hours a day or longer."
Noridian Healthcare Solutions, LLC	L24280	South Dakota	Botulinum toxin	"the prophylaxis of headaches in adult patients with Chronic MIGRAINE (≥ 15 days per month with headache lasting 4 hours a day or longer."
Noridian Healthcare Solutions, LLC	L24280	Idaho	Botulinum toxin	"the prophylaxis of headaches in adult patients with Chronic MIGRAINE (≥ 15 days per month with headache lasting 4 hours a day or longer."
Noridian Healthcare Solutions, LLC	L24280	Alaska	Botulinum toxin	"the prophylaxis of headaches in adult patients with Chronic MIGRAINE (≥ 15 days per month with headache lasting 4 hours a day or longer."

Medicare Contractor	LCD ID Number	Coverage Region	Covered Service	Coverage
Noridian Healthcare Solutions, LLC	L24280	Oregon	Botulinum toxin	"the prophylaxis of headaches in adult patients with Chronic MIGRAINE (≥ 15 days per month with headache lasting 4 hours a day or longer."
National Government Services Inc.	L26841	Connecticut	Botulinum toxin	"Coverage will only be allowed for those patients with chronic daily headaches (headache disorders occurring greater than 15 days a month - in many cases daily with a duration of four or more hours - for a period of at least 3 months) who have significant disability due to the headaches, and have been refractory to standard and usual conventional therapy."
National Government Services Inc.	L26841	New York	Botulinum toxin	"Coverage will only be allowed for those patients with chronic daily headaches (headache disorders occurring greater than 15 days a month - in many cases daily with a duration of four or more hours - for a period of at least 3 months) who have significant disability due to the headaches, and have been refractory to standard and usual conventional therapy."
National Government Services Inc.	L26841	Massachusetts	Botulinum toxin	"Coverage will only be allowed for those patients with chronic daily headaches (headache disorders occurring greater than 15 days a month - in many cases daily with a duration of four or more hours - for a period of at least 3 months) who have significant disability due to the headaches, and have been refractory to standard and usual conventional therapy."
National Government Services Inc.	L26841	Rhode Island	Botulinum toxin	"Coverage will only be allowed for those patients with chronic daily headaches (headache disorders occurring greater than 15 days a month - in many cases daily with a duration of four or more hours - for a period of at least 3 months) who have significant disability due to the headaches, and have been refractory to standard and usual conventional therapy."
National Government Services Inc.	L26841	Vermont	Botulinum toxin	"Coverage will only be allowed for those patients with chronic daily headaches (headache disorders occurring greater than 15 days a month - in many cases daily with a duration of four or more hours - for a period of at least 3 months) who have significant disability due to the headaches, and have been refractory to standard and usual conventional therapy."
National Government Services Inc.	L26841	New Hampshire	Botulinum toxin	"Coverage will only be allowed for those patients with chronic daily headaches (headache disorders occurring greater than 15 days a month - in many cases daily with a duration of four or more hours - for a period of at least 3 months) who have significant disability due to the headaches, and have been refractory to standard and usual conventional therapy."

Table 1. (Continued)

Medicare Contractor	LCD ID Number	Coverage Region	Covered Service	Coverage
National Government Services Inc.	L26841	Maine	Botulinum toxin	"Coverage will only be allowed for those patients with chronic daily headaches (headache disorders occurring greater than 15 days a month - in many cases daily with a duration of four or more hours - for a period of at least 3 months) who have significant disability due to the headaches, and have been refractory to standard and usual conventional therapy.'
National Government Services Inc.	L26841	Wisconsin	Botulinum toxin	"Coverage will only be allowed for those patients with chronic daily headaches (headache disorders occurring greater than 15 days a month - in many cases daily with a duration of four or more hours - for a period of at least 3 months) who have significant disability due to the headaches, and have been refractory to standard and usual conventional therapy."
National Government Services Inc.	L26841	Minnesota	Botulinum toxin	"Coverage will only be allowed for those patients with chronic daily headaches (headache disorders occurring greater than 15 days a month - in many cases daily with a duration of four or more hours - for a period of at least 3 months) who have significant disability due to the headaches, and have been refractory to standard and usual conventional therapy."
National Government Services Inc.	L26841	Illinois	Botulinum toxin	"Coverage will only be allowed for those patients with chronic daily headaches (headache disorders occurring greater than 15 days a month - in many cases daily with a duration of four or more hours - for a period of at least 3 months) who have significant disability due to the headaches, and have been refractory to standard and usual conventional therapy."
First Coast Service Options, Inc.	L29088	Florida	Botulinum toxin	"prophylaxis of headaches in adult patients with chronic MIGRAINE (≥ 15 days per month with headache lasting 4 hours a day or longer)."
First Coast Service Options, Inc.	L29103	Puerto Rico	Botulinum toxin	"prophylaxis of headaches in adult patients with chronic MIGRAINE (≥ 15 days per month with headache lasting 4 hours a day or longer)."
First Coast Service Options, Inc.	L29103	Virgin Islands	Botulinum toxin	"prophylaxis of headaches in adult patients with chronic MIGRAINE (≥ 15 days per month with headache lasting 4 hours a day or longer)."
CGS Administrators, LLA	L31855	Kentucky	Botulinum toxin	"Coverage will only be allowed for those patients with chronic daily headaches (headache disorders occurring greater than 15 days a month - in many cases daily with a duration of four or more hours - for a period of at least 3 months) who have significant disability due to the headaches, and have been refractory to standard and usual conventional therapy."

Medicare Contractor	LCD ID Number	Coverage Region	Covered Service	Coverage
CGS Administrators, LLA	L31855	Ohio	Botulinum toxin	"Coverage will only be allowed for those patients with chronic daily headaches (headache disorders occurring greater than 15 days a month - in many cases daily with a duration of four or more hours - for a period of at least 3 months) who have significant disability due to the headaches, and have been refractory to standard and usual conventional therapy."
Palmetto GBA	L31701	Virgina	Botulinum toxin	"Chemodenervation of procerus and bilateral frontalis, corrugator, occipitalis, temporalis, trapezius, and cervical paraspinal muscle group for the prophylaxis of headaches in adult patients with chronic MIGRAINE (≥ 15 days per month with headache lasting 4 hours a day or longer)."
Palmetto GBA	L31701	North Carolina	Botulinum toxin	"Chemodenervation of procerus and bilateral frontalis, corrugator, occipitalis, temporalis, trapezius, and cervical paraspinal muscle group for the prophylaxis of headaches in adult patients with chronic MIGRAINE (≥ 15 days per month with headache lasting 4 hours a day or longer)."
Palmetto GBA	L31701	South Carolina	Botulinum toxin	"Chemodenervation of procerus and bilateral frontalis, corrugator, occipitalis, temporalis, trapezius, and cervical paraspinal muscle group for the prophylaxis of headaches in adult patients with chronic MIGRAINE (≥ 15 days per month with headache lasting 4 hours a day or longer)."
Palmetto GBA	L31701	West Virgina	Botulinum toxin	"Chemodenervation of procerus and bilateral frontalis, corrugator, occipitalis, temporalis, trapezius, and cervical paraspinal muscle group for the prophylaxis of headaches in adult patients with chronic MIGRAINE (≥ 15 days per month with headache lasting 4 hours a day or longer)."
Cahaba GBA	L30025	Alabama	Botulinum toxin	"Prophylaxis of headaches in adult patients with chronic MIGRAINE (≥ 15 days per month with headache lasting 4 hours a day or longer)"
Cahaba GBA	L30025	Georgia	Botulinum toxin	"Prophylaxis of headaches in adult patients with chronic MIGRAINE (≥ 15 days per month with headache lasting 4 hours a day or longer)"
Cahaba GBA	L30025	Tennessee	Botulinum toxin	"Prophylaxis of headaches in adult patients with chronic MIGRAINE (≥ 15 days per month with headache lasting 4 hours a day or longer)"

CMS.gov. Medicare Coverage Database (2014). Retrieved from http://www.cms.gov/medicare-coverage-database/overview-and-quick-search.aspx

This has allowed acupuncture to flourish as a treatment option while revealing what impact obtaining insurance coverage could have on other treatments.

It is important to take insurance coverage and patient financial responsibilities into consideration when developing a finance policy for your migraine surgery program.

Since Medicare, Medicaid, and commercial insurances all have varying levels of coverage for these types of interventions, patients will often have more out of pocket costs for these procedures then they may have for interventions for other types of pathology. With that being said, these patients can have significant and frequent symptomology and as such may have a high propensity to take on the financial burden of care. In a recent study of patients suffering from tinnitus, 50.1% of surveyed respondents were willing to spend $10,000 or more in out of pocket expenses for Vagus Nerve Stimulation if it were to eliminate their symptoms while 23.9% of respondents were willing to spend as much if it reduced their symptoms by half. [16] Migraine sufferers may have a similar willingness if the treatment were to provide reasonable relief.

Cost-Effectiveness of Migraine Surgery

While the financial cost of migraine treatments should be secondary to the efficacy and safety of the patient [17] there is no doubt that the cost-effectiveness of the treatment is paramount to the growth of the treatment. For these treatments to become more commonly covered by insurance, it will be important to demonstrate that these invasive types of interventions are not only as, but possibly more, effective as medical management alternatives.

It has been reported that persistent migraine suffers represented high utilization of the Emergency Room. Chan and Ovens found that these patients visited the Emergency Room 42% more than other high utilizers. [18] Reducing this and other costs are crucial in demonstrating the value to Medicare and commercial payers what these interventions have on migraine sufferers.

Overall, there are many considerations for the type of care that is available to patients. Insurance status has shown to be an important consideration in the cost of care for patients receiving Neurostimulation procedures. In Huang et al.'s study on the impact of the type of insurance coverage on neuromodulation outcomes, they found that Medicaid patients had higher utilization of all services (LOS, ED visits, Meds, etc) but quality outcomes (complication rates) did not differ. [19] Interestingly enough, Huang found that commercially insured patients generated higher overall costs (charges) than these Medicaid patients. [19]

Some studies have shown that the implantation of Neurostimulation has as high as a 32% to 46% complication rate with 22% to 24% of those necessitating revision. [20] This is an area of worry since there is some concern that Spinal Cord Stimulators (SCS) and Intrathecal Drug Delivery Systems (IDDS) may be on CMS's radar for "never events" due to surgical site infection. [21] This is a significant challenge as 2% to 10% of cases present with surgical site complications due to infections. [22, 23] It is important to consider the possible costs of these complications when discussing plan of care with patients. Since many of these procedures require a large patient out of pocket expense, complication and revision rates can greatly impact the patients total cost of care.

Coding and Billing of Neurostimulation

Accurate coding of procedures is essential in the development and success of a surgical migraine program. The Centers for Medical and Medicaid Services' Office of Inspector General continually monitors medical and surgical claims submitted by Physicians to ensure they are medically necessary, are supported by documentation, and an allowable service under National Coverage Determination (NCD) and Local Coverage Determination (LCD).

It is important to understand that Neurostimulation has four parts: 1. Trial, 2. Implant, 3. Explant/Revision, and 4. Maintenance (battery changes). Each of these is a separate procedural incidence and should be treated as such.

Coding the use of Neurostimulation procedures for Migraine treatment must follow all applicable Medicare National Correct Coding Initiative (NCCI) guidelines. The available procedures codes should be used for medically necessary services (Table 2). It is imperative to keep in mind that NCCI edits should be followed for all payers who use these guidelines for their claims payment processing.

Table 2. Common Migraine Surgery Codes

CPT Code	Description
64553	Percutaneous implantation of neurostimulator electrode array; cranial nerve
64555	Percutaneous implantation of neurostimulator electrode array peripheral nerve (excludes sacral nerve)
64575	Incision for implantation of neurostimulator electrode array; peripheral nerve (excludes sacral nerve)
64585	Revision or removal of peripheral neurostimulator electrode array
64590	Insertion or replacement of peripheral or gastric neurostimulator pulse generator or receiver, direct or inductive coupling
64595	Revision or removal of peripheral or gastric neurostimulator pulse generator or receiver
L8680	Implantable neurostimulator electrode, each
L8681	Patient programmer (external) for use with implantable programmable neurostimulator pulse generator, replacement only
L8682	Implantable neurostimulator radiofrequency receiver
L8683	Radiofrequency transmitter (external) for use with implantable neurostimulator radiofrequency receiver
L8685	Implantable neurostimulator pulse generator, single array, rechargeable, includes extension
L8686	Implantable neurostimulator pulse generator, single array, nonrechargeable, includes extension
L8687	Implantable neurostimulator pulse generator, dual array, rechargeable, includes extension
L8688	Implantable neurostimulator pulse generator, dual array, nonrechargeable, includesextension
L8689	External recharging system for battery (internal) for use with implantable neurostimulator, replacement only
L8695	External recharging system for battery (external) for use with implantable neurostimulator, replacement only

Abraham, M. Glen, R. O'Heron, H. et al. (2014) Current Procedural Terminology: Professional Edition. Chicago, IL. American Medical Association CPT/ DBP Intellectual Property Services.

Surgeons removing the percutaneous trial electrode in the office should not bill for the removal of electrodes. [24] The removal CPT Codes (63661-63662) are intended for the intra-operative removal of the permanent lead that was placed via either percutaneous or laminectomy placement. [24]

One area of procedural coding for Neurostimulation that often causes confusion is whether the surgeon is billing for the number of electrodes placed vs. the number of arrays. Correct coding will necessitate that the surgeon bills by the number of neurostimulation arrays placed during the procedure. [24] This could possibly require the use of modifiers to note that multiple or separate procedures were performed. The surgeon should follow the coding guidelines of the insurance carrier to ensure that correct coding is followed as per their guidelines.

Key Components of a Robust Migraine Surgery Program

A robust migraine surgery program will require significant investment of resources in order to be successful, including a well-supported patient and program. The medical team often consists of a variety of health care practitioners and support staff (Table 3). The key will be integrating practitioners into a management model that is multi-disciplinary but is still patient centered. Neurologists, Neurosurgeons, Plastic Surgeons, Psychiatrist, and Dentists have typically been considered as vital team members in the treatment of migraine patients. As we move into more multi-disciplinary care, other providers could also play an important role. One area that is often overlooked when integrating care is pharmacological services. The introduction of ambulatory pharmacists to the treatment team will help to better screen patients, provide better instruction on their medication utilization, and potentially ward off complications or medication overuse. As the inclusion of pharmacists to the care teams grow, their potential to reduce the use of analgesic medications will help to improve the long-term outcomes and costs of migraine surgery.

Table 3. Migraine Surgery Team

Medical Staff	Program Support Staff
Neurosurgeon(s)	Patient Navigator
Neurologist(s)	Registered Nurse
Physiatrist	Insurance/Finance staff
Facial Plastic Surgeons	Surgical Coordinator
Anesthesia Pain Management	
Dentists	
Advance Practice Nurses	
Pain Psychologist	
Psychiatrist	
Acupuncturist	
Pharmacists	

Often times valuable information regarding the patient's medical or pharmacological history are not fully appreciated. Intractable migraine sufferers have the additional complexity of most likely being treated by multiple providers that may, or may not, know of the others treatment plan. This is especially true due to the high utilization of the Emergency Room for these patients, which makes it even more important to ensure proper and timely communication is maintained. Supporting the program with a patient navigator is crucial. Having one person serve as "gate keeper" for these patients will reduce unnecessary utilization and better coordinate care amongst the various specialists.

Beyond this primary team, the inclusion of Pain Psychologists, Physiatrists, Acupuncturists, and additional support staff are necessary to round out the medical team. Having a team that is comprehensive and collaborative will ultimately impact the success of the program as well as make communication with the patent's primary care doctors more efficient and improve patient safety.

Conclusion

There is immense opportunity for Surgical and Interventional treatment of migraines. The current status of insurance coverage for some of these procedures however presents challenges for both the providers and patients. It is important to understand the current insurance coverage issues as well as the financial impact to the patient and healthcare system when considering the plan of care. All of these issues impact the ability to pay for and support a comprehensive program. Care should be taken when considering the development of the program as well as the services that will be offered as part of that program.

References

[1] Goldberg, L. D. (2005). "The cost of migraine and its treatment." *Am. J. Manag. Care* 11(2 Suppl): S62- 67.

[2] 2. Hu, X. H., et al. (1999). "Burden of migraine in the United States: disability and economic costs." *Arch. Intern. Med.* 159(8): 813-818.

[3] Hazard, E., et al. (2009). "The burden of migraine in the United States: current and emerging perspectives on disease management and economic analysis." *Value Health* 12(1): 55-64.

[4] Munakata, J., et al. (2009). "Economic burden of transformed migraine: results from the American Migraine Prevalence and Prevention (AMPP) Study." *Headache* 49(4): 498-508.

[5] Faber, C., Garcia, R., Davis, J., and Guyuron, B. (2012). "A Socioeconomic Analysis of Surgical Treatment of Migraine Headaches" *Plastic and Reconstructive Surgery* 129: 871-877.

[6] Lanteri-Minet, M. (2014). "Economic burden and costs of chronic migraine." *Curr. Pain. Headache Rep* 18(1): 385.

[7] Mitchell, M. P., Schaecher, K., Cannon, E., Speckman, M. (2008). "Humanistic, Utilization, and Cost Outcomes associated with the use of Botulinum Toxin for

Treatment of Refractory Migraine Headaches in a Managed Care Organization." *Journal of Managed Care Pharmacy* 14(5): 442-450.

[8] Blue Cross Blue Shield of Kansas. (2013). "Medical Policy: Implanted Peripheral Nerve Stimulator (PNS) for Pain Control." Current Procedural Terminology: 1-6. Retrieved from: (http://www.bcbsks.com/customerservice/providers/MedicalPolicies/policies/policies/ImplantedPeripheralNerveStimulator_PainControl_2013-03-13.pdf)

[9] Guyuron, B., et al. (2009). "A placebo-controlled surgical trial of the treatment of migraine headaches." *Plast. Reconstr. Surg.* 124(2): 461-468.

[10] Blue Cross Blue Shield of Rhode Island (2014). "Medical Coverage Policy: Surgical Deactivation of Migraine Headaches." Medical Coverage Policy 1-6. Retrieved from: (https://www.bcbsri.com/sites/default/files/polices/surgical_deactivation_migraine_headache_trigger_sites.pdf).

[11] Mathew, P. G. (2014). "A critical evaluation of migraine trigger site deactivation surgery." Headache 54(1): 142-152.

[12] Aetna. (2014). "Acupuncture." Clinical Policy Bulletin. Retrieved from: http://www.aetna.com/cpb/medical/data/100_199/0135.html

[13] Excellus. (2001). "Acupuncture" Medical Policy. 1-11. Retrieved from: https://www.excellusbcbs.com/wps/wcm/connect/e4b9a340-9564-4284-ae52-80f5d664b15d/mp+acupunc+mpc3+14.pdf?MOD=AJPERES&CACHEID=e4b9a340-9564-4284-ae52-80f5d664b15d

[14] Cigna (2014) "Acupuncture." Cigna Medical Coverage Policy. 1-22. Retrieved from https://cignaforhcp.cigna.com/public/content/pdf/coveragePolicies/medical/mm_0024_coveragepositioncriteria_acupuncture.pdf

[15] Ambrosio, E. M., et al. (2012). "Costs and consequences of acupuncture as a treatment for chronic pain: a systematic review of economic evaluations conducted alongside randomised controlled trials." *Complement Ther. Med.* 20(5): 364-374.

[16] Engineer, N. D., et al. (2013). "Willingness to accept and pay for implantable tinnitus treatments: a survey." *Neuromodulation* 16(2): 154-162.

[17] Jenkins, B. and S. J. Tepper (2011). "Neurostimulation for primary headache disorders: Part 2, review of central neurostimulators for primary headache, overall therapeutic efficacy, safety, cost, patient selection, and future research in headache neuromodulation." *Headache* 51(9): 1408-1418.

[18] Chan, B., & Ovens, H. (2004). "Chronic Migraineurs: An Important Subgroup of Patients Who Visit Emergency Departments Frequently." *Annals of Emergency Medicine* 43(2): 238-242.

[19] Huang, K. T., Hazzard, M.A., Babu, R., Ugiliweneza, B., Grossi, P. M., Huh, B., Roy, L. A., Patil, C., Boakye, M., & Lad, S. (2013). "Insurance Disparities in the Outcomes of Spinal Cord Stimulation Surgery." *Neuromodulation.*

[20] Deer, T. R. (2013). "Neurostimulation should be used as a method of reducing or eliminating opioids in the treatment of chronic pain: the digital drug revolution." *Expert Rev. Med. Devices* 10(6): 697-699.

[21] Welch, M. and J. Attalah (2013). "Centers for Medicare and Medicaid Services will stop payment for infected cardiac implantable devices; will implantable pain therapy be next?" *Pain Pract.* 13(2): 171.

[22] Ubbink, D. T., et al. (2004). "Systematic review and meta-analysis of controlled trials assessing spinal cord stimulation for inoperable critical leg ischaemia." *Br. J. Surg.* 91(8): 948-955.

[23] Spincemaille, G. H., et al. (2000). "Technical data and complications of spinal cord stimulation: data from a randomized trial on critical limb ischemia." *Stereotact. Funct. Neurosurg.* 74(2): 63-72.

[24] Hayek, S., Levy, R. (2012) A Volume in the Interventional and Neuromodulatory Techniques for Pain Management: *Neurostimulation for the Treatment of Chronic Pain*: 1.

Index

G

H

I

L

M

N

O

P

Q

R

S

T

V

W